TEXT BOOK OF FRACTURES AND DISLOCATIONS

TEXT BOOK OF FRACTURES AND DISLOCATIONS

Manzoor Ahmad Khan

Professor of Orthopaedic Surgery
Khyber Medical College, Peshawar
Visiting Orthopaedic Surgeon
Khyber Teaching Hospital, Peshawar

Formerly:
Professor of Orthopaedic Surgery (King Edward Medical College, Lahore)
Visiting Orthopaedic Surgeon (Mayo Hospital, Lahore)

Copyright © 2015 by Manzoor Ahmad Khan.

Library of Congress Control Number: 2015915416
ISBN: Hardcover   978-1-5144-4066-7
               Softcover   978-1-5144-4065-0
               eBook   978-1-5144-4064-3

All rights reserved. No part of this book may be reproduced or transmitted in any form or by any means, electronic or mechanical, including photocopying, recording, or by any information storage and retrieval system, without permission in writing from the copyright owner.

Any people depicted in stock imagery provided by Thinkstock are models, and such images are being used for illustrative purposes only.
Certain stock imagery © Thinkstock.

Print information available on the last page.

Rev. date: 09/24/2015

To order additional copies of this book, contact:
Xlibris
1-800-455-039
www.Xlibris.com.au
Orders@Xlibris.com.au
719081

CONTENTS

Preface ix

Chapter 1	Definition, Signs, Symptoms, And Treatment............1
Chapter 2	Types Of Fractures 8
Chapter 3	Complication Of Fracture 12
Chapter 4	Compound Fracture 25
Chapter 5	Plaster Of Paris Technique...28
Chapter 6	Traction...40
Chapter 7	Healing Of Fracture 47
Chapter 8	Radiographic Changes In Fracture-Healing................58
Chapter 9	Union Of Fractures 61
Chapter 10	Injuries Of The Upper Limb 70
Chapter 11	Fracture Of The Clavicle 72
Chapter 12	Dislocation Of The Shoulder Joint 81
Chapter 13	Fracture Of The Scapula 89
Chapter 14	Fracture Of The Humerus..92
Chapter 15	Fractures And Dislocations Of The Elbow 104
Chapter 16	Fracture Of The Shafts Of The Radius And Ulna....119
Chapter 17	Fractures Of The Wrist And Hand............................128
Chapter 18	Fractures And Dislocation Of The Spine 143
Chapter 19	Fracture Of The Pelvis..157
Chapter 20	Injuries Of The Lower Limb......................................170
Chapter 21	Fracture And Dislocations Of The Hip Joint...........172
Chapter 22	Fracture Of The Neck Of The Femur 185
Chapter 23	Fracture Of The Shaft Of The Femur 199
Chapter 24	Fractures Of The Shaft Of The Tibia & Fibula........209
Chapter 25	Injuries Of The Ankle 214
Chapter 26	Injuries Of The Foot 232
Chapter 27	Chest Injuries 246
Chapter 28	Facial Fractures..254

Chapter 29	Fractures In Children	268
Chapter 30	Fractures Of The Long Bones	274
Chapter 31	Internal Fixation Of Fractures	280
Chapter 32	Rehabilitation	290
Chapter 33	Occupational Therapy	312

Index 315

DEDICATED TO

Dr Abdul Hakeem Khan,
former consultant surgeon,
Lady Reading Hospital, Peshawar.

PREFACE

In presenting this volume, I am not unaware of the number of books dealing with this subject already available. It speaks of voluminous efforts taken by me to complete it over many years. This shows my immense love for the subject of orthopaedic surgery.

During the active period of service of teaching of this subject, I had received widespread approval by many students, and many have expressed the desire that I should write it down.

I take pleasure in acknowledging this encouraging words of the students and some well wisher colleagues as well.

In my professional life as an orthopaedic teacher/surgeon, I have been guided by these golden principles. These principles are what do you want to do, why do you want to do it, when do you want to do it, how do you want to do it, and are you doing it.

These words may appear meaningless to some, but for me, they have been the guiding principles in my treatment of fractures since the beginning of my orthopaedic career from 1956 to 1972 at King Edward Medical Collage, Lahore, and from 1972 to 1992 at Khyber Medical Collage, Peshawar, and up-to-date.

To write a book is not an easy task, in view of the fact that every now and then a new book on fracture appears somewhere in the world. However, I have written this book for which writing was started as early as 1967 and completed it in 2010. Perhaps no one might have given so much time to write a book on fracture while involved in active professional work. I hope this humble work finds its due place with orthopaedic teachers and orthopaedic surgeons including future doctors being trained for orthopaedic surgery.

I wish to acknowledge the support and encouragement I have received from my wife and children (Dr Fawad, Faisal, and Faiqa) because without their worlds of encouraging sentiments, this book would not have seen the light of the day.

Prof. Dr Manzoor Ahmad Khan

Orthopaedic surgery is that branch of surgery, which is to be seen and learnt, not to be read and learnt. But sound basic knowledge helps to develop sound orthopaedic surgery.

Manzoor

CHAPTER 1

DEFINITION, SIGNS, SYMPTOMS, AND TREATMENT

Definition

Fracture is a forcible solution of the continuity of the bone. In layman's term, it is known as the breaking of bone.

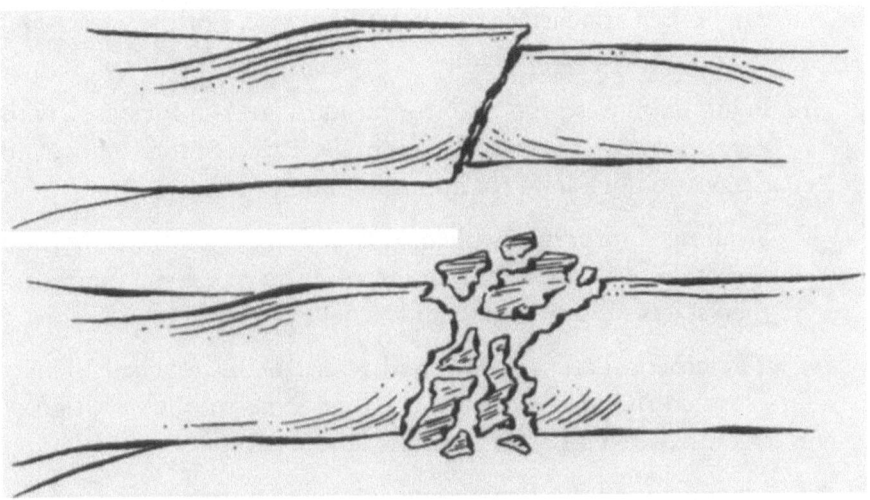

Fig. 1: Fracture.

Fracture can be caused by:
  i. direct trauma
  ii. indirect trauma.

Direct Trauma

The fracture occurs at the site of injury.

Indirect Trauma

The fracture occurs away from the site of injury (e.g. the patient falls on outstretched hand, and he gets a fracture of the wrist, elbow, or shoulder).

Signs and Symptoms

i. History of the injury: Patient volunteers the statement of having sustained an injury or a fall to his limb or his body. He can usually describe the exact mechanism of the fall or injury.

ii. Signs of injury: Usually at the site of injury, dirt, sand, or mud can be seen attached to the part. Otherwise, a bruise, laceration, or wound will be present.

iii. Pain: Pain is severe and continuous, and it increases with movements of the part or the body. Pain is more marked in dislocation of a joint than in fracture.

iv. Swelling: The part is swollen, and swelling extends well beyond the site of fracture. Swelling increases up to 24–48 hours and then starts subsiding gradually.

v. Tenderness: Part is tender and resists being touched. It may be noted that persistent localized tenderness is a classic sign of fracture when all other signs are absent.

vi. Loss of function: The patient is unable to move his limb. In case of lower-limb injury, he may not be able to raise himself from the ground.

vii. Deformity: The normal configuration of the part is lost. The deformity may be angular or rounded, depending upon the type and force of injury.

viii. Unnatural mobility: movement appears at the site where they are, in normal circumstances, not present.

ix. Crepitus: When the fracture fragments rub against each other, it produces a sound which is called crepitus. It is a confirmatory sign of fracture. It may be heard during the course of examination; otherwise, effort should not be made to elicit it because these extra movements may convert a simple fracture into a complicated one.

   x. Radiological examination: Radiological examination of the part must be done as a matter of routine. X-ray examination is indicated:

      a. to confirm the diagnosis (if in doubt)

      b. to demarcate the line of treatment

      c. to see the success of the treatment

      d. to see the progress of the fracture

      e. to confirm the healing of fracture.

To see the progress of treatment, X-ray examination must be done at a monthly interval because only then can a visible change (improvement or deterioration) be seen.

The difference between clinical and radiological union of fracture to take place is three weeks. Clinical union takes place early, and radiological union appears late because of the deposition of calcium salts in the bone, which are radiopaque.

Amongst the signs and symptoms mentioned above, pain, swelling, and loss of function can be caused by something else other than fracture injury. However, these symptoms disappear in other injuries but are likely to persist in fracture for a longer time. These are called indefinite signs of fracture.

The definite signs of fracture are:

    i. deformity

   ii. unnatural mobility

  iii. crepitus.

These signs present from the time of injury, either alone or together, confirm the diagnosis of fracture.

Treatment: First Aid

The following are immediate treatments of a fracture:
   i. rest to the part
   ii. rest to the body.

Rest to the part is provided by application of a splint. The splint should be well covered with cotton wool. The limb is placed with comfort on it, covered with cotton wool, and tied down snugly with an ordinary bandage. Tight bandaging must be avoided. The joint above and joint below must be immobilized. In case of injury of the upper limb, cuff, and collar, sling must be given.

If an open wound is present, it should be covered with clean dressing, and then bandage is applied.

Rest to the body is provided by giving a warm comfortable bed and administrating analgesics to relieve the pain. If the patient can swallow, he may be given a warm sweetened drink.

If the patient is in shock, the feet of the bed should be raised by blocks. If the patient has lost blood, it should be replaced, or if fluid loss is present, it should be rectified.

It may be noted that shock is more marked in fracture of the bone, and shock is usually primary or neurogenic in type to begin with. Later on, it may pass on to a secondary or haemorrhagic type.
   i. primary shock (neurogenic shock)
   ii. secondary shock (haemorrhagic shock).

Primary shock lasts from 1¼ to 2¼ hours. In a primary shock, the patient appears pale. Pulse is slow and low in volume. Respiration is slow and shallow. But after a lapse of an hour or so, beads of perspiration appear on the forehead. This is an indication that the patient is passing from primary to secondary shock. The pulse becomes full and bounding.

Respiration becomes rapid and deep. As shock advances, the pulse becomes rapid and thready. The volume of pulse falls, and respiration becomes rapid and shallow (if haemorrhage continues). Immediate blood replacement becomes essential.

The usual blood loss for individual bone fracture is as follows:

- femur: 500 cc
- tibia and fibula: 400 cc
- humerus: 400 cc
- radius and ulna: 400 cc
- radius or ulna (alone): 200 cc each.

In case of secondary shock, the shock may be reversible. This state depends upon the blood pressure. The kidneys function well at 80 mm Hg. If the blood pressure falls suddenly and rises suddenly, it is a reversible shock. If the blood pressure falls down and rises slowly or if it does not rise again, it is an irreversible shock. Hence, it is the state of the blood pressure which determines the outcome of the shock. Below 60 mm Hg, the kidney cannot function, and the shock becomes irreversible.

Fluid loss along with blood loss occurs according to the site of fracture.

- fracture of the femur: 500 cc + 500 cc = 1,000 cc
- fracture of the tibia: 400 cc + 250 cc = 650 cc
- fracture of the humerus: 400 cc + 200 cc = 600 cc
- fracture of the radius and ulna: 400 cc + 200 cc = 600 cc
- fracture of the radius or ulna alone: 200 cc + 100 cc = 300 cc

If the patient has double fractures or multiple fractures, the shock will be greater due to the loss of blood and fluid inside the tissues. In case of compound fracture, the loss will still be greater, and the shock will be more marked. The chances of irreversibility of shock increases unless treated immediately.

Treatment of fractures:
i. closed
ii. open

Closed Method

The three principles involved are the following (fig. 2):
i. reduction of fracture to restore the anatomy
ii. immobilization of fracture to maintain the anatomy
iii. restoration the function to preserve the physiology.

All fractures should be treated by closed method except when it fails. More than 2,000 years ago, Hippocrates said, 'Let there be two strong men to pull the limb in opposite direction and the fracture be reduced.'

The downward pull is called traction, and the upward pull is called counter-traction. This allows the muscle to be overstretched and get relaxed. Immediately after the fracture, there is muscle spasm, which can be overcome by this method. The traction and counter-traction must be maintained for three minutes to allow the spasm of muscles to disappear (e.g. to reduce fracture in the forearm, traction is applied to the hand, and counter-traction is applied to the elbow). Since the traction and counter-traction are applied separately by assistants, the surgeon is free to manipulate and reduce the fracture.

During the reduction of fracture, steady force is applied in traction and counter-traction. Jerky movements and frequent interruptions of pull must be avoided. Having manipulated the fragments in position, the limb is immobilized in plaster of Paris cast. The golden principle must be followed—that is, the joint above and the joint below must be immobilized. The period of immobilization depends upon the site of the fracture:

- femur: 12–14 weeks
- tibia: 10–12 weeks
- humerus: 8–10 weeks
- radius and ulna: 6–8 weeks

- metacarpals/metatarsal: 4–6 weeks
- phalanges: 3–4 weeks.

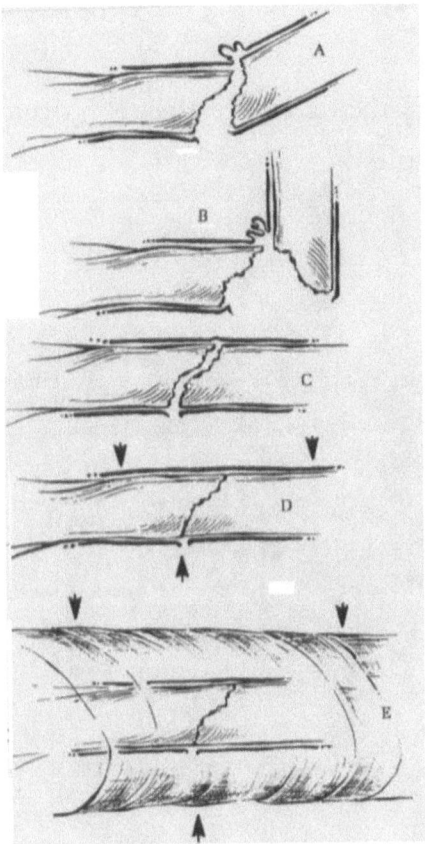

Fig. 2: Reduction of fracture.

Indications of open reduction:
a. compound fracture
b. complicated fracture
c. when closed reduction fails
d. certain special sites (e.g. fractured patella, olecranon process)
e. when closed treatment may not be successful (e.g. fractured forearm or femur).

CHAPTER 2

TYPES OF FRACTURES

Clinically speaking, there are three types of fractures:
1. simple fracture
2. compound fracture
3. complicated fracture (fig. 3).

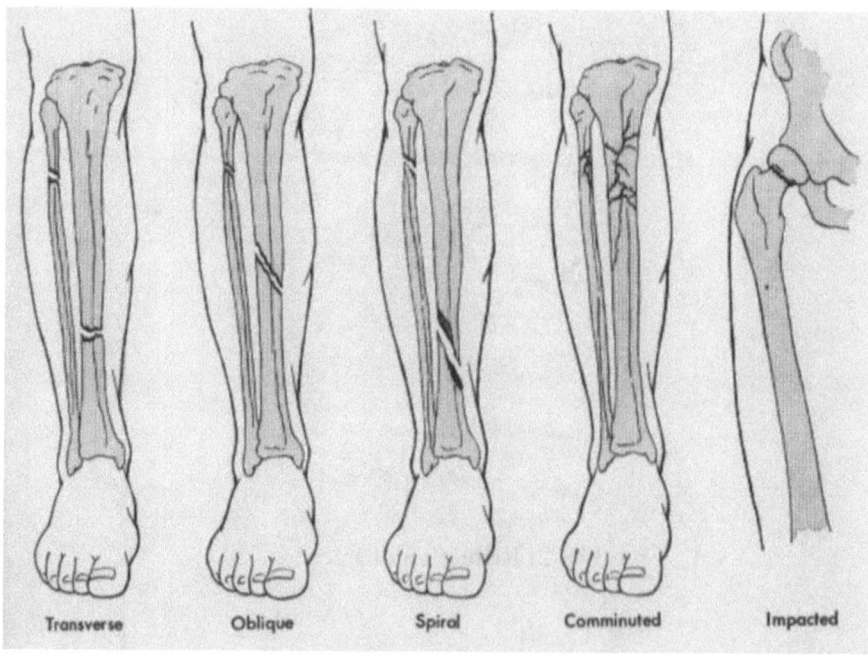

Fig. 3: Types of fractures.

Simple fracture is when only the bone is broken. In each and every fracture, there is an injury to the surrounding tissues (i.e. muscles), but they are labelled as simple fracture.

Compound fracture is that in which there is a wound in addition to the fracture, and the fracture site communicates with external air.

When the bone is seen through the wound, when it is felt through the wound, or when it comes out through the wound, then it is called a compound fracture. If there is a fracture at the lower end of the thigh and a wound at the upper end of thigh and they are not communicating, it is not a compound fracture.

Complicated fracture happens when, in addition to fracture, there is an injury to the vessel or nerve. For example, when there is a fractured humerus along with an injury to the radial nerve, it is called complicated fracture.

Radiological classification based on X-ray findings is as follows:
1. greenstick fracture
2. comminuted fracture
3. transverse fracture
4. oblique fracture
5. spiral fracture
6. impacted fracture
7. double fracture
8. multiple fractures
9. pathological fracture
10. fatigue fracture
11. avulsion fracture.

Based on clinical and radiological classification, the fracture can be described as a simple oblique fracture of the left femur or a compound transverse fracture of the left femur or a complicated double fracture of the left tibia or a compound, complicated, comminuted fracture of the right humerus.

Greenstick Fracture

When a branch is broken from a tree, it never completely breaks down. Half of it is broken transversely, and half of it longitudinally.

This is the same in a greenstick fracture, and it occurs in children under 10 years of age. The bones are soft. They bend under pressure, and therefore, fracture is not complete.

Comminuted Fracture

When the bone at the fracture site is broken in more than three or four fragments, it is called a comminuted fracture. This is caused by a direct blow or a crushing force.

Transverse Fracture

When the fracture line is transverse to the long axis of the bone, it is a transverse fracture. This is caused by a bending force.

Oblique Fracture

When the fracture line is oblique, it is called an oblique fracture. This is caused also by a bending force applied to a long line.

Spiral Fracture

When the line of fracture is spiral, it is a spiral fracture. The difference between a spiral fracture and an oblique fracture is that, in an oblique fracture, the fracture line is equidistant from one end to the other. In a spiral fracture, the fragments overlap at one or another portion of the fracture line. It is caused by a torsion or twisting force.

Impacted Fracture

When the fracture fragments are driven into one another after a fracture and they get locked, it is called an impacted fracture. It is caused by a compression force applied along the long axis of the bone.

Double Fracture

When two fractures occur in one bone, it is called a double fracture.

Multiple Fractures

When more than one bone is fractured, it is called multiple fractures.

Pathological Fracture

Pathological fracture occurs due to minimal trauma, a trauma insufficient to break a normal healthy bone. It is caused by some underlying disease of the bone, such as tumour of the bone or secondary deposits.

Fatigue Fracture

A healthy bone may be fractured with repeated minor trauma. Such fractures are called stress or fatigue fractures. The commonest example is a fracture of the second metatarsal after a long march, where moderate stress that is repeated thousands of times ultimately breaks the bone.

Avulsion Fracture

A violent muscle contraction may produce an avulsion of a portion of the bone where tendon is attached.

CHAPTER 3

COMPLICATION OF FRACTURE

Complications of fractures are:
1. immediate
2. late.

Immediate complications are:
i. shock
ii. haemorrhage
iii. fat embolism
iv. pulmonary embolism.

Fat Embolism

Fat is liquid at body temperature. Fat is present everywhere in the body, and it is present in bones. Fat embolism occurs within three hours after an injury, manipulation, or operative treatment, wherein fat is pushed into the circulation. It produces two types of symptoms:

v. pulmonary symptoms
vi. cerebral symptoms.

The patient coughs fat globules in sputum. If such sputum is stained with black ink, the fat globules are stained black, but the rest of the tissue is not stained. Also, laboratory investigation shows that there is a sudden fall in haemoglobin level in fat embolism. The reason is that when the fat enters the circulation, it joins with the haemoglobin portion, and thus, its level falls.

Pulmonary symptoms will be dyspnoea, cyanosis, and patchy consolidation. When the fat globules passes the lung barrier and reaches the brain, the patient becomes unconscious, may get hemiplegia (hemiparesis), then passes into stupor, coma, and death.

This complication is much less common. The treatment of fat embolism is prophylactic (i.e. move the limb as little as possible, and be gentle while reducing the fracture). Once the embolism occurs, the treatment is symptomatic.

The first evidence of fat embolism may be noted within 24 hours of injury. Temperature elevation to 102 °F is common, and the heart rate may be above 100 beats per minute. Headache, irritability, lethargy, or delirium may appear.

The late complications which occur due to fracture are as follows:

1. joint stiffness
    a. periarticular adhesions
    b. intra-articular adhesions
    c. muscular adhesions
    d. periarticular ossifications
    e. Sudeck's syndrome
2. injury to the nerve
3. injury to the artery
4. slow and delayed union
5. malunion
6. non-union
7. avascular necrosis
8. osteoarthritis.

1. Joint Stiffness

Some stiffness after fractures and dislocations is inevitable. The incidence can be reduced if good primary treatment and aftercare of fracture is carried out.

Periarticular Adhesions

Every injury is followed by swelling of the part due to capillary haemorrhage and extravasation of fluid. Normally, fluid is removed with activity, but it accumulates when the limb is splinted. Fibrin is deposited and is converted into fibrous tissue if left undisturbed. In the periarticular region, because of close proximity to joint capsule, lack of muscle belly, and lack of space for expansion, the chances of adhesions are greater.

Usually, joint recovers function even if it is fixed in a plaster cast for a few weeks, but if the capsule has been damaged, stiffness is likely to persist.

The best treatment is to encourage activity by constant repetition of a particular movement (e.g. if stiffness of ankle after tibial fracture develops, it can be treated by exercises of plantar flexion and dorsiflexion). It is important that the movement must be done every hour (with a minimum of five minutes), day and night, for a sufficiently long time, with perseverance and patience. Only then will the function of the joint be restored.

Manipulation under anaesthesia may be helpful, and fixed deformity sometimes can be corrected by wedge plaster method. However, both these methods require knowledge and experience and should only be carried out carefully in stages. Complete correction at one stage is not possible, nor is it recommended.

Intra-Articular Adhesions

There is always haemarthrosis after dislocation, fracture traversing the joint, and severe ligamentous injuries. Synovial membrane does not have the capacity to absorb portion of the blood; therefore, the fibrin content of the blood sticks to the articular ends and is converted into fibrous tissue. This leads to limitation of movement. In such a case, a prophylactic injection of hyaluronidase (Hyalase) into the joint shortly after the injury, which is then repeated after a few days, prevents the onset of adhesions in the joint.In late stages, manipulation may be carried out especially in the case of knee, ankle, elbow, and shoulder joints, but it must be remembered that manipulation of smaller joints, particularly joint of fingers, usually does more harm than good, and it must never be carried out under anaesthesia. In these joints, it is advisable to allow the movements to recover by active exercises only.

Muscular Adhesions

Injury to the muscle, whether caused by the scalpel of the surgeon or due to vehicle trauma, ends in fibrosis of the muscle with adhesions to the surrounding parts. This is due to the organization of haematoma of fracture. The commonest example is limitation of knee movements following the fracture of the middle and lower third of the femur.

In such cases, prevention is always better. And no matter what type of treatment is carried out, the active static contraction of corresponding muscle must be carried out (e.g. in a fractured femur, it is always profitable to start quadriceps exercises from the very start of the treatment of the fracture of the femur).

Manipulation at a later stage is strongly contraindicated. Fracture of the bone, avulsion of the muscle, or tear of the tendon may occur due to injudicious manipulation. Active exercises are more helpful. The more active treatment, if disability is severe, is to free the muscle belly from the scar tissues, but recovery of full movements is unusual even after surgery.

Periarticular Ossification

Periarticular ossification commonly follows dislocation or fracture–dislocation of the elbow joint and hip joint. In the elbow, it usually forms on the anterior aspect, and in the hip, it forms on the posterolateral side.

It always follows the tear of capsule of the joint and occasionally occurs after muscle damage. But it is not true myositis ossificans and can be easily differentiated from it by the fact that new bone is laid down in the muscle fibres and not subperiosteally as in the case of myositis ossificans. Diagnosis is confirmed by radiography. Manipulation is strongly contraindicated and must never be attempted. Rest to the part is absolutely essential and must be carried out till serial X-ray films show no evidence of bone.

In late stages, when bone has been sufficiently organized, it may be excised. But results of operative interference are not good and should be undertaken only when there is marked limitation of movements.

Sudeck's Syndrome

Sudeck's syndrome is rather a serious affair and a difficult problem to treat. It is a troublesome cause of joint stiffness in which both the soft tissue and bones are involved.

It most often follows injuries of the wrist, fingers, or foot. The cause is unknown. Many theories regarding its aetiology have been put forward, but not one has wholly explained the symptomatology. The most plausible one has been neurovascular imbalance.

Symptoms of Sudeck's atrophy are so characteristic that once the complication has been seen in its most developed form, it cannot be mistaken for any other condition. Usually after injury, when the splint or plaster cast is removed, the wrist or foot becomes stiff and painful instead of regaining movements gradually. The skin presents a characteristic of having a smooth, shiny look, and bone shows a mottled radiological appearance.

Prolonged immobilization makes the matter worse. The best form of treatment is active exercises of the part while it is elevated and warmed by means of a rubefacient. It is a fact that no one can say which patient is going to develop this syndrome, but if active movements of parts not immobilized in the plaster cast are carried out, the chances of developing this syndrome are markedly reduced. Once the condition has developed fully, recovery is very slow and protracted, but it does take place in due course of time (may be many months). Hence, it is worth the trouble to continue the treatment for many, many months. It must be remembered that the condition is very painful and demoralizing in nature, and suicidal tendency has been seen in patients in his condition.

Hence, repeated assurance and encouragement to the patient is very necessary and must be given.

Hormonal treatment has been tried but without any definite effect on the disease itself. Cervical and lumbar sympathectomy has also been done to relieve the patient of pain. Although effective in early stages, pain returns again after some time, and the results are not worth the surgery. It is considered that probably somatic sensation of pain is so highly ingrained that no method of treatment succeeds except time, which is the great healer.

2. Injury to the Nerve

Injury to the nerve may be one of the three types generally described:

1. Neuropraxia (interruption of conduction): the nerve has been contused or compressed, but there has been no actual disruption of the axons.
2. Axonotmesis (damage to the axon): The nerve has been contused or compressed. There has been no physical division of the axons, but the injury has been severe enough that Wallerian degeneration has taken place or will take place. Since there has been no actual division of the fibres, regeneration may be expected to take place by axonal growth along its original pathway.
3. Neurotemesis (complete division of the nerve): The nerve has been completely or partially divided. Regeneration cannot be expected to take place until the nerve division has been repaired. If repair is successful, axonal growth will then proceed at a uniform rate, generally estimated at 1–2 mm per day. By this formula, one can roughly estimate the time to be taken for complete recovery of the nerve.

The following peripheral nerves are injured with fracture or dislocation:

1. axillary nerve
2. radial nerve
3. median nerve

4. ulnar nerve
5. sciatic nerve
6. lateral popliteal nerve.

Axillary Nerve

In about 15% of humeral head dislocation, evidence of injury to the axillary nerve may be found. This consists of sensory impairment over the superficial distribution of this nerve on the lateral side of the shoulder and upper arm and weakness or paresis of the deltoid muscle. The lesion is evidently due to traction on the nerve by the displaced head of the humerus. Recovery is usually spontaneous and complete within several months. Occasionally, the recovery may not happen, causing loss of function of deltoid muscle.

Radial Nerve

The radial nerve may be injured in the groove of the humerus when that bone is fractured. Injury is manifested by the inability to extend the wrist, the thumb, and the metacarpophalangeal joints of the fingers. This injury is usually one in which the nerve retains continuity, and recovery is generally apparent by the third or fourth month. If (as it infrequently occurs) recovery is delayed beyond this period, exploration with the expectation of repairing the nerve should be carried out. During the period in which muscles supplied by the nerve are paralysed, support should be given to these muscles in the form of an active splint, usually by a cock-up splint.

Median Nerve

The median nerve may be injured at the elbow, especially in supracondylar fractures of the humerus or at the wrist in dislocations of the lunate. With the injury occurring at the wrist, sensory loss over the thumb, index finger, middle finger, and one-half of the ring finger is noted. The abductor brevis and opponens are paralysed. With injury occurring at the elbow, the forearm muscles supplied by the nerve are involved additionally. This is demonstrated clinically by loss of flexion of the interphalangeal joint of the thumb. The nerve at either level is seldom lacerated, and relief from a compressing agent will usually permit recovery.

Ulnar Nerve

Injury to the ulnar nerve is not as common as injury to other nerves. It may be seen in the injuries around the elbow, especially those that force the forearm into valgus or displace it forward. The nerve injury is almost always left in continuity, and complete recovery occurs in a few weeks or months.

Sciatic Nerve

Injury to sciatic nerve is seen occasionally in association with posterior dislocation of the head of the femur and rarely with fracture of the pelvic ring. Paralysis of all muscles below the knee indicates this lesion. As the nerve is rarely lacerated, recovery is usually complete in three months' time.

Lateral Popliteal Nerve

The lateral popliteal nerve may be injured in fractures of the proximal tibia and fibula in various injuries of the knee with rupture of the lateral soft tissue and, probably most commonly, through the compression of the nerve at the neck of fibula by improperly applied casts and splints. Sensory loss is noted over the dorsum of the foot and the peroneal muscles, and the muscles of the anterior compartment are paralysed. If the compression is promptly relieved, complete recovery is expected. Foot drop should be prevented by the use of a splint or brace during the period of recovery. It is to be noted that amongst all nerve injuries, lateral popliteal nerve has got the worst prognosis.

Nerve Injury with Open Fracture

At the time of original wound debridement, injured nerve will probably be seen. If the injury is that of contusion or compression, recovery may be expected. If the nerve has been divided, primary repair is not advisable. The nerve ends may be marked by suture, and repair must be delayed until all wound swelling has subsided. Repair can then be accomplished without danger of wound sepsis, which might jeopardize the anastomosis.

The injury to the nerve may be partial (nos 1 and 2) or complete (no. 3) and may occur as a result of traction, compression, or tear of the nerve.

To avoid later regrets, it is always advisable to test the sensation and motor power distal to the site of injury (e.g. in fracture humerus, the sensation on the dorsal surface of hand and extension of wrist joint should be tested).

In a partial injury, the recovery usually sets in after a few days and is complete in a few weeks' time.

In a complete injury, if recovery does not set in after three to four weeks, it is always advisable to explore the nerve. If a tear is found, suture can be carried out.

It is to be noted that failure of nerve function may occasionally be due to its involvement in the callus, and if proper precaution in testing the nerve function at the time of injury has been taken, much worry and suffering can be avoided.

3. Injury of the Artery

The main artery is occasionally severed at the time of injury. When this happens and the collateral circulation is inadequate, recovery lies in immediate repair, if necessary, with a graft.

The common sequel to arterial injury is ischaemia, which is due to complete or partial obstruction. This is either due to compression or irritation by fracture fragments or, more often, by a tight plaster cast. Early diagnosis is essential. Certain fractures like supracondylar fracture of the humerus, fracture of the forearm, and fracture of the upper end of the tibia demand special attention because of the danger of getting this complication.

The appearance of any of the five *P*s—i.e. pain, pulselessness, pallor, paralysis, and puffiness—has an urgency that must not be ignored.

Any pain which persists after a good dose of analgesic and sometimes hypnotic medication demands immediate attention. The treatment should be immediately carried out, preferably in the operation theatre. First of all, the position of the fracture should be changed, and see if the pulse returns. If not, a ganglionic block should be given. If it does not work, then proceed to explore the artery. Sometimes only exposure helps to relieve the spasm, and at other times, it is necessary to infiltrate the artery with 1–2% novocaine solution. It has been noted that the spasm in the artery is not sympathetic but myogenic in origin. Therefore, the vessel should be given a bath in a 2% solution of papaverine. It is further seen that it takes some time for the spasm to disappear; hence, the papaverine solution should be allowed to remain in contact with the artery for 30 minutes so that it penetrates the muscular coat of the artery. As a last resort, the spastic or damaged portion of the artery should be resected and replaced by a graft or direct suture.

It is to be remembered that such arterial injury is responsible for many ischaemic contractures in patients, who have been treated by long-setters, and it is difficult to find a solution of such problem of ischaemic contracture.

4. Slow and Delayed Union

The slow and delayed union are the same entity, but the difference is that in slow union, the process of healing takes place slowly while in delayed union, the healing stops and starts again after some time. It is difficult for those who see occasional cases of fractures to decide between slow and delayed upon. Therefore, one can safely say that slow and delayed union is that stage in which the fragments are in perfect apposition but are still not united after due date and fragments may be movable. If given time, this fracture will unite. However, it must be noted that union and non-union of fracture are definite entities, but slow and delayed union is an intermediate stage and may end in one or another. In certain sites (e.g. fracture of the lower third of the tibia), one would be inclined to supplement the rate of union by a bone graft because this is the common site of delayed union and the effect of the prolonged immobilization in plaster cast usually leads to stiffness of the ankle joint.

5. Malunion

Malunion is the stage in which fracture fragments unite in a distorted or angular position. In children, 10–15 angulation or rotational deformity and overlapping by 1 cm are permissible, but under no circumstances should rotational or angular deformity be allowed to persist in adults because they interfere markedly with the function of the limb. In children, angulation is corrected by gradual growth process, but in adults, it will not be straightened. If function of the limb is good after malunion, it is unnecessary to interfere with it (e.g. in fracture of the tibia, if there is malunion but the leg is strong for weight-bearing purposes, then the malunion should be allowed to remain). Also, malunion should be allowed to remain if it is feared that the procedure necessary to correct it will do more harm than good and will lead to further complications (e.g. fracture of the surgical neck of the humerus). Since this is a fracture which is difficult to manipulate and repeated manipulations may endanger the life of the head of humerus and perfect alignment may not be attained, some malunion may be allowed to persist. Usually, this does not hinder the function of the shoulder joint.

6. Non-Union

Non-union means that the fracture will not unite unless aided. Amongst the many causes of it, disturbance of the primary haematoma, whether by the trauma or by the injudicious treatment, is the most important single factor. To prevent this complication to occur, one must use manipulation as gentle as possible, and excessive force must be avoided. Furthermore, repeated manipulations and frequent change of plaster cast should not be practised, for these often lead to this complication.

Non-union is present if fracture fragments are mobile (may be painless) and the X-ray shows sclerosis (rounding of bone ends) and/or obliteration of medullary cavity.

Such cases should be treated by cancellous bone graft taken from iliac crest. There are many who still believe that excision of the fibrous union and replacement by graft is to be done. But study of cases treated by onlay cancellous bone grafting without excision of fibrous union has given good results.

7. Avascular Necrosis

Avascular necrosis is the condition in which part of or the whole of the bone dies when it has been deprived of its blood supply. The four common sites are the head of the femur, following subcapital fracture of the neck of the femur scaphoid, following fracture of the scaphoid; lunate (after dislocation of lunate and talus), following fracture–dislocation of the neck of the talus. Occasionally, the head of the humerus may become necrosed, following fracture–dislocation of the neck of the humerus or too extensive operation on the shoulder in which all the attachments of the capsule of the shoulder joint have been cut off from the head of the humerus.

Diagnosis is not easy, and usually, some time must elapse before radiological signs appear. No hard and fast rule can be drawn. Sometimes the bone may show signs of necrosis only a week after the injury, while in other cases, the necrosis may not be apparent for many months after the injury. But a good practical rule is that if it is suspected that necrosis will occur, especially at the sites mentioned above, have always an X-ray examination after one month and repeat it at a monthly interval. There is no occasion to be surprised if necrosis is detected six months or a year after the injury because it can occur after this time.

The treatment is not easy. Suffice it to say that in some cases and at certain sites, it is necessary to leave the patient and the fracture at rest, and in other cases, it will be necessary to resort to surgery. However, if patient is seen only when necrosis has fully developed, surgery is required to replace the necrosed portion of the bone.

8. Osteoarthritis

Osteoarthritis commonly occurs after fractures involving the joints, but its onset can be often delayed much longer. Osteoarthritis is a degenerative process in the primary form. It occurs with the passage of time. Only in old age do the many minor symptoms of wear and tear affecting the joints manifest. The degenerative process is usually initiated in the articular cartilage, and if the changes are already present, an injury will accelerate the disease process. But if the fracture line is a linear one and the joint is healthy at the time of injury, the symptoms will not develop for many years. However, osteoarthritis sets in early if the articular cartilage is crushed or when the subarticular area has poor nutrition.

Radiological signs are not a definite proof that osteoarthritis is causing symptoms. On the contrary, we often see many patients walking about and doing their normal duties in spite of marked radiological evidence of osteoarthritis. Therefore, symptoms in secondary type of osteoarthritis are probably due to periarticular adhesions and may respond to various measures as described earlier for stiffness of joint. It is necessary that this type of patients should be excluded before osteoarthritis is held responsible for symptoms. Osteoarthritis that is causing symptoms should be treated as if it were not associated with injury.

The commonest joint affected is the knee joint, following fractures around knee joint. The onset is marked since it is a weight-bearing joint and comparatively more exposed. Although the treatment is difficult and many old methods have become obsolete, nowadays the commonly practised method is the intra-articular cortisone injections or Hyalase injection (hyaluronidase). Results are variable, but it does seem to work. The patient is relieved of the pain, and the range of movements increases. But the relief is temporary, and relief is there as long as injections are given in the joint. Permanent relief can be obtained after surgery, and severe symptoms do warrant its use. After surgery, movements are sacrificed, but painless stability is attained by arthrodesis. Knee joint replacement can also be carried out, but results are variable. These abovementioned complications do demand a vigilant and correct approach to the treatment of fractures. Thus, the patient's suffering is reduced to a minimum, and the patient may be protected from suffering its effects for months or sometimes for years.

CHAPTER 4

COMPOUND FRACTURE

Compound fracture is that where the fracture site communicates with the external air (fig. 4).

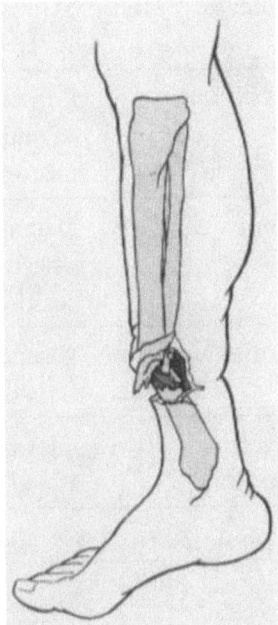

Fig. 4: Compound fracture of the tibia and fibula with laceration of the skin caused by the sharp edge of proximal fragment.

Compound fracture is of two types:
 i. compound from within
 ii. compound from without.

Compound from within is the one where the bone fragments pierce the skin and come out.

Compound from without is the one where the skin is damaged first and fracture occurs later.

Compound from Within	Compound from Without
i. It is necessarily a clean fracture. Because the fragments of bones come out from inside, they are clean.	i. It is basically an infected fracture.
ii. Skin is clean cut and not damaged.	ii. Skin is damaged, and margins are lacerated.
iii. Primary suture of the skin may be carried out.	iii. Primary suture of skin is not advisable, or it is not possible to suture the skin.
iv. Skin margins need not be cut.	iv. Damaged margins of the skin have to be cut to allow clear healthy margins to come out.
v. Wound heals quickly and with primary intentions.	v. Wound healing is delayed.
vi. Internal fixation of fracture may be carried out.	vi. Internal fixation of fracture is not advisable.
vii. Results are generally good.	vii. Results are generally poor.

Treatment of Compound Fracture

The patient should be taken to the operation theatre. The patient should be anaesthetized under general anaesthesia. The wound should be washed thoroughly with soap and water. All the sand or dirt should be removed. The limb should be shaved well and prepared with antiseptic solution. The procedure of debridement should be performed upon the wound. The skin margins are excised with a clean knife. The fascia and muscle portion which are damaged are excised. Blood clots are removed. Pieces of bone which are lying free should be excised, but no piece of bone which has periosteal attachment should be excised. If advisable or permissible, the fracture should be fixed with a screw, plate and screws, or intramedullary nail (i.e. internal fixation is carried out). The muscle should be approximated by interrupted sutures. Fascia must never be stitched. The skin should be stitched by interrupted sutures placed at a distance from one another.

A wound treated in this manner will not allow the fluid collection to occur and will not be put under tension. Wound healing will progress satisfactorily. The wound should be covered with dressing pads. The limb should be padded with cotton wool, and plaster cast should be applied. It must be remembered that a skintight plaster must never be applied because it will not have space for swelling; hence, compression of vessels will take place, leading to complications like gangrene.

The wound in the following types of compound fractures must never be stitched:

i. roadside accidents
ii. industrial fractures
iii. gunshot injuries
iv. crush injuries or badly lacerated wounds
v. wounds received after golden period has passed (i.e. later than six hours).

In all compound fractures where plaster cast has been applied, it should be removed after 7–10 days. Wound should be cleaned and dressed, and a new plaster cast should be applied, which may be maintained according to required time.

Every case of compound fracture is watched after operative treatment, and if there is marked soaking with blood, the plaster should be slit open immediately and kept open. At the end of 24 hours, the limbs are made bare, wound cleaned, dressing applied, and a new padded plaster cast or posterior plaster slab applied. However, plaster of Paris cast must not be applied immediately after the injury and after operative procedure. Instead, a back plaster slab should be applied and completed into plaster cast after 24–48 hours.

CHAPTER 5

PLASTER OF PARIS TECHNIQUE

Since ages, plaster of Paris has remained the best form of external fixation for fractures. Various methods, such as wooden and plastic splints and leather support, have been used for treatment of fractures. However, in due course of time, it has been found that they cannot replace the plaster of Paris (fig. 5).

The plaster of Paris is used for the following types of applications:

1. shoulder spica
2. arm cast
3. above-elbow cast
4. below-elbow cast
5. fingers cast
6. hip spica
7. above-knee cast
8. below-knee cast.

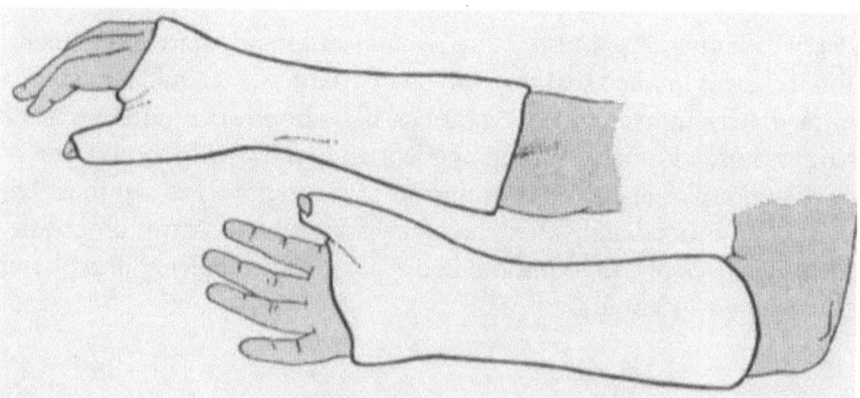

Fig. 5a: Plaster gauntlet for fracture scaphoid and Bennett fracture.

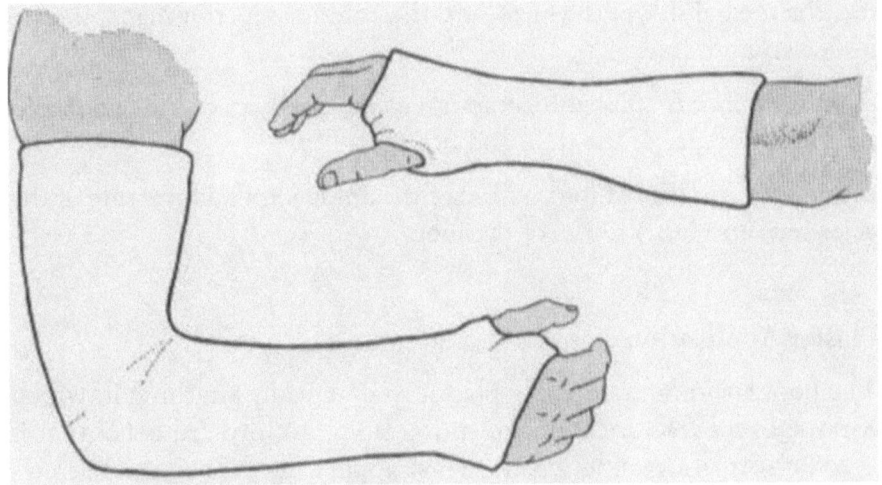

Fig. 5b: Types of plaster casts: above-elbow plaster cast and below-elbow plaster cast.

Shoulder spica is applied for injuries and diseases of the shoulder girdle. The position of the shoulder spica is 45 degrees abduction, flexion is 30 degrees, and external rotation is 15 degrees.

Arm cast is applied for fractures of the humerus. It extends from the shoulder to the elbow and surrounds both these joints.

Above-elbow cast is applied for injuries of the elbow joint, which means fractures of the lower end of the humerus and upper end of the radius and ulna and fractures of the forearm. It extends from the mid arm to the fingers.

Below-elbow cast is applied for fractures of the lower end of radius and ulna. It extends from the elbow to the fingers.

Fingers cast is applied for fractures of the hand and fingers (metacarpal and phalanges). It provides immobilization to the finger only. If one finger is fractured, another finger close to it should also be included in the plaster cast to provide support to the injured finger.

Hip spica is applied for dislocated hip joint and fractured neck of the femur, trochanter, and shaft of the femur. It extends from around the pelvis to the whole length of the affected limb up to the foot. The hip spica should be applied in such a manner that the medial side of the big toe, the medial side of the knee, and the anterior superior iliac spine are in one straight line.

Above-knee cast is applied for fracture of the condyles of the femur and tibia and fracture of the tibia and fibula.

Below-knee cast is used for fracture of the ankle joint and fracture of the calcaneus and other bones of the foot.

Plaster Application

The popular impulse to apply plaster to practically anything in which X-ray shows a fracture seems to spring from an unvoiced belief that it is some sort of dressing which, when applied to the skin, accelerates the healing of the underlying bone. It is true that liberal application of plaster to minor fractures encountered daily can do no serious harm to any and may do good to many. Treatment of fractures without rigid external fixation may be practised easily, and it does work, but there is no method of external splintage which could fulfil the criteria of immobilization, which is to prevent even microscopic movements between the bone ends during the process of healing. This can all be achieved by some form of internal fixation, such as plate and screws, intramedullary nailing, and bone grafting.

A walking plaster for fractures of the tarsus or metatarsus is not effective as the soft tissue in the sole of the foot is compressed and springs back again when the weight is relieved. Hence, a walking plaster for such fractures is no more effective than a leather boot.

It is a fact that a spontaneous increase in deformity occurs if fractures of long bones are left without artificial support. However, such displacement may not occur in fractures of short bones. Hence, there is always the possibility that what has been an undisplaced fracture in the initial radiograph may have been grossly displaced at the time of treatment, and in the process of first aid, splintage may have been reduced to an almost perfect position.

The following are the general misconceptions regarding plaster fixation:
1. The fragments of a fresh fracture are always mobile unless fixed by artificial means.
2. A plaster cast will prevent such mobility.
3. Displacement will increase if the limb is not splinted.
4. Plaster fixation accelerates fracture-healing.
5. The quality of the end result will be better after treatment with plaster than without it.

It is to be noted that plaster fixation cannot accelerate fracture-healing; plaster merely ensures that the limb is retained in good alignment when healing takes place. The healing of fracture cannot be accelerated, and it can easily be inhibited by unfavourable external conditions, such as faulty blood supply or gross and continuous movements. The aim of fracture treatment is to eliminate all deleterious influences rather than to accelerate the union. After plaster application, static muscular contractions will maintain the blood supply and, thus, accelerate the union. They will also enable the patient to regain the movements of the joint involved in the plaster cast soon. However, although plaster application is a good method of treatment of the fracture, it can cause delayed union of the fracture and joint stiffness. Late oedema is a frequent complication following removal of the plaster splint.

Cases Suitable for Treatment without Plaster

The following list comprises those fractures which are suited to early mobilization without plaster fixation:
1. olecranon (if undisplaced)
2. elbow fracture
3. tuberosity of carpal scaphoid
4. other carpal bones (excluding waist of scaphoid)
5. shaft of fibula
6. tibial condyles (in the aged)
7. patella (if stellate or transverse without separation)

8. tarsal bones
9. march fracture
10. styloid process of the fifth metatarsal
11. phalanges of toes, metatarsals
12. os calcis
13. thoracic spine
14. mild compression fractures of the lumbar spine
15. central dislocation of the hip
16. pelvis without displacement.

Positive indications for the treatment of fractures by plaster might be stated in the following terms:

1. to maintain a position secured by reduction.
2. to 'immobilize' if movements are likely when adjacent joints are moved.
3. to 'immobilize' when one fragment is prone to ischaemic necrosis.
4. to permit weight-bearing in order to stimulate bony union in delayed union of long bones.
5. for economic reasons (i.e. to evacuate hospital beds or make a patient ambulant for his personal convenience).

Pressure Bandage

A carefully applied pressure bandage provides some degree of splintage by reason of rigidity, and at the same time, it allows movements through a restricted range.

The bandage is applied by alternate layers of cotton wool and bandage over the injured part. This type of dressing, for majority of knee injuries, is infinitely better than any form of plaster cast because plaster cast is incapable of applying continuous gentle pressure once an effusion in the knee joint has started to diminish. As soon as the efficacy of this simple but highly scientific dressing is appreciated, it will be found that very few plaster cylinders need to be used for the non-operative treatment of knee injuries or fracture of the patella.

Plaster Application Method

Usually, 6 in. or 9 in. plaster bandages are used for immobilization of fracture.

The bandage is removed from its cover and is placed in a bowl full of water. Cold or hot water should not be used. Best results are obtained when lukewarm water is used. The bandage is placed in the water. When submerged gradually in water, bubbles come out of it. When bubbles stop coming out, it shows that the bandage is completely soaked. The bandage should be lifted out of the water, and excess water should be allowed to drip out of it. Bandage should never be squeezed to remove excess water. Doing so will harm the application of bandage as it will get dry quickly, and setting or smoothening will not be possible as it will set quickly. After lifting the bandage from the water, the bandage should be applied around the limb. The bandage should be rolled over the arm or leg according to the contours of the limb. During the application of plaster bandage, it should not be pulled or pressed against the limb. This will produce pressure on the limb, leading to complication of the circulation and oedema, which will affect the functions of the limb. The time taken to set the plaster is three minutes; therefore, the limb should be held in the right position for this period till the plaster cast is completely dry. For the upper limb, a sling should be given from the elbow to the wrist joint to hold the limb at right angle. For the lower limb, the patient should not be allowed to walk with a plaster cast for 48–72 hours (till plaster cast has become dry completely). If the patient walks with the plaster cast in initial stages, the plaster cast is likely to break down, and it may cause injury to the limb skin.

Plaster cast can be divided into two types:
   i. unpadded plaster
   ii. padded plaster.

It is to be noted that the skintight plaster is not recommended for general use. Unless properly applied, the padded plaster is just as efficient as an unpadded one. It is much more comfortable and has certain subtle advantages. Unless extreme attention is given to the detail in using the padding correctly, it is likely to produce a badly padded plaster.

There are two contraindications to unpadded plaster:
  i. immediately after trauma
  ii. immediately after bone operation.

Unpadded Plaster

Unpadded plaster is a type of plaster made by applying the turns of wet bandage directly to the skin without intervention of any cotton. The closeness of its application to the limb and, to some extent, the actual adhesion to the skin are believed by some to enhance the fixation of a fracture. Even if stockinet is used, the plaster for all practical purposes is still the unpadded plaster cast. It is important that the bandage should never be pulled tight. In the unpadded technique, the bandage should be made to roll itself around the limb. By laying the wet roll of plaster on the skin and pushing it around the curves of the limb with the flat of the hand, it will find its own way without causing tight ridges. In no circumstances should the roll of plaster bandage be lifted off the limb and pulled. This technique is considerably easier to acquire than the padded plaster technique.

In the following fractures, an unpadded plaster is required (all plaster strips or slabs should be applied directly to the skin):
  i. the Colles fracture.
  ii. fracture of the scaphoid of the wrist
  iii. the Bennett fracture.

However, skintight plaster is not recommended for general use.

Padded Plaster

In a padded plaster, a layer of cotton wool is interposed between the skin and the plaster, which is then firmly compressed against the limb by applying the wet plaster bandage under tension. Instead of the wool rendering the plaster loose, the elastic pressure of the wool actually enhances the fixation of the limb by compensating for slight shrinkage in the tissues after the application of the cast. The amount of tension used in pulling tight individual turns of plaster is difficult to describe; it can be surprisingly high, yet it never appears to cause any harm to circulation. If properly applied, such plasters grip the limb more firmly and keep this grip for a longer time than skintight plasters do.

In padded plaster technique, the cotton wool is carefully applied as an even layer of rolled cotton wool. This roll having a thickness of almost half an inch is used. It will be later on compressed by the overlying plaster to thickness of almost an eighth of the inch. This will make it lighter and become easy to be retained by the patient, for the time required for healing of the fracture. The care with which this layer of wool is applied is essential for success; it must not obscure the shape of the limb by being put on in careless and ugly lumps. The sheet of cotton wool, if it is not already rolled, should be carefully prepared in rolls before application.

The roll of bandage remains in contact with the surface of the limb almost continuously, but instead of being lightly applied around the limb, it is pressed and pushed around the limb by the pressure of the thenar eminence under a strong pushing force to produce a smooth surface. Each turn is applied slowly and is settled in position, in the natural inclination of the bandage without forcing it unduly in any weary direction. If required, the ends of bandage can be tucked in to accommodate the tapering parts of the limb.

The durability of the plaster cast and its strength for given lightness depends on smoothening of the individual turns of plastic bandage by the required movements of the hand. As such, the whole cast is built up from circular bandages, and when evenly applied, it can tolerate sufficient tension. The hallmark of a good plaster is that it should be of even thickness from end to end. A cast of even thickness is produced if, during the application of plaster, two turns are not applied at the same place except at the ends. This can be easily done by doing a forward and backward movement from the top to the bottom of the plaster.

One of the commonest causes of defective reduction is when the plaster is allowed to reach the consistency of wet cardboard before the final turn has been applied. Therefore, using a quick-setting plaster is a serious mistake because this type of plaster always takes a little longer time to apply.

Frequent change of plaster is neither needed nor desirable. It produces more cases of delayed and non-union of fractures. A cast should never be applied with the idea that it can be changed next month if it turns out to be imperfect.

Plaster Application

The process of reduction and fixation is regarded in three distinct phases:

 a. examination and planning

 b. reduction and holding

 c. plastering.

Examination and Planning

In the examination and planning phase, the effect of gravity on the displacement of fracture must be remembered as it is often of great importance. The limb should be placed in such position so that undesirable effect of gravity can be eliminated. The amount of force required and the range of motion from the position of greatest deformity to the position of reduction must be visualized. Sometimes, with minimal force applied at a key point, the reduction of fracture can be obtained. It is very easy to find this key point by palpation.

Reduction and Holding

Sufficient plaster should be applied just to hold the fracture when it is being set. With the plaster wet and soft the reduction of fracture, can be adjusted and realigned if necessary. During the last few minutes of the setting, the hands should be moved over the plaster to obliterate any abrupt local impression which might cause a pressure sore. The plaster cast is now completed to its required thickness, and the upper and lower ends are shaped to the required limits.

Plastering

To do the plastering, the limb is held by the assistant in the position of approximate reduction. The cast is applied as quickly as possible so that it is still completely soft by the time the last turn is applied. For it, a slow-setting plaster is to be used. If the cast is of large size, sufficient plaster should be applied to hold the reduction position temporarily. The plaster can later on be made thicker and completed at its both upper and lower ends.

Function While in the Plaster

When the decision is made to remove a plaster, it is unwise to do so if the patient is not by this time already capable of good function in the plaster. If the plaster is removed before the fixed time, the patient may need two sticks to walk or even be unable to walk at all. There are three common causes of defective function in a walking plaster:

i. An uncomfortable plaster or bad walking heel: The plaster may have been uncomfortable for weeks as a result of being badly applied. The patient often thinks that pain is to be expected from the fracture and does not report it. If the plaster is a bad one, the patient may never be able to learn to walk while he is in the cast.

ii. Failure of psychic rehabilitation: The patient may not have received the encouragement necessary to show him that he can walk, or he may not have seen other patients in the same type of plaster who are playing games or doing similar robust function. The importance of cheerful rehabilitation in close contact with the doctor and pleasant services in hospital cannot be overemphasized.

iii. Bone atrophy: Post-traumatic osteodystrophy, though rare, does occur. In these cases, after the removal of plaster, the limb swells and may become even more painful than before. They are possibly the result of treatment in plasters which have been too tight or plasters which have been painful for many weeks and have induced a superadded hysterical state of disuse.

Errors in Applying the Padded Cast

The following errors may occur in padded cast application:

1. attempting to plaster at the same time as attempting to hold a precise reduction
2. applying wool carelessly and in shapeless lumps instead of having it previously neatly prepared in rolls and bandaging it on with great care to give an even layer
3. not bandaging tightly enough, with the result that the finished plaster is loose
4. not bandaging the fleshy proximal part with greater tension than in the bony distal part, resulting in a below-knee plaster of the boot effect
5. failing to recognize the sensation of reduction through plaster as a result of using quick-setting plaster, which becomes stiff too quickly
6. failing to recognize the sensation of reduction from inadequate examination during the initial phase of reduction
7. applying the plaster carelessly on the supposition that there is no harm in changing it any time.

Windowed Plasters

Generally speaking, the making of windows in plaster is not a policy to be encouraged. There is a danger of oedematous tissues herniating through a window, especially in plasters of lower extremity. However, there are numerous occasions on which it can be of advantage, although the advent of antibiotics has probably made these occasions less frequent than formerly. There may be a time when decomposing discharge accumulating in plaster become irritant and damage the skin, preventing the growth of new epithelium and producing unhealthy granulation tissue. In these cases, plaster is windowed, and a few daily dressings performed. A remarkable improvement in the conditions of tissue is noticeable in a few days.

In windowed plaster, the patient should be told not to hold his limb in a suspended position for a long period. It is also important to apply a dressing properly designed to give pressure to the aperture of the window because maintenance of this local pressure has a beneficial effect on wound-healing. It is important that windows should be kept as small as possible and compatible with their purpose, and for this reason, they should be centred accurately over the discharging sinus. A useful technical hint is to apply a piece of wool of a sufficiently large size over the centre of the wound before applying plaster bandage. The result is that, when the plaster cast is complete and is allowed to dry, the top of this protrusion can be cut off with a saw and then the centre of wound will become visible in the windowed plaster for dressing and treatment.

CHAPTER 6

TRACTION

Traction, literally speaking, means 'pull', but technically, it describes a process by which the fracture fragments are brought together in apposition gradually and steadily. Based on the principle that for every action there is an equal and opposite reaction, traction on a limb requires a fixed point from which to work or to apply an equal counter-traction in the opposite direction.

Objectives

The main objectives of traction are:

a. to gain or maintain bony alignment in fracture or dislocation
b. to secure immobilization of an inflamed joint
c. to correct deformity.

Types

There are two main types of traction:

i. Fixed traction: It is traction between two fixed points, and it is usually employed when the aim is to give rest to the limb. In Thomas's splint, the traction is exerted by extension tapes tied to the end of the splint while counter-traction is applied by the pressure of the ring against the ischial tuberosity.

ii. Balanced traction: It is traction exerted against a weight. The aim here is to secure reduction of fracture fragments. The extension tapes are tied to a cord which carries a weight running over a pulley fixed to the elevated foot end of the bed; counter-traction is applied by the weight of the patient's body.

The following are two additional types of traction:
  i. Combined fixed and balanced traction: In a fixed traction, Thomas's splint is applied in the usual way, and extension tapes are tied. The splint is then fastened to the raised foot end of the bed, or traction is applied to it by a weight and pulley system in a balanced traction.
  ii. Sliding traction: The patient is placed on a wooden surface or board which slides on roller bearings over the bed itself. The feet of the bed are elevated, and extension tapes are tied to its fixed part.

Methods of Application

The following methods are employed for traction:
  i. skin traction
  ii. skeletal traction
  iii. pulp traction.

Skin Traction

In skin traction, the traction is applied to the skin (whence it acts on muscles) and then to bones.

Indications:
  a. fracture of the neck and shaft of the humerus
  b. fracture of the neck of the femur
  c. fracture of the shaft of the femur
  d. fracture of the tibia and fibula
  e. tuberculosis of the hip and knee joints
  f. contractures of the hip and knee

g. fracture of the spine with paraplegia

h. tuberculosis of the spine with paraplegia

Contraindications:

Skin traction must not be done in old and weak patients whose skin is atrophic and inelastic and cannot withstand constant irritation.

Procedure

For the purpose of understanding, traction as applied to fracture of the shaft of the femur is described below.

An adhesive plaster reel of 3 in. wide is taken and is unfolded. The plaster is then applied as a continuous layer starting from above downwards on the outer side of the limb, covering the whole surface. It stops short of lateral malleolus, and there it spreads apart on a wooden square piece. It is then turned inwards and is applied to the inner side of the limb in the same manner, but the upper end does not extend higher than the outer side. The outer strip should be centred slightly behind the midline of the limb; the inner strip slightly in front so that, when the tapes are fixed, the tendency for the lower limb to roll into external rotation is controlled.

In application, the condyles of the femur, tibia, and malleoli are protected by cotton wool. Spiral strips may be applied to the front and back of the thigh and leg, but it should be remembered that day after day as the strapping is pulled down, it tends to slide down the limb and over a period of six or eight weeks, it may slide as much as 2 in., and these spiral or transversal strips may cut into the skin and cause sores.

The danger is omnipresent and more real than can be imagined. Then the whole strap is tied with a soft bandage from below upwards, starting from above the malleoli and ending at the upper end. A cord is passed through the central hole of the wooden piece, and the extension is applied to the weight after placing the limb in a Thomas's splint. After some weeks, it may be necessary to replace the adhesive strapping and apply a new traction, but there should really be no difficulty in controlling pressure sore by covering the sides of the joints with cotton wool.

Skeletal Traction

In skeletal traction, the traction is applied directly to the bone. Hence, it acts more powerfully. It is used when stronger pull is required to be applied to the patient because of the strong muscles or when the patient's skin is atrophic and inelastic or when the skin is sensitive to adhesive plaster. It should not be used in children and adolescents because of the danger of epiphyseal damage and stunting of growth. The sites for skeletal traction are as follows:

i. greater trochanter: 1 in. inside the lateral portion from anterior to posterior side (for central dislocation of hip joint)

ii. lower end of the femur: ¾ in. in front and ¾ in. above the adductor tubercle

iii. upper end of the tibia: 1 in. below the tibial tubercle

iv. lower end of the tibia: 1–2 in. above the ankle joint

v. calcaneus: 1 in. in front of posterior surface and 1 in. above the inferior surface of calcaneus

vi. elbow: 1 in. in front of the posterior surface of olecranon process

vii. forearm: 1–2 in. above the lower end of radius and ulna.

In addition, traction may be applied through the temporal bones of the skull by a special calliper applied at 1 in. in front and 1 in. above the external auditory meatus.

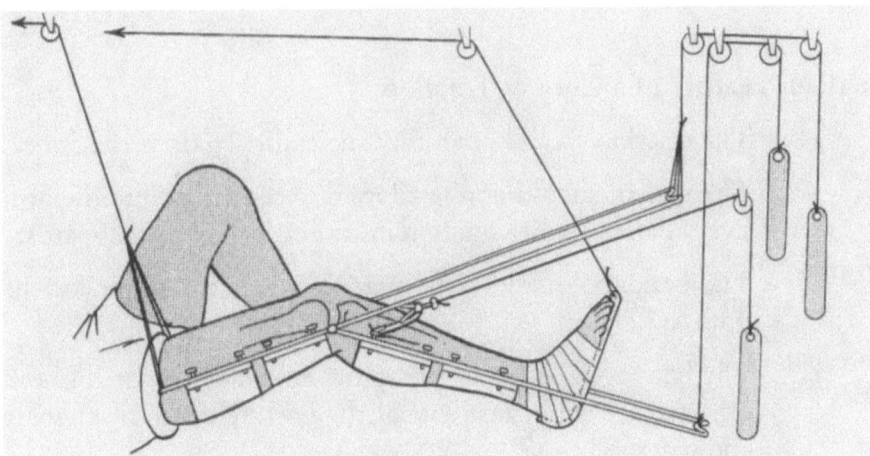

Fig. 6: Skeletal traction applied through upper end of the tibia.

A Steinmann pin or Kirschner wire is inserted through one of these sites as required, usually under local anaesthesia, in a horizontal plane at right angle to the long axis of the bone. It is better to use Steinmann pin because it gives a firm hold on the bone. A stirrup is then mounted over the ends of the pin and tightened. A cord is attached to the centre of the stirrup, and weight is applied to it after placing the limb in a splint. An antiseptic dressing is applied to both the sides of the pin track. It is very important that every precaution of aseptic surgery is taken while inserting the pin, and a stab incision should be employed for the skin. The danger in this method is that it results in such a low-grade infection. Whatever precaution is taken, a serous discharge will come out from the pin track, and it usually persists for many days. It should not arouse any anxiety as it subsides itself. The danger is real when the pin gets loose in its track and the infection of the surrounding tissues occurs or when the site of the pin is near the joint which may get infected and lead to stiffness and subsequent limitation of movements of the joint.

Pulp Traction

Pulp traction is usually employed in the fractures of fingers (i.e. metacarpals and phalanges). A pin is passed through the pulp of the finger ½ in. proximal to the tip of the finger, and stirrup is applied to it. The cord exerts traction from this stirrup by incorporating it in the plaster cast.

Salient Feature of a Correct Traction

i. The traction should be in the longitudinal axis of the bone.

ii. The patient should not be allowed to sag down into the bed. Every patient under traction must be given fracture boards.

iii. The bandage should form a trough with the splint for the limb to lie in it.

iv. The bandage applied to the splint should stop short of heel; otherwise, it will cause sore at the heel by constant pressure and irritation.

v. The ring of Thomas's splint must rest against the pubic bone and ischial tuberosity to exert full traction.

vi. The splint should be suspended by cords from an overhead beam. It should increase the comfort of the patient, provide him freedom of movement, and help him to attend to his daily toilet.

vii. Every splinted patient must be attended every 4 hour for the first 24 hours, 6 hours during the next 48 hours, and twice daily afterwards to prevent the development of sores. The area under the ring of Thomas's splint should be rubbed with methylated spirits and dusted with dusting powder.

viii. The foot of the bed must be raised by 18 in. to provide sufficient counter-traction.

ix. The patient should not be given any pillow while lying down.

x. Weight applied should not touch the end of the bed.

xi. The splint should be tied to the end of the bed.

xii. The patient's limb must not be allowed to touch the bar of the splint, for it may injure the lateral popliteal nerve by constant irritation and produce palsy and foot drop.

xiii. The foot must be supported by a foot piece to prevent foot drop and also to take off the weight of the sheets.

xiv. In skin traction, the adhesive straps should extend well above the site of fracture to get a firm hold on the muscles around the bone.

xv. The adhesive straps should not cover the bony points because friction will lead to the development of sores. Hence, these should be protected by cotton wool.

xvi. The adhesive plaster must never encircle the whole limb as it will lead to oedema below the plaster.

xvii. The adhesive plaster should spread apart at the end of the foot at a considerable distance below it so that the maximum traction is exerted higher up on the bone.

xviii. The adhesive plaster should be tied to the limb by soft cotton bandage so that it does not come off.

xix. Sufficient cotton wool should be placed underneath the upper end of the leg to avoid development of subluxation of the knee joint.

xx. The back of tendo-Achilles should also be protected by cotton wool to avoid pressure sore.

It may be noted that many faulty unions of fractures can be avoided and correct reduction of fracture attained if the simple traction is applied correctly. Moreover, the traction should not be traction on the first day only, but it should work and be maintained every minute, every hour, and every day up to the end when radiological reduction is attained and clinical union is established. It is very important to attain perfect reduction and union of fracture because one cannot appreciate the mental anguish these patients suffer with their deformed limbs.

Traction is applied simply to maintain the reduction rather than in any way an attempt to reduce the fracture slowly over several days by increasing the amount of weight. With some exceptions, the method is generally not satisfactory for the treatment of fractures in the young or in the old. In younger individuals, great difficulty is often experienced in maintaining the proper traction arrangement. In older persons, any method of treatment that requires recumbency in a certain position for a long time will be difficult and will often be followed by pressure sores and pulmonary complications. However, any type of treatment by traction suspension methods must provide not only for a method of traction but for a method of counter-traction as well.

CHAPTER 7

HEALING OF FRACTURE

The healing or union of fracture takes place in three stages:

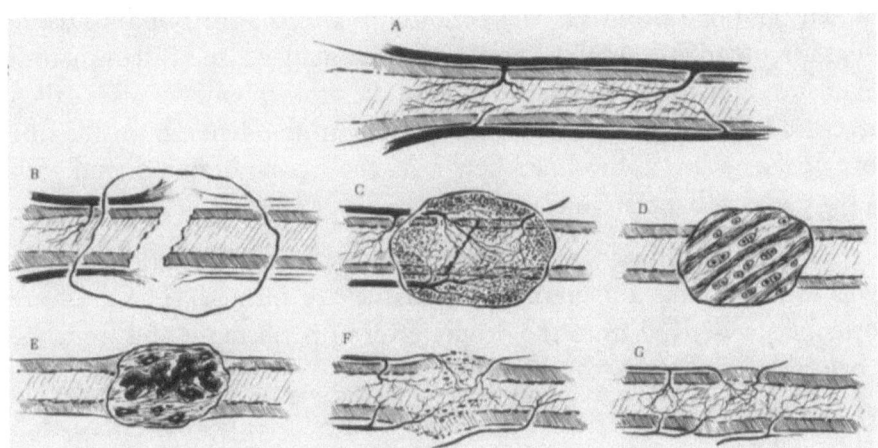

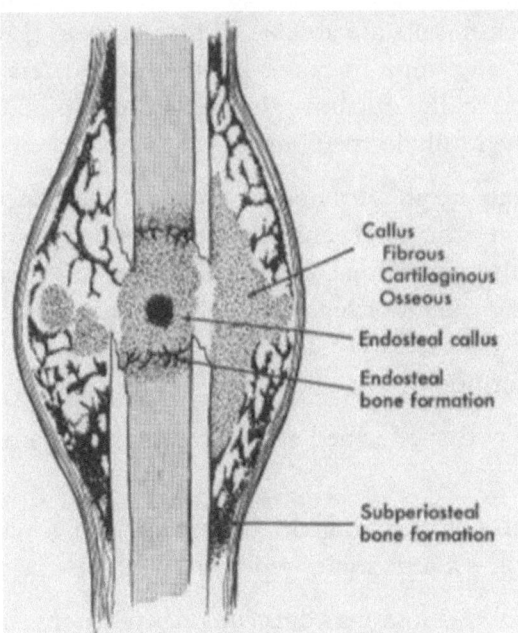

Fig. 7: Stages of healing of fracture.

i. Granulation tissue forms in the exudates between the broken ends of the bones.
ii. This becomes converted into osteoid tissue.
iii. Calcium salts are deposited in the osteoid tissue with the formation of bone.

When the bone is broken, the periosteum and the surrounding tissue are torn, blood is poured out, and a mixture of blood and inflammatory exudates is formed between and around the broken bones. This is called fracture haematoma. The amount of haematoma depends on the line of fracture. With a thin line, there is less collection of blood, and with a big gap, the haematoma is bulky.

The exudate is quickly invaded by cells, and new capillaries (usually within 24 hours) and granulation tissue are formed. The cells are osteoblasts, derived from the deeper layer of periosteum and from the cortical layer of bone.

In four to five days, this granulation tissue becomes converted into osteoid tissue, which resembles bone in its homogenous matrix structure except that calcium salts are absent. At first, osteoid tissue is scattered in clumps, but later on, it increases in amount and acts as an efficient internal splint. Finally, calcium salts are laid down, and the ends are knit together by a fully formed bone.

In the immediate neighbourhood of fracture, the bone cells die, and near the fracture, the osteogenic cells proliferate massively and may form cartilage instead of bone. The cartilage formation is more marked when there is movement or separation of fragments. The new cartilage is invaded and replaced by bone; failure of this process may lead to delayed union or non-union.

The mass of new tissue formed at the fracture site is known as callus. The callus may be:

- external—ensheathing the broken ends as a plumber's solder unsheathes a junction of pipes
- intermediate—forming a direct union between the fractured surfaces
- internal—filling up the marrow cavity.

The intermediate callus is the only form which persists. The internal and external calluses are removed in due course of time. Failure of this process may also lead to non-union.

Such a callus, if left to it, may give the deceptive radiological appearance of the union of fracture, but when put to test, these fractures fail to bear the strain of weight on them.

The process of healing is not finished even when the gap has been patched and the ends united. A slow process of moulding ensues, which may last for years. The internal and external calluses are absorbed, and this work is done by the large multinucleated osteoclast. Ultimately, the bone is moulded to a required form so as to bear the stresses and strains to which the part may be subjected.

In fractures, through the metaphysis, osteogenesis begins from the endosteum of the injured cancellous bone as early as the third or fourth day. In fractures of the shaft, new periosteal bone develops between the fifth and tenth day. A lag period exists in the calcification of the callus. After the callus has reached a maximum size, the osteoid is rapidly converted into bone, and from then onwards, new bone formation is simultaneous with calcification. The new bone does not become visible in X-ray film for 10 to 14 days after its formation because of lack of calcification.

Influence of Systemic Factors

In all average individuals fed on normal diets, the repair of a fracture is purely a local phenomenon, and the haematoma sac may be regarded as an isolated vital chemical factory.

Low blood calcium produced by deficient diet does not slow the rate of healing or lead to non-union. Also, vitamins, proteins, and hormonal deficiency are not accepted as a causative factor of delay in union.

However, sometimes a patient's fractures have responded favourably to dietetic treatment, correction of protein deficiency, and administration of vitamins and calcium.

It is true that a certain amount of delay in the healing of fractures can be avoided, but as far as diet (i.e. the minerals, vitamins, and hormones) is concerned, its correction definitely prevents the development of non-union and leads to early healing of fractures.

Senility and starvation do delay the union of fractures. This state may occur with nutritional cachexia attained in certain compound fractures. Cachexia is accompanied by haemoconcentration, hypoproteinaemia, a negative nitrogen balance, malnutrition, and anaemia. These factors may delay the union of fractures.

Syphilis and cardiovascular diseases may delay the union of fractures.

Ossifiable Medium

The organization of the coagulated extravasation depends upon:

1. maintenance of an adequate local blood supply
2. union by interfragmentary granulation tissue
3. proliferation of osteogenic cells (histosynthesis).

If these factors are not available, the lag period and time required for repair are increased. Thus, the distance to be traversed by the invading granulation tissue is of prime importance. Separation of the fragments is commonly associated with extensive periosteal damage and consequent local anaemia. Thus, large wound surfaces due to the displacement of fragments are commonly associated with vascular and cellular death. The parent structures are themselves damaged. The response is therefore not infrequently poor, and delayed union is quite common.

The degree of local necrosis, local anaemia, and separation of surfaces, dehydration, and infection intimately affect the rate of healing. The most important single factor in healthy individuals is the immobilization of the wound area with consequent protection of the fibrin and granulation tissue until the collagen shows maturation. In widely separated wound surfaces, serum collections devoid of fibrinogen are encountered not infrequently, which do not organize and lead to delay or non-union.

Bone Marrow

Fragments of bone marrow are found in the hematoma, which undergo fatty degeneration while the marrow reticulum is infiltrated with extravasated blood. Necrosis and autolysis are followed rapidly by organization.

Injured Muscles

Incorporated muscle fragments undergo necrosis if isolated or fibrous degeneration if viable. An isolated muscle shows endomysial haemorrhages and inflammatory changes. Within 5–10 days, with consequent autolysis, interposed muscle flaps show subacute cellular infiltration in place of haemorrhage, terminating in fibrous degeneration of the involved muscle fibres, with the formation of a fibrous capsule considerably retarding the progress of osteogenic process.

Adjacent Soft Tissue

Inflammatory reaction that persists in the soft tissue around the fracture site is readily seen at operations.

Cartilage ossification is predominant in the following:

1. if the bone ends are widely separated
2. about the compact ends of long bones (even without displacement)
3. when the periosteum is lacerated or destroyed throughout the subperiosteal callus.

The medullary callus is usually cartilaginous when a compact bone end is displaced opposite to the medullary cavity of the other fragment.

The subperiosteal mass of callus is the characteristic feature of the union of tubular long bones and is an expression of the relative avascularity of the subperiosteal and cortical zones of the bone ends.

The Condition of the Bone Ends

In fractures in which union rapidly occurs, the bone ends which have become necrotic as a result of trauma and the adjacent living compacta undergo resorption. The necrosis of compacta in the metaphysical region is much less then in diaphyseal fractures. The living part of the shaft enclosed in the callus undergoes progressive resorption, and in rapid anaplasia, the process is so extensive that the compacta is deeply perforated with vessels and cells. The cortex under these conditions resembles the spongy bone.

Chemistry of the Fracture Site

It is found that if fluid is aspirated from between the fragments on the first day, it is largely composed of blood and has the same pH value as blood—that is 7.4. As the days pass, the reaction becomes more acid. In some cases, by the fourth day, it registers a pH of 4.5. Thereafter, up to the 10th or 12th day, the haematoma becomes more alkaline and ultimately reaches a pH of 8.2 or more. The acidity of the haematoma is brought about by the exudation of CO_2 from the dead and the dying cells around, from the lactic acid in the damaged muscles, and from the conversion of blood sugar. The acidity of haematoma absorbs salts from the bone ends and gives the moth-eaten appearance seen in the radiograph. At certain stages, the lactic acid content is 15 times the normal. By the 10th day, the calcium content has increased to 10 times the normal. It seems reasonable to state that the formation of bone is due to the action of hypercalcaemic haematoma fluid and the chemical alteration in the fluid around the ends of a fractured bone which takes place in a sealed-off cavity which has no immediate relationship with the surrounding body fluid.

If a good reduction is carried out after a fracture, sealed-off chemical factory surrounds the ends of the broken bone, and the processes indicated above take place. Anything which interferes with the position of the fractured bone, with the chemical activity in the factory, or with the living walls of the factory will lead to delayed union or non-union.

Changes at the Fracture Site after the Trauma

After the trauma, the following changes may occur:

1. necrosis
2. separation
3. impaction
4. comminution
5. sclerosis
6. infection
7. organization of the callus
8. rate of healing of fractures.

1. Necrosis of Bone Ends

When compact bone is cut off from its blood supply, it shows necrosis except where the cells are in contact with a good supply of lymph or close to the normal vascular supply of adjacent compacta, endosteum, or periosteum.

2. Separation of Bone Ends

There is a definite relationship between the surface area of the fracture site and the rate of healing. Loss of substance in soft-tissue wounds may prevent healing.

Separation of fragments may also result in the interposition of the soft tissue between the fragments. The interposition of avascular periosteum prevents the ingress of vascular tissue to the enveloped compacta and occupies a portion of the haematoma sac from which the ossifiable medium is thereby excluded. This results in the formation of fibrous tissue at the fracture site which contributes to the delay in union.

3. Impaction of Bone Ends

Union occurs rapidly by granulation tissue without interruption. The damage to the blood supply is negligible, and the callus is small in amount.

4. Comminution

Comminuted fractures unite quickly provided there is no interposition of soft tissue or loss of substance and provided that immobilization is adequate. However, occasionally, comminution may unite, leaving behind a single line of fracture which may fail to unite, thus producing non-union.

5. Sclerosis

The ends of fragments may result in the smooth round contours and a white radiopacity of the compacta, thus hindering union.

6. Infection

Infection definitely hampers the progress of healing of the fracture and may lead to delayed or non-union.

7. The Organization of the Callus

The callus becomes firm subperiosteally and endosteally so that the callus resembles a plumber's joint.

Organization of the callus is, therefore, of the highest significance and involved the following elements:

a. The production of an ossifiable medium from the interfragmentary haematoma: this process of tissue repair is characteristic of mesenchymal response to injury throughout the body; it is preceded by inflammatory and autolytic activity in an acid tide and is consummated by proliferation in an alkaline tide.

b. The calcification of the tissues so produced with mineral salts mainly derived from the bone ends.

c. The amalgamation of this primary bone with the bone ends which have been converted from secondary lamellar compacta to a porous type of bone for this purpose.

d. The conversion of this tissue into secondary lamellar bone between the cortices of the bone fragment: the necessary calcium for this final reorganization is derived mainly from the resorption of the subperiosteal and endosteal callus, for the secondary bone contains two to three times as much calcium as primary callous bone.

8. Rate of Healing of Fractures

In simple fractures, strength is absent before the 6th day, but it mounts rapidly until the 21st day. The period of callus reconstruction and the reorganization of the primary bone begin after the 25th day. This reorganization diminishes the strength of the union until the 30th day, but later, it rises subsequently to a new high level. This diminution in strength is further related to a macroscopic reduction in the size of the callus to that of the diameter of the shaft. At this time too, the bone ends show their maximal translucency, the lamellar bone ends reach their maximal resorption and resemble primary bone, and added reconstruction continues in repair of the bone.

The rate of repair in fractures might be considerably slower under clinical conditions, which is based upon the lag period.

The lag period is an index of the degree of trauma, of the rate of restoration of the collateral circulation at the fracture site, and of the duration of the inflammatory and autolytic phases. The greater the degree of injury (whether traumatic or inflammatory), the slower the circulatory restoration and the longer the lag period.

There is no clinical or radiographic method of determining the duration of the lag period. It corresponds to the acid tide, and although decalcification is inaugurated during this phase, no radiographic decalcification is registered, despite a tenfold calcium concentration in the haematoma. From the intrinsic factors which affect this period (circulatory deficiency and the autolytic problem due to interposed soft-tissue fragments), it is evident that a long lag period is commonly followed by long subsequent phases, so delay in union is to be expected.

If blood supply is not destroyed, the resorptive process is established in the second week after the fracture. If the collateral circulation has not been efficiently restored, the resorption process may not be prominent in some diaphyseal fractures, even by the fifth month.

The Reconstructive Phase

At the stage of union, two types of fractures are encountered:
1. metaphyseal fractures, which, if properly reduced, heal without external callus
2. diaphyseal fractures, which heal by external and internal callus.

It is evident that this phase may be much longer in diaphyseal than in metaphyseal fractures because of the greater mass of callus to be remodelled. The external callus is reduced to the shaft diameter, and the medullary cavity is reconstituted while the vascular intercortical bone is reformed.

Healing of Infected Fracture

Infection is not all detrimental, but a certain amount of infection at the site of fracture stimulates new bone formation, and the cortex between the points of infected erosion produces numerous and exuberant callus buds. Provided that sequestra do not obstruct the process of union, the efforts at union are widespread and effective.

Callus produced in the presence of sepsis is more loosely constructed and laciform than the ordinary callus. Owing to the diffusion of the reparative process in the presence of sepsis, there is a widespread production of vascular granulation tissue. The adjacent soft tissue is involved, and bone is formed on the vascular zone between the vessels, which are in great profusion. Primary bone so produced is extremely porous, and porosity remains an index of vascularity of a living bone.

If this infection is widespread and sequestra are present, a biopsy of the area will show that the internal inflammatory reaction with the substantial tissue reaction (consisted mainly of inflammatory granulation tissue) overlies the zone of osteogenesis. The zone is poorly defined, and localization is prevented by virulent sepsis.

When the infection is quiescent or controlled, the zone of inflammatory granulation tissue is narrow, the fibrin barrier well defined, and broad zone of hyalinized fibroblastic tissue separates the inflammatory from the loose neurovascular zone in the deeper portion of which osteogenesis progresses. Localization with the demarcation of the zone is a prominent feature in a chronic indolent condition (sequestration without much sepsis). The local epidermal reaction and the prominent and the predominant lymphocytic reaction are seen with moderate demarcation of the zone.

The presence of intense local reaction in the granulation tissue zone along with the demarcation of the layers indicates the persistence of the sepsis, a condition which does not prevent union but terminate in an unstable ulcerated scar which often overshadows the bony problem.

CHAPTER 8

RADIOGRAPHIC CHANGES IN FRACTURE-HEALING

The following are the stages of repair:
1. A thin clear line is seen at the site of fracture.
2. The line or space between the fragments has widened, and the bone edges present a moth-eaten appearance.
3. Callus is joined—wide at the site of fracture and narrowing as it extends up and down the shaft. The line of fracture is still visible.
4. The callus, shaped like a plumber's joint, is denser, and the fracture line is obliterated.
5. The excess of new bone inside and outside has been removed, and the marrow cavity is restored.

Calcification of the cartilaginous callus provides the first radiographic evidence that the process of union by primary bone is progressing. Calcium is not demonstrable in the early stage throughout the haematoma sac because any mobilized calcium is probably in solution, as the soluble salt, in an acid medium. Deposition, however, occurs during the alkaline tide. In human fractures, the calcification of the callus tends to be delayed until the callus is of the maximal size, then it proceeds rapidly.

In fractures, without impeding factors (separation of the fragment, inadequate immobilization, inadequate blood supply, or sepsis), the radiographic evidence indicates that the fracture site should be bridged by primary bone in the majority of cases in the following periods:

Type	Upper Limb	Lower Limb
Spiral fractures	3 weeks	6 weeks
Transverse	6 weeks	12 weeks

Fractures through the spongiosa of the metaphysis without displacement and some fractures of the shorter long bones may show no external callus, but at the stages indicated above, they should show loss of definition and density (i.e. resorption) in the compacta of the fracture surface.

On the other hand, diaphyseal fractures may manifest external callus, which becomes maximal when resorption of the adjacent compacta is demonstrable radiographically. Failure to demonstrate resorption of the compacta at the periods stated should stimulate a close enquiry into the etiology of the delay in the union of the fracture.

Unrestricted function should be permitted only when the clinical signs of sound union are supported by X-ray evidence that the interfragmentary bone is accompanied by the reduction in the external and internal callus. Until this stage is reached, refracture is to be feared, and the fracture must always be protected. It is very important that such radiographic evidence should be available in clear films not taken through the plaster splints.

Radiograph, therefore, should be taken in the following stages:

1. The diagnosis of the fracture.
2. The assessment of the degree of displacement and the condition of bone ends.
3. The determination of the efficacy of the reduction of the fracture and the retention of the fragments and the tendency of redisplacement.
4. The subsequent progress of union by primary bone in:
    a. calcification of the callus
    b. resorption of the compacta of the bone ends.

5. The chronological study of these radiographic changes. necessitates a review of the treatment of all fractures, in which the optimal rate of progress is not maintained.

6. The determination of the reorganization of the callus and the conversion of the interfragmentary primary bone into secondary lamellar bone. Combined with clinical tests, the picture presents an index of the degree of permissible function.

CHAPTER 9

UNION OF FRACTURES

The union of fracture depends on the following factors:
1. age of the patient
2. nature of injury
3. site of fracture
4. type of fracture
5. general health of the patient
6. intercurrent or systemic diseases
7. presence of infection
8. hormonal or mineral deficiency
9. disturbance of local haematoma
10. length of lag period.

1. Age of the Patient

It has been proved beyond doubt that the younger the patient, the quicker is the union of a fracture and the greater is the remodelling power. There is greater incidence of delayed union and non-union of fractures in adults and old age group.

2. Nature of the Injury

With severe trauma, there is greater damage to blood supply of bone fragments and little callus formation. So union of fracture is delayed. The reverse happens with fractures sustained after a mild trauma.

3. Site of the Fracture

Fractures through metaphyseal region progress rapidly and unite quickly than diaphyseal fractures. The former fracture passes through spongiosa, which has greater osteogenic power than the latter, in which the fracture line traverses the compact bone.

4. Type of Fracture

In oblique and spiral fractures, union is quicker than in transverse fractures because a much bigger and a much broader surface is in apposition and is available for callus formation.

5. General Health of the Patient

It is an important factor to be remembered that in countries where poverty and ill health are in abundance and the general health of a man in the street is at a low ebb, the specified period for union of fractures cannot be accepted as a standard time for this country. As the time factor is not the subject under discussion, it is sufficient to say that the general health of a patient does affect the union of the fracture. As a robust and good physique can determine the type and the extent of trauma, similarly, this physical characteristic may alter the time required for union of the fracture.

6. Intercurrent and Systemic Diseases

Diabetes, cardiovascular diseases, and syphilis delay the union of fractures.

Carcinoma with secondaries and certain bone diseases also delay the union process. Hypoproteinaemia, anaemia, and cachexia due to any cause may delay union of fractures.

7. Presence of Infection

A simple fracture unites earlier than a contaminated compound fracture. And if the treatment of a compound fracture is delayed for any reason, the union of fracture is also further delayed.

8. Hormonal or Mineral Deficiency

Hormonal imbalance or deficiency retards the union of a fracture (e.g. in cretinism, there is an arrest of both endochondral and subperiosteal new bone formation). This is not due to the lack of calcium salts, but it is due to the arrest of proliferation of the cartilage and arrest of osteoblastic activity.

Deficiency of the levels of calcium and phosphorus in the blood produces an imbalance of the chemistry of bone salts. The calcium and phosphorus are mobilized from the bone to maintain this level. Therefore, in fractures, the normal process of repair is hampered. Hence, the union of fracture is delayed.

9. Disturbance of Local Haematoma

If due to repeated manipulation or unwanted operative procedures the primary haematoma is disturbed, the process of repair of fracture is interfered, and the union is delayed. It may also lead to non-union.

10. Length of Lag Period

The time elapsed between the time of injury and the start of process of ossification depends on all the factors enumerated above. But the greater the lag period, the more time taken by the fracture to unite. Sometimes a delay in calicification may occur due to the failure in the supply and transport of bone minerals rather than the lack of calcifiability in the bone matrix.

Non-Union of Fracture

Union and non-union of fracture are definite entities, but slow or delayed union is a dynamic state of healing of fracture which may end in either of these.

Delayed union is a condition in which clinical and roentgenographic examination shows that repair is going on slowly although the fracture is still un-united. *Delayed union* is a term applied to un-united fractures in which:

1. X-ray examinations at any time from 4 to 18 months of healing showed inadequate callus
2. the individual judgement of the surgeon led him to advise a surgical operation to stimulate healing of fracture.

Non-union is said to have taken place when the clinical examination and roentgenographic study indicate that the fracture is still un-united and that there is no attempt at repair.

The terms *delayed union* and *non-union* as commonly used refer to the delay in or failure of the process of calcium deposition in this healing tissue to form bone. The underlying basis of non-union is a deficiency in the concentration of the inorganic bone-forming elements of the blood.

Diagnosis of non-union is based on the following criteria:

i. false motion at the fracture site
ii. sclerosis of bone ends
iii. rounding of bone ends
iv. obliteration of the medullary canal
v. presence of a bone defect.

There are three types of non-union, namely:

i. typical pseudarthrosis with sclerosis of the ends of the fragments.
ii. fibrous union with osteoporosis of the fragments
iii. fibrous union with disuse atrophy of the fragments.

More cases of non-union of fractures are seen which are due to a general increase in the number of fractures, which in its own turn is due to:

1. an increase in the severity of fractures as evidenced by more compound fractures and more trauma to soft parts, bones, nerves, and vessels

2. the occurrence of a greater number of multiple fractures which makes a greater demand on the callus output of the individual as evidenced by defective union at one or more sites

3. incompetent and often inadvisable surgery which has been caused by evolution in the treatment of fractures to meet the demands of the X-ray picture (i.e. perfect alignment).

The causes of non-union are:

i. constitutional

ii. local.

Constitutional

Constitutional factors have nothing to do with the union of fractures, which is evident that we do have constitutional ailments which prevent union. However, they are so rare that (except in those fractures which are infected) union occurs in 95% of the cases and that non-union of fracture is undoubtedly caused by local interference with the physiological or nature's attempt at producing union.

It is a fact that calcium and phosphorus index cannot be used as a prognostic index of union and non-union. Local causes are far more significant in the development of non-union of fracture than general or systemic causes, and the chemical analysis of blood to determine the calcium and phosphorus content is valuable in a small number of cases.

It is to be noted that in normal healing of fractures, the catabolism of calcium shows but little change. There is a marked loss of nitrogen, phosphorus, and sulphur—the main excretory path for these catabolites being the kidneys. However, metabolic analysis did not throw any light upon the problem of un-united fracture. A catabolic loss of sulphur, nitrogen, and phosphorus may result from injury to the tissues other than bone.

Diseases such as tuberculosis, osteomalacia, and rickets only delay but do not prevent union. It is also a fact that non-union after fractures of shaft is often found in powerful and healthy individuals and is disproportionately more common in men than women.

In spite of all these facts, it can be briefly stated that the following constitutional factors predispose to the non-union of fractures:

a. circulatory disturbances
b. deficiency in the quality of tissues as induced by excessive scar tissue and dense eburnated bone
c. many diseases, especially syphilis
d. a congenital deficiency (present in some persons) in the quality of the bone that does not permit normal ossification (just what element is deficient is not known)
e. deficiency in the inorganic elements of the blood as denoted by calcium–phosphorus index.

Local

It is interesting to note that as early as the tenth century, Avicenna (Ibn Sīnā, 980–1037) advanced the following causes of non-union of fractures: 'Multiple embrocation with warm water, and frequent changing; haste and moving the part when there is little viscous blood; or too great, stricture, which prevents the limb from being nourished; or the presence of pieces of bone.'

In the modern era, the common causes met with in the daily practice are as follows:

a. gross separation of the fragments
b. interposition of soft tissue between the fragments
c. lack of immobilization
d. inadequate immobilization
e. compound condition of the fracture
f. secondary sepsis
g. damage to the nutrient artery
h. damage to the vessels of the limb
i. damage to the nerves of the limb

j. injudicious operations (e.g. metal plates)
k. pathological bone.

a. Gross Separation of Fragments

When the fragments are too far apart, the granulation tissue fails to bridge the gap; hence, non-union occurs. It is to be noted that the gaps fill up at the rate of 0.5 cm per year and fractures with defect of 1 cm or more in length require at least 18 months (2 years) to heal.

b. Interposition of Soft Tissue

Interposition of soft tissue prevents the granulation tissue from joining together from either side because the latter cannot penetrate the soft tissue.

c. Lack of Immobilization

By movements, the granulation tissue is degenerated into scar tissue before the ossification has been established.

d. Inadequate Immobilization

Inadequate immobilization does not allow the granulation tissue sufficient time to get calcified. The young tissue cannot bear the weight. It gives way and leads to non-union. The early granulation tissue may be so disrupted by manipulation or inadequate immobilization. Because of the stress exerted on it by the muscles or the strain of early weight-bearing, the repair process may not occur.

e. Compounding of Fracture

The primary haematoma is disturbed, and the granulation tissue is completely disrupted. With the added tissue, necrosis, and delayed process of repair, non-union may result.

The local process may be normal, but the reaction of the surrounding tissues to the excessive trauma may be such that invasion of granulation tissue with development of fibrous tissue may overcome the natural process of bone repair.

f. Secondary Sepsis

In pyogenic infection, there is a fluid formed, which dissolve the callus and bone, considerably delays and often prevents union of fracture.

g. Damage to the Nutrient Artery

Since the nutrient artery is the main source of blood supply, when it is cut off, this may lead to non-union.

h. Damage to the Vessels of the Limb

An intense reaction from excessive damage to tissue vessels may induce an inflammatory reaction with coincident increased or decreased blood supply in callus formation. Formation of blood clot is present. Bone atrophy ensues, and adult fibrous tissue is formed between the fragments.

i. Damage to the Nerves of the Limb

Gross injuries to the nerves do not apparently impair callus formation, but the nerve is usually traumatized at the site of fracture and not above. Probably, imbalance of the vasomotor system may impair osteogenesis. This may be the reason why the union of un-united fractures occurs after sympathectomy.

j. Injudicious Operations

An injudicious operation disturbs the primary haematoma. By loss of blood clot and defective circulation, the bone production may be limited to the extremities of the fragments; thus, there is condensation of the bone with highly developed connective tissue and cartilage between the fragments.

Sometimes the internal fixation by wires, plates, and screws may prevent the union of fractures because they repel the callus. However, the chances of success with either method have been observed to be the same.

k. Pathological Bone

In pathological conditions such as Paget's disease, there is already an imbalance of the normal biochemical status of the bone. The demand put by the fracture cannot be met with as this fracture is the result and not the cause of pathology. Hence, non-union occurs.

Mechanism of Non-Union

Actually, no definite process can be stated, but fibrinoid degeneration of connective tissue is the universal mechanism of non-union. This fibrinoid degeneration occurs inside the callus and is a continuous process. The function of the fibrinoid and mucinous fluid, which forms when the callus splits, appears to be to create and to preserve the false joint space. Glycoprotein, hyaluronates, and other polysaccharides are found at the site of pseudarthrosis, but their origin is not known. Some consider it to be the degradation products of ground substance and fibrinoid. The cellular and chemical changes which accompany these substances closely resemble those in chronic adventitious bursitis except that they occur in bone ends. These changes arise with injury and necrosis of the connective tissue. They are sustained by inflammation, infection, motion, and friction and result in an extracellular effusion of mucinous tissue fluid. The process is inhibited and reversed by immobilization of the part.

Sites of Non-Union in Long Bones

The following are the common sites of non-union in long bones:
  i. tibia (lower one-third)
  ii. femur (middle one-third)
  iii. radius and ulna together (middle one-third)
  iv. radius alone (lower one-third)
  v. ulna alone (middle one-third)
  vi. humerus (middle one-third and lower one-third).

CHAPTER 10

INJURIES OF THE UPPER LIMB

Injuries of the upper limb are divided into two types:
 i. common
 ii. less common.

Common injuries are:
 1. fracture of the clavicle
 2. subluxation and dislocation of acromioclavicular joint
 3. dislocation of shoulder joint
 4. fracture of the neck of the humerus
 5. fracture of the shaft of the humerus
 6. supracondylar fracture of the humerus
 7. fracture of lateral condyle of the humerus
 8. fracture of the head of the radius
 9. fracture of the olecranon process of ulna
 10. Monteggia fracture–dislocation
 11. fracture of the forearm
 12. Colles fracture
 13. fracture of the scaphoid
 14. fracture of the metacarpals and phalanges.

Less common injuries are:
 1. dislocation of the sternoclavicular joint
 2. fracture of the neck of the scapula

3. fracture of the body of the scapula
4. fracture of the acromial process of the scapula
5. fracture of the glenoid cavity of the scapula
6. fracture of the greater tuberosity of the humerus
7. fracture of the lesser tuberosity of humerus
8. *T-;* & *Y-;* shaped fractures of the lower end of the humerus
9. fracture of the coronoid process of the ulna
10. fracture of the styloid process of the ulna and radius
11. fractures of the small bones of the hand.

CHAPTER 11

FRACTURE OF THE CLAVICLE

The fracture of the clavicle is caused by transmitted or indirect violence. Although clavicle is subcutaneous throughout its length, fracture of the clavicle is rarely compound. This is partly due to the mobility of the overlying skin and also because the breaking force is seldom transmitted directly to the clavicle except in firearm injury.

Fracture commonly occurs in the middle third of the shaft, and sometimes, it is comminuted, but more often, only one separated fragment is present.

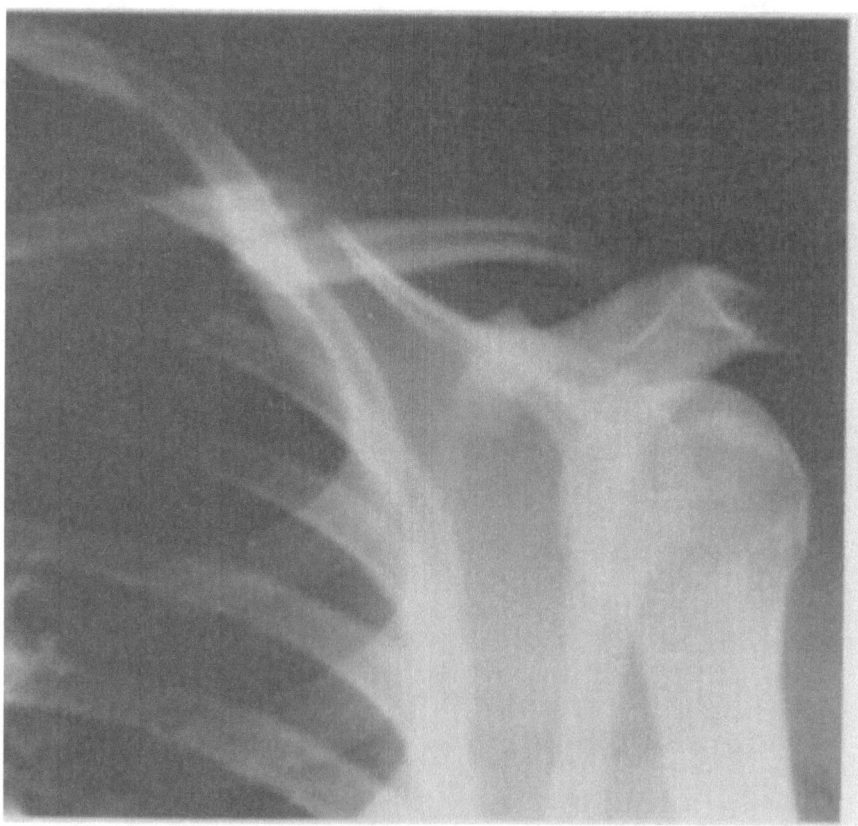

Fig. 8: Fracture of the clavicle (middle portion).

The proximal half of the shaft to which the sternomastoid is attached is pulled upwards and backwards, causing the separation of the fragments, and an obvious change in the shape of the clavicle is visible. Less commonly, the fracture occurs in the outer third of the bone, between the acromioclavicular joint and the attachment of coracoclavicular ligaments. Displacement is then minimal, for these ligaments (unless damaged) hold the inner end of the clavicle down and prevent deformity.

Diagnosis is never difficult. The patient usually supports the arm across his chest, holding it with the other hand. The head usually leans to the side of the fracture, and there is visible deformity, tenderness, loss of function, and easily palpable crepitus, which the patient will usually notice himself.

Treatment

Fortunately, non-union of clavicle is very rare. In spite of poor immobilization, malalignment, and even radiological evidence of a small gap between bone ends, union does occur.

It is fortunate that the two features of this fracture overlap, and angulation (even if allowed to persist) may cause only slight alteration in the appearance and no functional disability. However, when there is too much overlap of bone fragments or for cosmetic reasons, the open reduction may be undertaken.

Fracture of the Middle Third

The traditional method of treatment with figure-of-eight bandage is still the best and most popular.

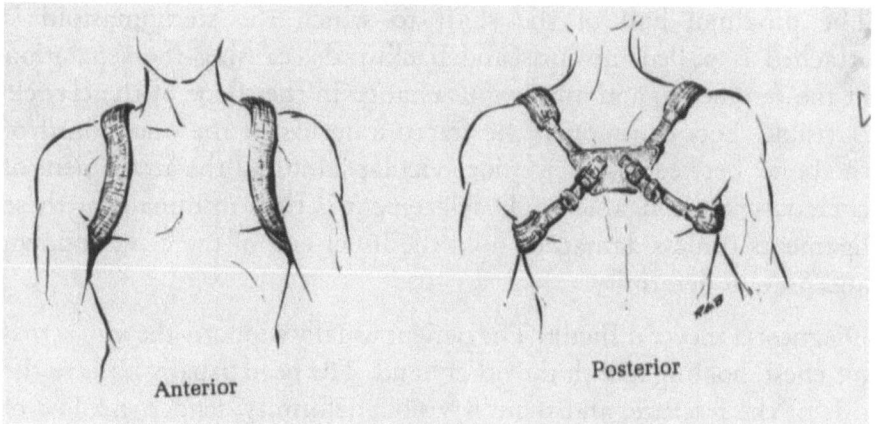

Fig. 9: Fracture of the clavicle treated by calendar rings tied together.

The patient sits on a stool with his back to the surgeon, who first must apply pads of cotton wool to either shoulder, covering the anterior, superior, posterior, and axillary aspects. Next, with the patient's shoulder braced well back, with the support of knee placed on the back between shoulder blades and hands placed on his head, the bandage (usually of crepe) is applied over the shoulder, then across the back of the patient, and taken over to the opposite shoulder in the same manner so that a figure of eight is formed on the back of the patient. Firm application is essential, and cuff-and-collar sling should be given on the affected side. The bandage is likely to get loose; hence, reapplication or tightening of the bandage should be done at least every second day or when necessary. However, frequent change of bandage must be avoided. Some people prefer to use padded slings held together across the back, and certainly, this method has the advantage of simplicity and is probably just as effective.

The advantage of the figure-of-eight bandage is that the arms are free during treatment. Usually, a period of three weeks is required for the union of fracture; however, sometimes it may need to be extended for further three weeks.

In young patients in whom cosmetic consideration is supreme, reduction and immobilization in a full shoulder plaster cast is a satisfactory method of treatment. But it is a cumbersome method of treatment, and not many patients can tolerate it.

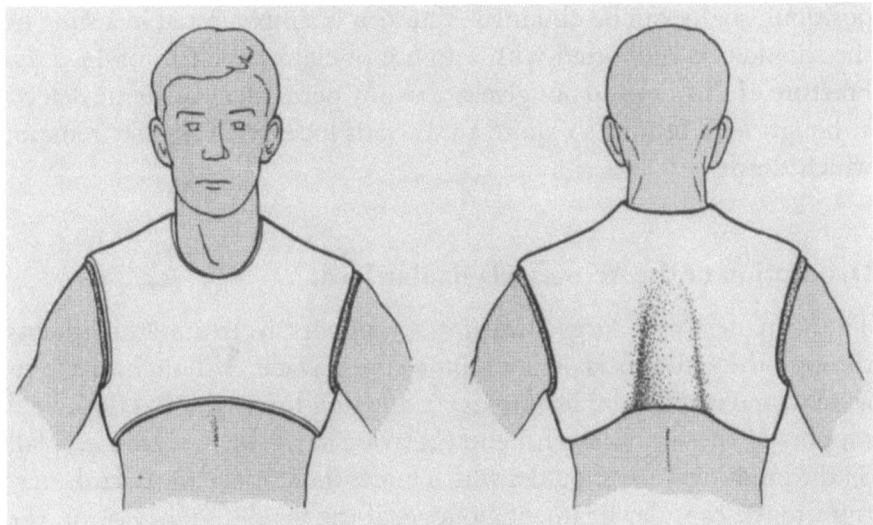

Fig. 10: Plaster jacket applied for fracture of the clavicle.

Fractures of the Outer Third

Unless the coracoclavicular ligaments, the main connections between the scapular and clavicle, are torn, displacement of fracture is minimal.

Treatment required is mainly for the relief of discomfort only, and for it, rest in a cuff-and-collar sling or especially designed elbow sling works well. It relieves the pain and discomfort.

When ligaments are torn, the situation is akin to acromioclavicular dislocation; therefore, a good reduction can usually be achieved and maintained by the use of supportive strapping alone. This is designed to exert a downward thrust upon the clavicle while at the same time supporting the scapula by an upward pressure on the flexed elbow. The strapping is kept in place for three weeks, by which time the fracture has usually become firm enough to support the weight of the shoulder girdle and prevent recurrence of displacement.

Fractures in Children

In early childhood, fracture of the clavicle is often of greenstick variety, with the disruption of one side of the cortex and bending of the other fragment. Quite often, marked angulation occurs, but acceptable position usually can be obtained. The arm is simply rested in a sling or the shoulder is supported with a figure-of-eight bandage for 14 days. Fracture of this type do not give rise to any permanent cosmetic defect, although for a year or so, quite an obvious local swelling may remain, which slowly subsides.

Dislocation of the Acromioclavicular Joint

The arm derives a large measure of support from its attachments through the acromioclavicular joint to the clavicle. Although this joint is small and its capsular ligaments are apparently weak, it has the added support of the very powerful coracoclavicular ligaments. Hence, a fall on the prominence of shoulder which forces the scapula downwards may rupture the capsular ligament alone, or if the force is more violent, the coracoclavicular ligaments are ruptured as well.

The former produces only subluxation of the acromial end of the clavicle, the main strain being taken by the attachment of the coracoid process. With the more severe injury, this attachment ruptures, and complete dislocation occurs.

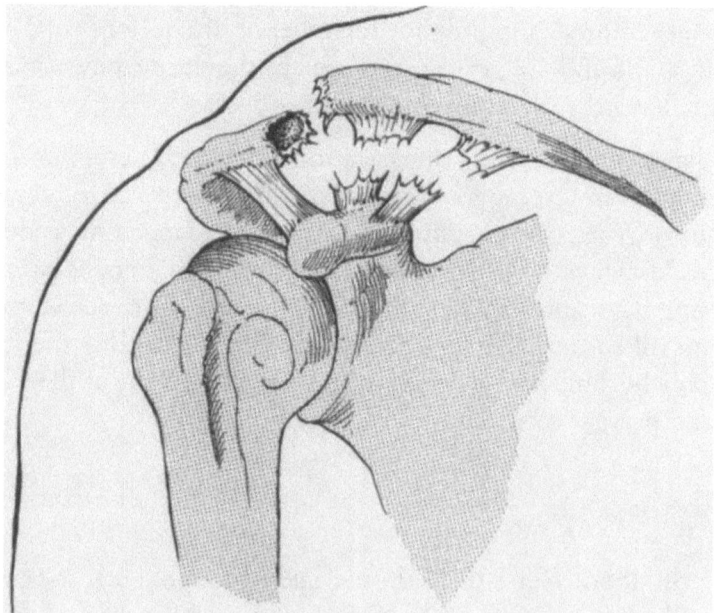

Fig. 11: Complete acromioclavicular dislocation with complete ruptures of ligamentous structure (attachments).

Diagnosis is not difficult if there is a history of injury to the shoulder and the patient feels pain in the region of the joint. There is always local tenderness and swelling. Displacement with dislocation shows an obvious step in the contour of the shoulder with prominence of the acromial end of the clavicle.

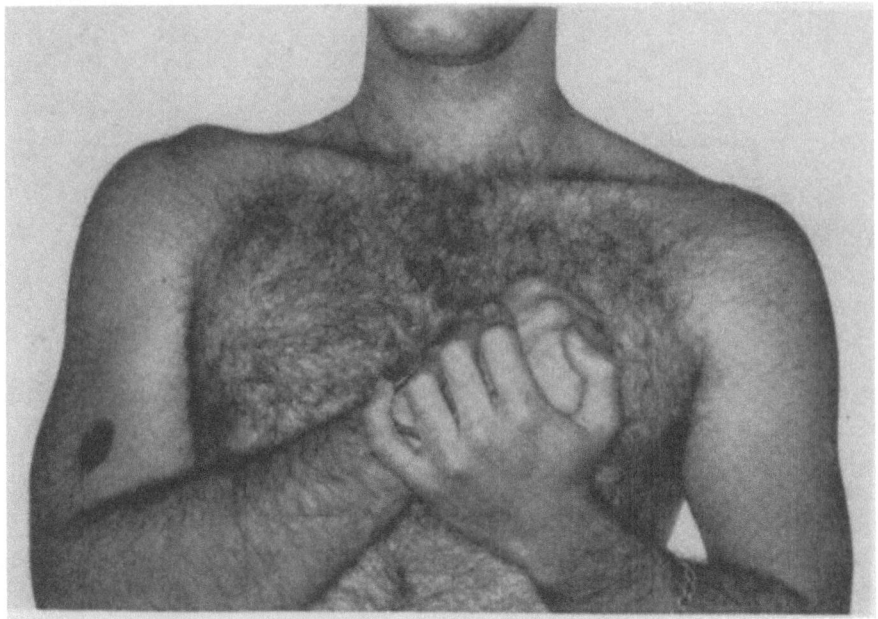

Fig. 12: Acromioclavicular dislocation prominence of the acromial end of the clavicle is visible.

X-ray is taken in a standing position, which will show an obvious disruption of the acromioclavicular joint.

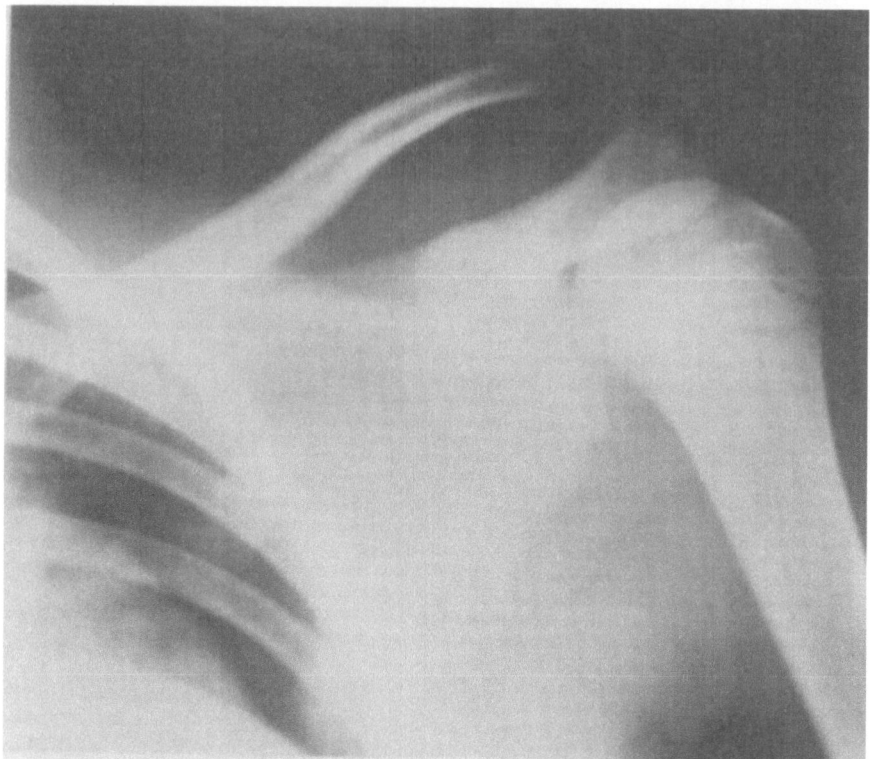

Fig. 13: X-ray film shows the dislocation of acromioclavicular joint.

Treatment

Subluxation: With the main ligament intact, quite adequate support remains, and slight displacement of the joint causes no functional disability. The support in a sling with strapping for a few days is sufficient to relieve the initial acute discomfort and allow the joint to be restored to its place.

Dislocation: The more severe injury is characterized by marked displacement of the acromioclavicular joint, with a clearly visible step in the line of the shoulder due to elevation of the clavicle and drooping of the acromial process. The aim of the treatment is to restore both the anatomy and function to normal. However, in this joint, function is not markedly disturbed in the presence of unreduced dislocation. This is fortunate because it is very difficult to maintain reduction of the dislocated acromioclavicular joint, owing to its inherent instability and dependence upon intact ligament.

The treatment is largely governed by cosmetic consideration, but it must not compromise the function. Primary operative procedure should not be considered because it may hold the joint but may produce painful joint stiffness. Unless open repair of the damaged ligaments is undertaken, it is doubtful whether any treatment will result in permanent reduction of the dislocation, and to do so is usually unwise.

By tradition, acromioclavicular strapping is more usually advised, and it does work in majority of cases.

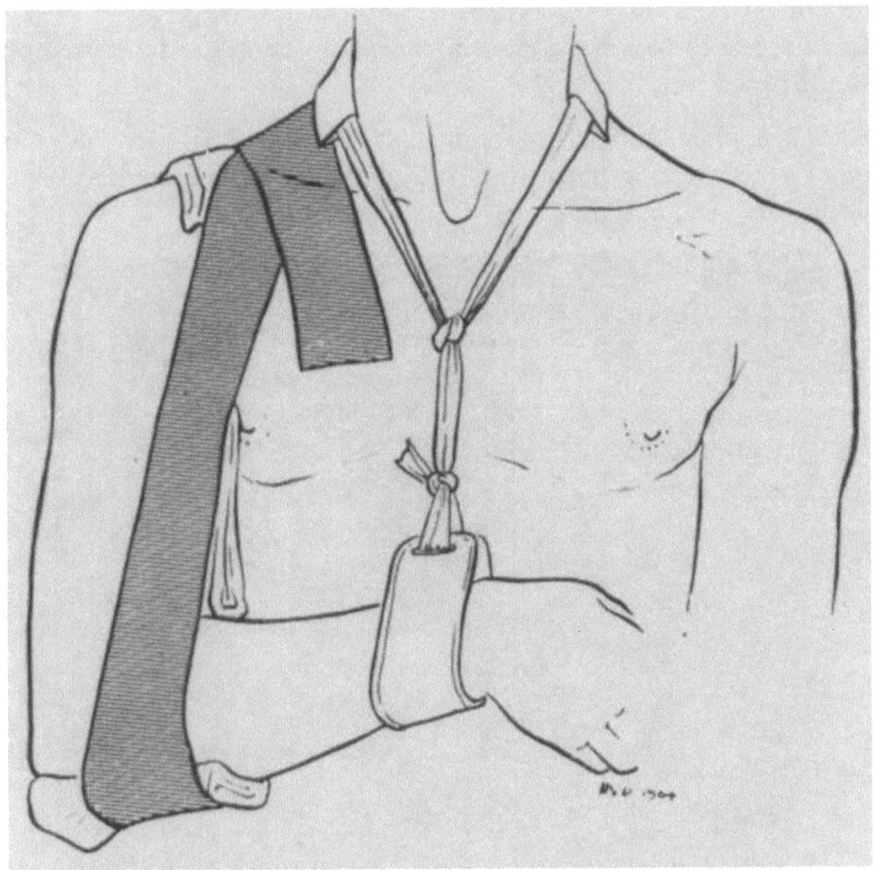

Fig. 14: Treatment by pressure strapping and cuff-and-collar sling.

But the bandage is certainly more difficult to apply, and it often produces excoriation of the skin and great discomfort, often leading to abandonment of the method. After the application, the strapping must be kept for six weeks, and to keep the joint fully reduced, it is important that the strapping should be applied tightly. The arm is supported in a cuff-and-collar sling, and thick pads are laid on the upper outer end of the clavicle and the undersurface of the flexed elbow. These two points are encircled by several layers of inextensible adhesive strapping applied with sufficient tension to pull the clavicle downwards while at the same time supporting the arm and thus preventing the scapula from descending. This strapping must be tightened at frequent intervals if required, and if it is to be effective, it should not be removed until the healing is complete (in about six weeks' time).

In complete displacement, the fracture–dislocation can be treated by transfixation pins.

Although uncommon, but occasionally, a patient may develop pain many years after the injury. In such cases, the best treatment is excision of the outer end of the clavicle.

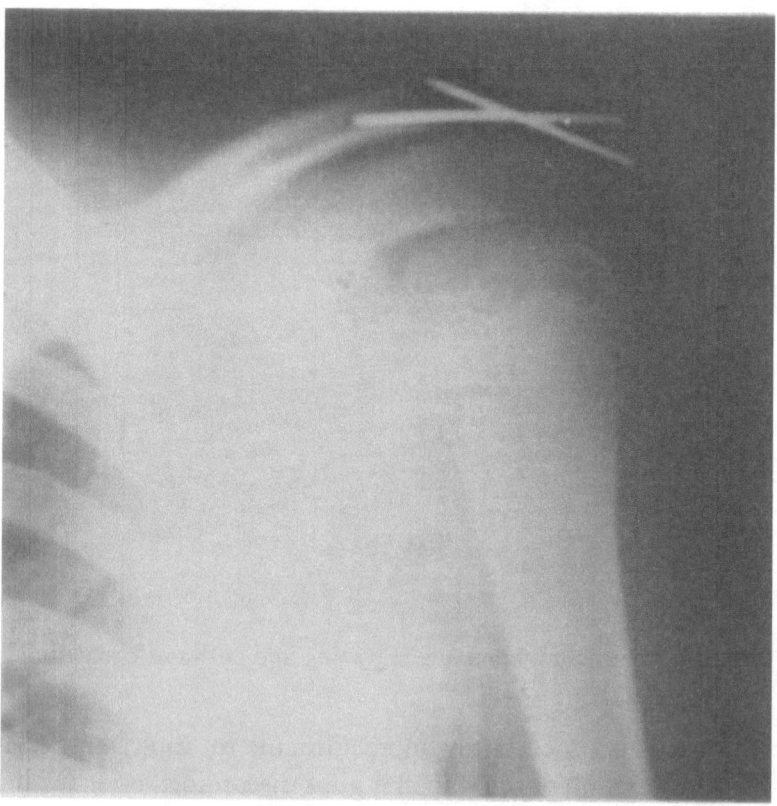

Fig. 15: Treatment by transfixation pins.

CHAPTER 12

DISLOCATION OF THE SHOULDER JOINT

Dislocation of the shoulder joint is a frequent injury of adults, rather more common in the young and athletic because of the more active life. It does occur in all ages and both sexes and old age as well. It is uncommon in children.

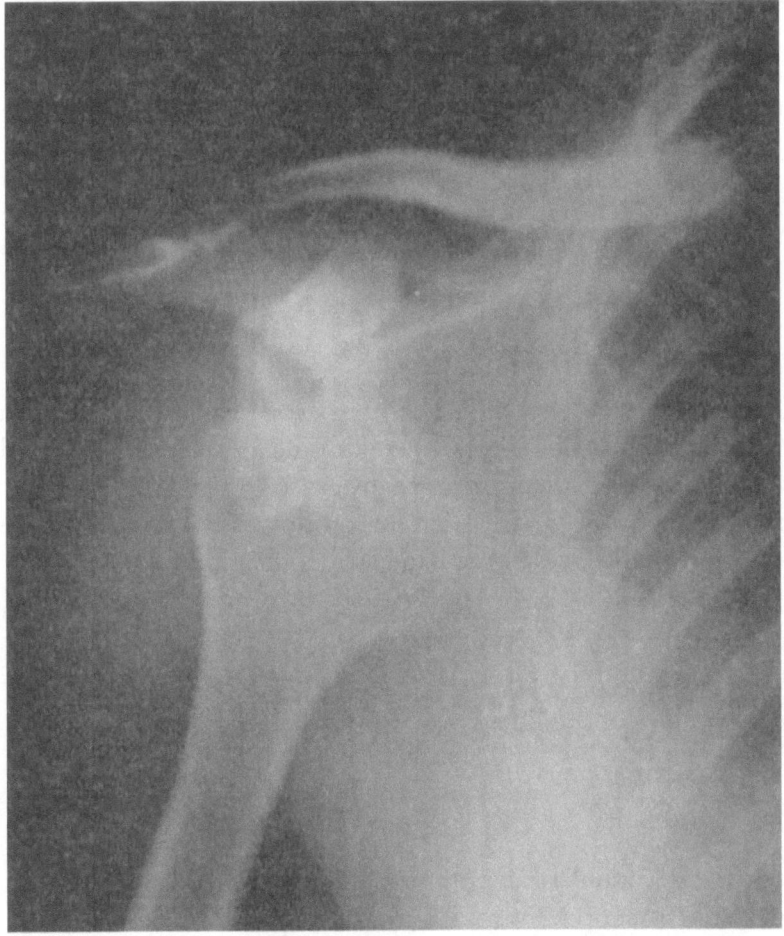

Fig. 16a: Dislocation of the shoulder joint (anteroposterior view).

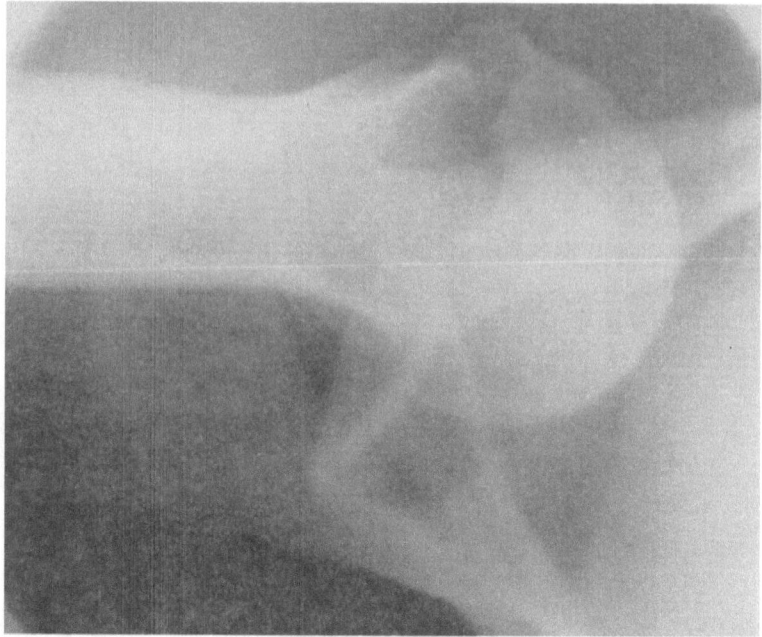

Fig. 16b: Axial view.

Mechanism of Injury

Shoulder joint is the most mobile joint in the human body. The weakest part of the joint lies inferiorly where capsule alone covers the head of the humerus. The dislocation is usually caused by a fall on outstretched hand. The thrust is greater to produce dislocation if the abduction of arm is more marked when the hand strikes the ground.

Types

The dislocation of shoulder is of two types:

 i. anterior
 ii. posterior.

Posterior dislocation is least common and is usually the result of a direct blow on the front of the joint. It may also be produced by a fall with the out-stretched arm in front of the body.

Luxatio Erecta

Luxatio erecta is a rare type in which the head of the humerus is driven downwards and is trapped below the glenoid and the arm cannot be lowered. This type of dislocation is the result of a fall with the arm fully abducted. The downward thrust is due to the combination of the fall and forcible protective muscular contraction at the moment of impact.

Anterior Dislocation

Anterior dislocation is the commonest variety and occurs in 95% of the cases. The following types of anterior dislocations occur.

i. subglenoid: stopped by the triceps muscle

ii. subcoracoid: stopped by the coracobrachialis muscle

iii. subclavicular: stopped by the clavicle bone.

Pathological Anatomy

The injury may produce two types of pathology:

A. The stripping of the capsule and labrum glenoidale from the anterior portion of glenoid cavity of scapula. This injury never heals and is bound to produce recurrent dislocation of the shoulder.

B. There is simple tearing of the capsule which heals rapidly, and hence, dislocation does not recur.

Unfortunately, there is no way to find out as to which patient will have recurrence and which will not have. Probably it depends on the degree rather than type, and in both cases, there is damage to the capsule and soft-tissue attachments on the glenoid margin. The dislocation which becomes recurrent is partly due to the greater degree of damage to the attachment of capsule and labrum and also partly due to a shorter period of immobilization after the reduction and frequent change of bandage, resulting in the incomplete healing of the injury.

Diagnosis

Anterior dislocation is easily diagnosed because the normal contour of the shoulder is lost and the shoulder appears flat on its outer aspect. The contraction of deltoid is tested by asking the patient to attempt the abduction of the arm so that the damage to axillary nerve is detected. A small area of skin hypoesthesia below the acromion will also be found when this nerve is damaged.

Posterior Dislocation

Besides being rare, the diagnosis of posterior dislocation is very difficult. However, radiograph taken in anteroposterior view reveals an appearance of the overlap of the humeral head and glenoid cavity, but an axial view will always confirm the diagnosis of posterior dislocation of the shoulder joint.

Luxatio Erecta

Inferior dislocation of the humeral head, with the position of the arm held in abduction, and the absence of palpable humeral head below the acromia are definite signs of this dislocation and are not seen in any other condition.

Treatment of Anterior Dislocation

There are two methods by which anterior dislocation can be treated:

1. Kocher's method
2. Hippocratic method.

Kocher's Method

With full general anaesthesia and muscle relaxation, the doctor stands on the affected side of the patient. The arm is held with the elbow flexed while the hand holding the elbow exerts traction in the long axis of the humerus as it lies by the side. Gradually the arm is externally rotated as the traction is maintained, and slowly the resistance of the surrounding muscle is overcome. When external rotation reaches 60 degrees, the arm is adducted and rotated inwards by bringing the elbow across the chest and carrying the hand to the opposite shoulder. There may or may not be a palpable snap or thud sound at the moment of reduction. But this method is gentle and will result in full reduction of the dislocation without injury to the surrounding tissue. Sometimes it can be tried in the playground immediately after the injury, and it can be successful as well.

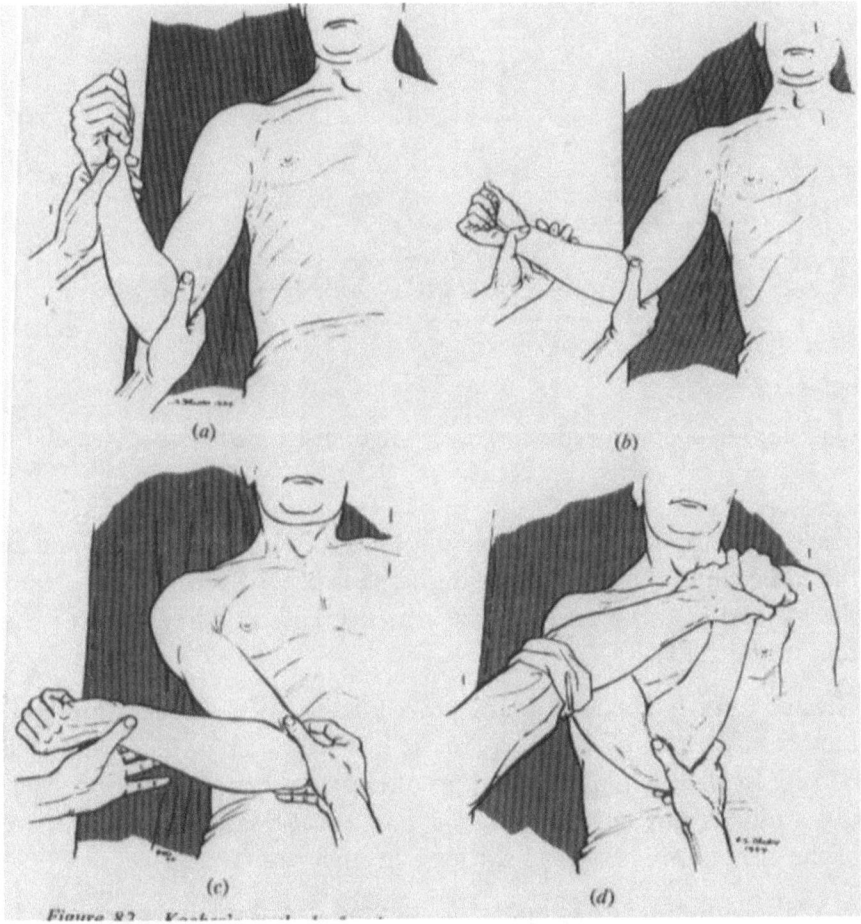

Fig. 17: Kocher's method of reduction of dislocation of the shoulder joint.

Hippocratic Method

In Hippocratic method, stockinged foot is used as a fulcrum placed between the chest wall and the upper part of the arm. This method is used if the Kocher's method fails to reduce the dislocation.

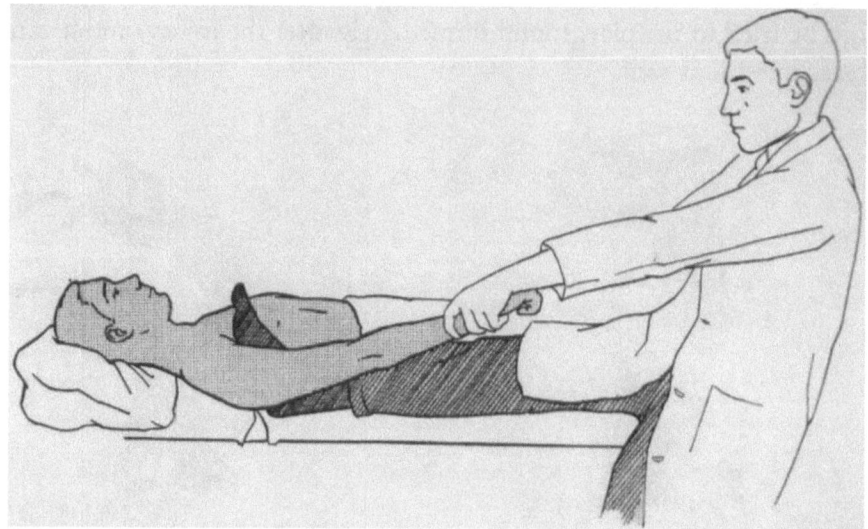

Fig. 18: Hippocratic method of reduction of dislocation of shoulder joint.

Traction is applied to the whole upper limb with both hands, and at the same time, the head of the humerus is levered outwards and into the glenoid fossa by bringing the arm medially as a lever against the foot in the axilla.

Greater force is applied in this procedure than in Kocher's method. However, with care, the procedure is free from risk of damage to the nerves. Indeed, it is the procedure of choice for rare occasions when dislocation is two to three weeks old, and it is also safer to avoid fracture of the osteoporotic bones of the joint in such cases.

A modification of the Hippocratic method can sometimes be used. It consists of traction on the arm with one hand while at the same time the fingers of the other hand are placed deeply in the axilla. Gently and by direct pressure, the head of the humerus is pushed over the edge of the glenoid into its socket.

Prone Method

In prone method, only sedation is required. The patient lies prone, and the dislocated arm is lowered over the edge of the table to hang vertically for several minutes. Reduction occurs slowly and is not accompanied by an uncomfortable sensation. Occasionally, reduction does not occur, and reduction by one of the other methods can be performed by manipulation under anaesthesia.

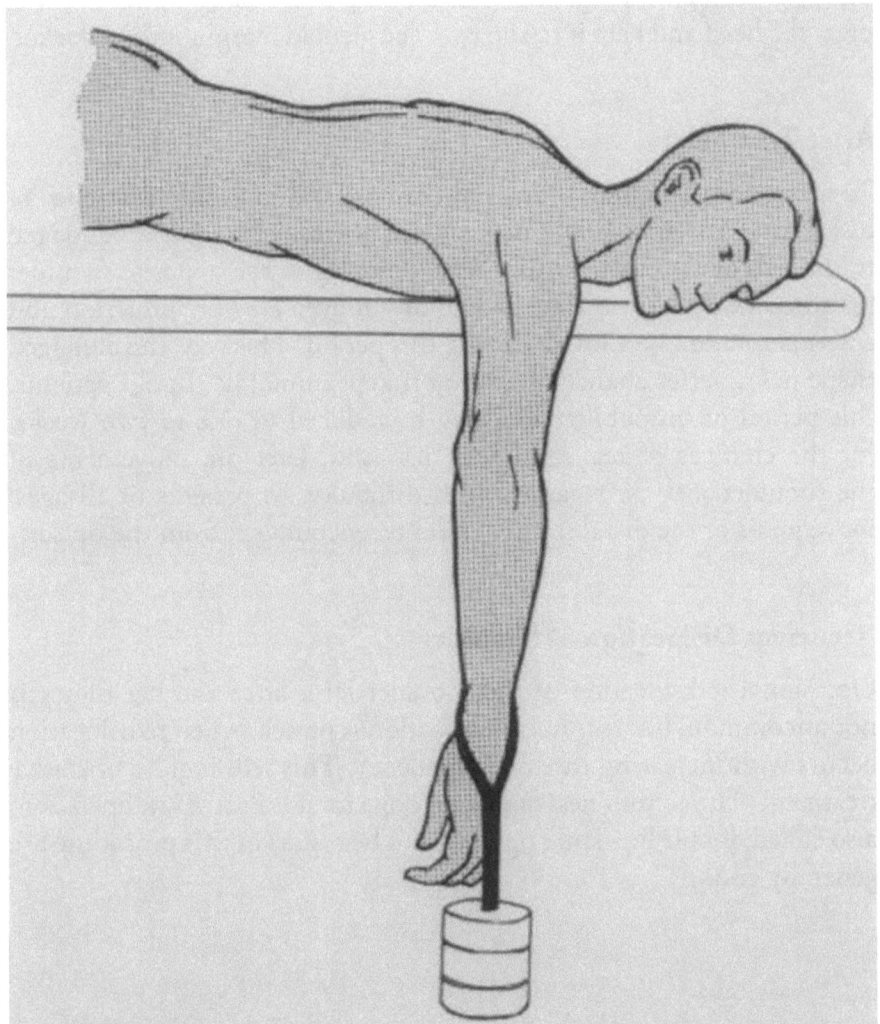

Fig19: Reduction of dislocation of the shoulder joint (prone method).

Posterior Dislocation

Though rare, reduction of posterior dislocation is simple. Traction in the long axis of arm and external rotation will reduce the dislocation.

Luxatio Erecta

Under full anaesthesia, luxatio erecta can be reduced by traction in the long axis of arm, together with the help of the hand in the axilla to press the head and help it to slip over the glenoid margin into its socket.

After Treatment

To allow the pathological anatomy to heal and to avoid recurrence of dislocation, the arm should be kept tied down in a sling and bandaged to the side of chest wall with fingers pointing to the opposite shoulder for three weeks. At no time should any movements of abduction and external rotation be allowed during this period. This way, the damaged tissue has a better chance of healing if kept immobile. In old patients, this period of immobilization may be reduced to one to two weeks, for the chances of recurrence are less and, later on, movements of the shoulder may be regained with difficulty. In patients of all ages, movements of the distal joints should be encouraged from the outset.

Recurrent Dislocation of Shoulder

Occasional redislocation of the shoulder joint after another injury is not uncommon, but recurrent dislocation is present when redislocation occurs with increasing ease and frequency. This will require operative treatment. The commonest operation done for it is Putti-Platt operation, also called double breasting operation. The results of this procedure are generally good.

CHAPTER 13

FRACTURE OF THE SCAPULA

Almost any part of the scapula may be fractured, and usually it is caused by a direct blow. However, the common fractures are:

i. neck of the scapula
ii. body of the scapula
iii. coracoid process of the scapula
iv. acromion process of the scapula.

Avulsion fracture also occurs, and injury to the neck of the scapula occurs due to a fall on the arm. Sometimes fracture of the blade or body of the scapula may be associated with an injury to the underlying ribs; otherwise, they present no problem. Fracture of the coracoid process is the result of sudden and uncontrolled contraction of the three muscles attached to it.

The acromion is fractured by a fall or fall of weight over the front of the shoulder, but displacement does not occur. The only fracture which presents difficulty is the one in which the fracture line starts just below the glenoid cavity and extends upwards to the coracoid process.

Diagnosis

Fractures due to direct violence are associated with superficial evidence of injury. In the rest of the injuries, such as in the acromion process and the spine of the scapula, local tenderness and swelling are present.

In fracture of the neck of the scapula, an acutely painful shoulder is present.

Fractures of the body of the scapula are often difficult to diagnose by anteroposterior radiography. Further X-rays may be required to be taken in patients who complain of pain and limitation of movements though routine X-rays appear to be normal.

Treatment

In majority of cases, there is no displacement, but pain is felt, which can be treated with analgesic. A cuff-and-collar sling is given for four to six weeks to allow the fracture to heal well. Active movements of the shoulder are allowed to prevent joint stiffness. Minor displacement of the neck of the scapula may be accepted, but marked displacement may require closed reduction and application of bandage to the scapula to provide efficient fixation. Too much interference may cause stiffness of the shoulder joint, which should be avoided.

Marked displacement of the glenoid cavity or coracoid process may require open reduction. In addition, gross displacement of the acromion fracture may be treated by excision of the outer end of the acromion process.

Fracture of the Body of the Scapula

Fracture of the body of the scapula is caused due to a direct blow on the scapula. It may be associated with fracture of the ribs. The fracture may be transverse or stellate. There is no displacement due to the splinting by subscapularis and infraspinatus.

The treatment is strapping with arm in a sling. Active movements are encouraged at an early date.

Fracture of the Neck of the Scapula

Fracture of the neck of the scapula may be caused by a direct blow or a fall on the side of the shoulder or on an outstretched hand. The fractured bone extends from the infraglenoid region to the base of the coracoid process. There may be slight downward and inward displacement by the weight of the arm, but it so slight, and it causes no disability.

The arm is supported in a sling, and active movements of fingers and hand are encouraged early, when the pain subside.

Fracture of the Coracoid Process

Fracture of the coracoid process may be caused by muscular violence or by a direct blow. This fracture may involve only a fragment or the base of the coracoid process.

The treatment required is support of the arm in a cuff-and-collar sling and encouragement of active movements.

CHAPTER 14

FRACTURE OF THE HUMERUS

The following sites are involved in the fracture of the humerus:
1. head of humerus
   a. greater tuberosity
   b. displaced
   c. undisplaced
2. neck of the humerus
3. shaft of the humerus
4. lower end of the humerus.

Fracture of the Head of the Humerus

Fracture of the greater tuberosity may be:
   i. displaced
   ii. undisplaced.

Undisplaced

The following are two distinct types of undisplaced fractures, but in both, the displacement is minimal.
   i. Contusion fracture: It is commonly caused by direct violence, such as a blow on the shoulder, or forcible impaction against the acromion in abduction. It is called contusion fracture, and sometimes, a large fragment is fractured but the fragment is seldom displaced. Sometimes it may be associated with fracture of the neck of the humerus, and the fragment is large and comminuted.

ii. **Avulsion fracture:** In this type, an undisplaced fracture of the top of the greater tuberosity is produced by a powerful contraction of the supraspinatus. This fragment may be displaced, but in majority of cases, the displacement is minimal, and management is the same as that of undisplaced contusion fracture. However, sometimes it may impinge into the joint surface and cause limitation of function. Then it may require removal of this small fragment by operation.

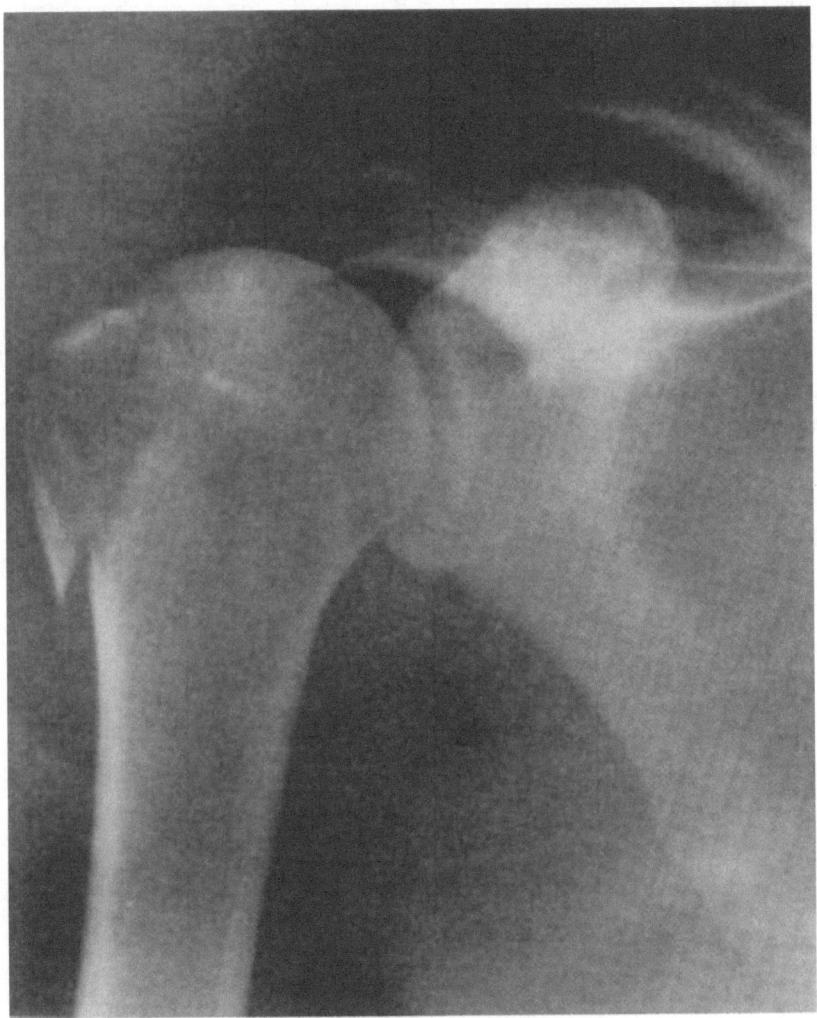

Fig. 20: Fracture of the greater tuberosity of the humerus.

Displaced

Avulsion of a small fragment from the top of the greater tuberosity by contraction of supraspinatus occurs. Complete displacement of the whole tuberosity is uncommon, but complete disruption of the surrounding soft tissue allows the wide separation of the fragment from its bed. As a result, the action of supraspinatus function suffers. This injury is often accompanied by the dislocation of the shoulder joint, but after the reduction of the dislocation of the shoulder joint, the fragment of greater tuberosity may be replaced by itself. The rest of the treatment is the same as for avulsion fracture without displacement.

Treatment

Undisplaced fracture of the greater tuberosity will require treatment by a triangular cuff-and-collar sling with analgesics to relieve the pain. This sling, in the initial stages, may be supplemented by a firm crepe and cotton wool bandage for 7–10 days, applied over the affected arm so as to give complete rest to the shoulder joint. While applying the bandage, a layer of cotton wool is placed between the arm and chest wall to make the bandage comfortable to the patient (figs 21 and 22).

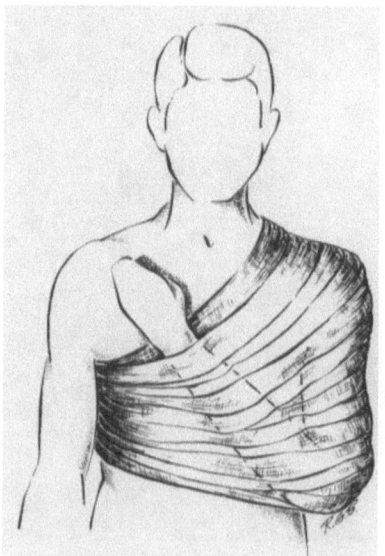

Fig. 21: Crepe bandage dressing applied to maintain adduction and internal rotation of the shoulder joint after reduction of the dislocation.

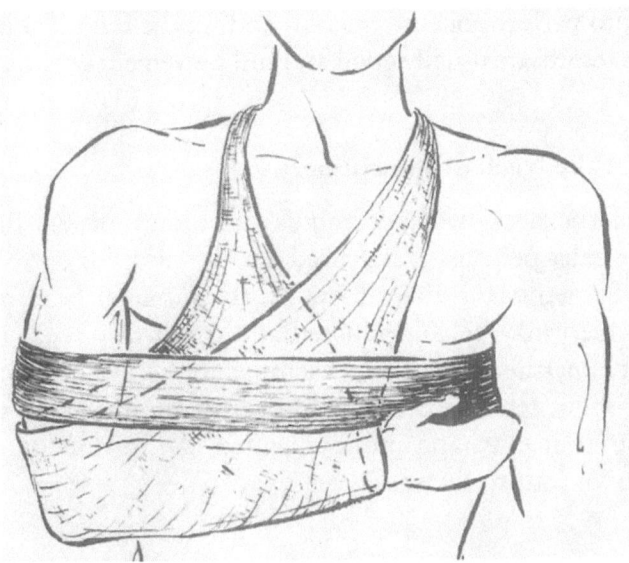

Fig. 22: Double-sling method of immobilization is used in treating certain shoulder injuries.

The stiffness of the shoulder joint is treated by early movements of the shoulder joint. The movements should be started within a week and continued for months till full recovery.

Displaced

When displacement is only a few millimetres, no reduction is required, and management follows as that of an undisplaced fracture. Wide separation will require simple reduction, but it is often accompanied by shoulder dislocation. The reduction of the dislocation of the shoulder usually reduces the fracture as well. Then it can be managed as mentioned above.

Wide displacement necessitates reduction, for without perfect reduction, the power and movements of abduction will become limited. Reduction is sometimes obtained by holding the arm in a horizontal position with some 30 degrees of external rotation of the shoulder. This position is held for six weeks in a shoulder spica moulded and rested upon the iliac crest or an abduction frame, but these methods are cumbersome and produce joint stiffness.

It is better to perform open reduction and fix the fragment by a single screw. The results are usually good and full movement's recovery occurs.

Fracture of the Neck of the Humerus

Fracture of the neck of the humerus commonly occurs in younger age and in older persons. It is caused usually by a fall on to the hand or elbow. Sometimes a direct blow on the humeral head may cause fracture, which may be comminuted and is not displaced; rarely is it compound in nature. Due to the attachment of multitude of soft tissues, fracture without separation is much more common. Fractures in this situation unite readily, and immobilization can be done by cuff-and-collar sling for four to six weeks.

Fractures without Separation (Adults)

The fracture line usually passes across the surgical neck of the humerus, but sometimes, fracture line may run into the head itself or into the greater tuberosity. Most commonly, the shaft is adducted. The fracture line may be at different level at the front and back of the bone, producing an appearance of impaction. In fact, true impaction is rare, but the stability of fracture is present due to intact soft-tissue attachments, which hold the fragments together.

Treatment

In old patients, minor angulation at the fracture site is accepted because manipulation may produce more stiffness. A cuff-and-collar sling is the best method to treat this fracture. At first, the fracture should be placed in a cuff-and-collar sling, and the whole arm held firmly to the side of the trunk by several layers of crepe bandage applied over pads of cotton wool placed between the arm and trunk. Movements of the wrist and hand are started at once, but active and assisted movements of the shoulder are encouraged as soon as the pain has subsided and the bandages have been removed, usually after 7–10 days. However, the cuff-and-collar sling (fig. 23) is retained for four to six weeks.

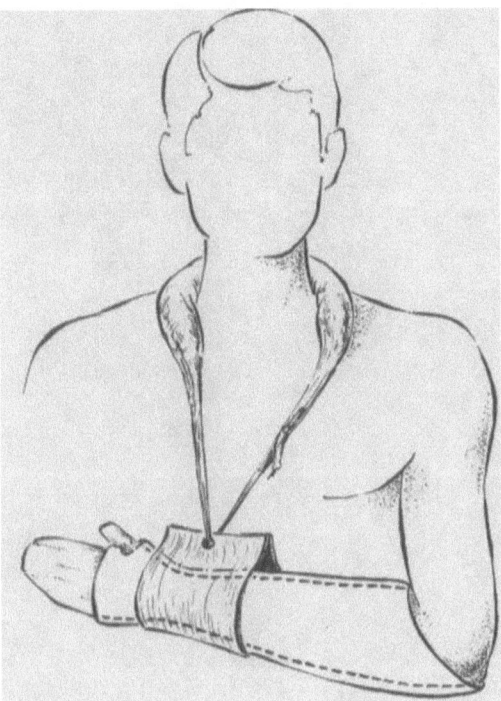

Fig. 23: Cuff-and-collar sling applied for support of arm and forearm.

Occasionally, when angulation is more than 30 degrees and the patient is under 50 years of age, it should be reduced by manipulation under general anaesthesia and then treated in a plaster cast for four to six weeks, with arm kept in a sling.

Fracture with Separation

Fracture with separation is an uncommon fracture. In this fracture, the head of the humerus is rotated into abduction by the rotator cuff muscles, and the shaft is displaced upwards and inwards by the action of the pectoralis major and muscles attached to the coracoid process.

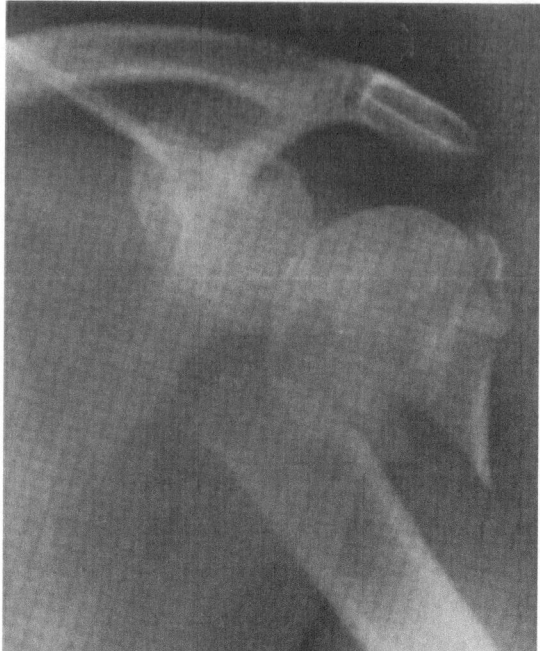

Fig. 24: Fracture of the surgical neck of the humerus with displacement.

Treatment

The fracture of surgical nock is a difficult fracture, and reduction by closed method is not possible. Rather, it should not be attempted because it may cause damage to the vessels, especially in an old person. Closed manipulative reduction is performed under general anaesthesia with full relaxation. Gentle traction is applied to the arm as it lies by the side. Then one hand is placed in the axilla, and by combination of outward pressure of fingers and adduction of the arm, it is sometimes possible to reduce the fracture in line with the head of the humerus. When this happens, the arm is immobilized by the side in a sling and trunk bandage. Immobilization in abducted position is avoided as it will redisplace the fracture. Instead, repeated X-ray is done every second or third day for the first week to ensure that loss of position has not taken place.

Open reduction is necessary when closed manipulation has failed or redisplacement has taken place. The reduction should be done under direct vision, and fixation should be carried out by an intramedullary nail. This may be supported by a plaster cast. The fracture unites in six to eight weeks' time.

Fracture of the Neck of the Humerus in Children

In children, the commonest fracture is of greenstick type with minimal displacement. The fracture line often runs near the epiphyseal line, which makes it difficult to make the diagnosis. In the majority of children, displacement is slight and consists of minor separation of the epiphysis or greenstick subtubercular fracture with less than 20 degrees of varus angulation.

Fortunately, the process of remodelling in the upper humerus with growth is good, but care should be taken not to accept great degree of displacement with this consideration.

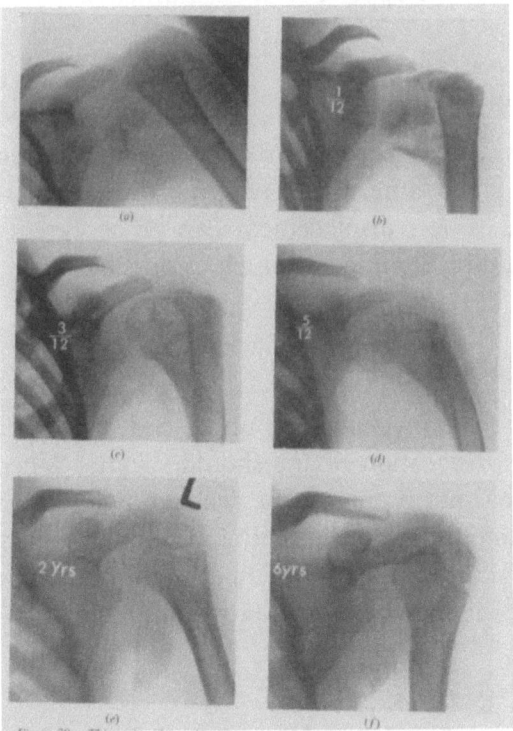

Figure 25: The remodelling process of fracture of the neck of the humerus in children is shown in these X-ray films.

Treatment

Subtubercular greenstick fractures is common in children up to the age of 7 years. The commonest site of fracture is just below the great tuberosity. It is usually a greenstick type with varus angulation which is often less than 30 degree. Such fracture can be provided comfort temporarily by a sling. When angulation is more marked, an acceptable position of correction can be obtained by a hanging cast. A plaster cast extending from below the shoulder to the wrist, with elbow at right angle, is applied and is supported by a cuff-and-collar sling. The weight of the plaster applies a mild continuous corrective traction force on the shoulder to correct the displacement.

If there is a complete separation of the fragments with complete fracture through the humeral neck, a similar method as stated can be used. In such cases, if perfect reduction is not possible, overriding up to 1 cm is permissible and does not cause any disability later on. However, open reduction should be avoided because there is every chance of damage to the epiphysis of the upper end of the humerus.

Separated Epiphysis

In older children, often it is epiphyseal fracture separation which occurs. The treatment is the same as the one given above except that as the age of child advances, less displacement can be accepted; hence, perfect reduction should be obtained as much as possible.

Fracture–Dislocation

Almost any fracture involving the upper end of the humerus may be associated with dislocation of the shoulder joint. When separation of the fragments has not occurred, the problem is not great because fairly accurate reposition usually occurs with reduction of dislocation alone. It is the separated fracture of the surgical neck of the humerus associated with a dislocation of the shoulder which provides a difficult problem to treat.

Diagnosis

Clinical diagnosis is difficult. It is always advisable to take X-ray when dislocation of the shoulder joint occurs. The usual method of reduction in the presence of fracture may cause injury to the axillary nerve or vessels or brachial plexus.

Treatment

1. Dislocation with Fracture of the Greater Tuberosity

Reduction is done by routine manner for an uncomplicated dislocation of shoulder. After reduction, X-ray film may show satisfactory reduction of the fragments, but sometimes replacement does not occur. It should then be treated by the usual manner as an isolated injury.

2. Dislocation with Unseparated Fracture of Surgical Neck

When the shaft and head of the humerus are in contact, the soft-tissue attachments are strong to withstand the stress of reduction. It can be reduced by placing the fingers deeply in the axilla while at the same time pulling gently on the arm in the line of trunk. A good relaxation makes this procedure successful. Afterwards, a cuff-and-collar sling or a plaster cast should be given for four to six weeks.

3. Dislocation with Separate Fracture of the Surgical Neck

Closed reduction can be carried out under general anaesthesia. The arm is abducted about 50 degrees from the trunk, and gentle traction is exerted while, at the same time, pressure with hand in the axilla reduces the palpable humeral head. If this method fails in the first attempt, then open reduction should be carried out. In open reduction, internal fixation can also be done. In elderly patients, excision of fracture portion may be considered, which will restore good shoulder movements.

Fracture of the Shaft of the Humerus

Fracture of the shaft of the humerus is easy to treat. A perfect anatomical position may not occur, but functional results are excellent. The fracture can be reduced without anaesthesia, but if displacement is marked, anaesthesia is required.

The limb is gently aligned, and plaster slab is applied, starting in the axilla and extending down around the elbow and up the outer arm over the shoulder to form a cap over the top of the joint. The slab is firmly bandaged on to the upper arm. The shoulder cap should be fixed with an adhesive tape, and the forearm supported in a cuff-and-collar sling. The movements of fingers and the rotation of the forearm can be started once the pain and swelling have subsided. The patient may need to sleep partly propped up in bed.

The fracture becomes clinically firm in four to five weeks, and full union takes place in six to eight weeks. Occasionally, this fracture is slow to unite, and if at the end of one month clinical and radiological union is not present, it will be required to apply shoulder spica for rigid fixation for three to four months.

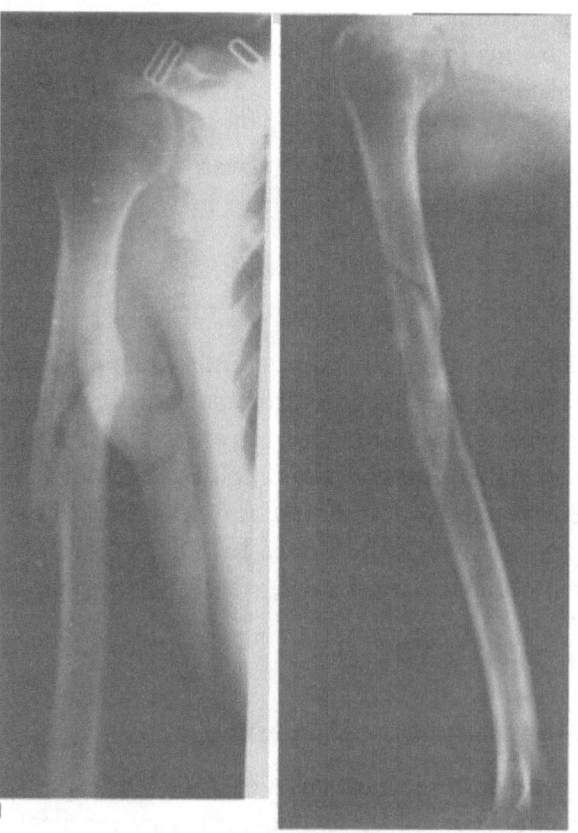

Fig. 26: Fracture of the humerus shaft
(shows union taking place).

Radial Nerve Palsy

The incidence of radial nerve palsy is fairly common in fracture of the shaft of the humerus. Fortunately, it always recovers in a few months' time without any treatment. To find this injury, the test of dorsiflexion of the hand at the wrist joint is helpful. The nerve is more likely to be injured in a spiral fracture about the junction of the middle and lower third of the shaft of the humerus, where it is in actual contact with the bone and adheres as it passes through lateral intermuscular septum. To avoid such injury to the nerve, open reduction of the fracture with removal of the nerve from between the bone ends and internal fixation with plate and screws should be done. If closed reduction of fracture has been done and if the fracture has united but there is wrist drop present after lapse of three months, the nerve should be explored, and if required, it can be sutured. The late results of this procedure are excellent. During the period of recovery, the wrist should be supported with a removable cock-up splint, but this should be taken off daily for passive wrist movements. The fingers should be left free and frequently extended passively.

Brachial Artery Injury

Brachial artery can be injured with penetrating wounds or closed crush injuries. In such cases, the artery should be explored and sutured if required, but the fracture will need to be fixed with plate and screws.

CHAPTER 15

FRACTURES AND DISLOCATIONS OF THE ELBOW

Aetiology

The majority of elbow injuries occur due to a fall on outstretched hand, but a fall on the point of the elbow can cause intercondylar fracture or fracture of the olecranon.

Dislocation and most displaced fractures involve tearing of the capsule, ligaments, and brachialis muscle. Early attempts at movement may cause ossification in these structures.

The complication of ischaemia and peripheral nerve injuries is common. It should be noted down in the initial examination. Ischaemia is an emergency, but reduction of displacement usually improves circulation, and exploration of brachial artery is rarely required.

Supracondylar Fractures

Supracondylar fractures are common in children between the ages of 5 and 8.

In fracture cases, 85% are of extension type, and 15% are of flexion type.

Extension Type	Flexion Type
• It occurs in 85% of the cases. • Fracture line runs from below upwards and backwards. • Lower fragment is displaced backwards. • Injury to the brachialis, brachial artery, or median nerve may occur. • Fracture is reduced in flexion. • It gives good results.	• It occurs in 15% of the cases. • Fractures line runs from below upwards and forwards. • Lower fragment is displaced forwards. • Injury to the brachial artery and median nerve is uncommon. • Fracture is reduced in extension. • It may cause limitation of function.

The supracondylar fracture is common cause of Volkmann's contracture, which is denoted by signs and symptoms of the five *P*s (i.e. pain, pallor, pulselessness, paralysis, and puffiness).

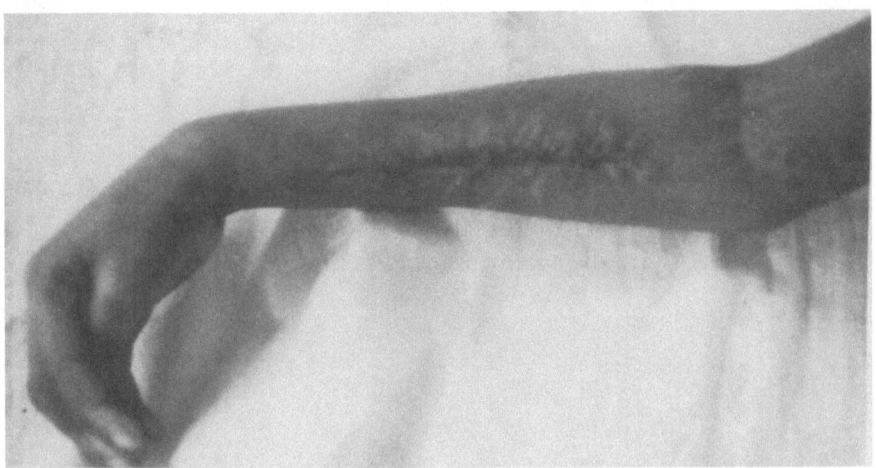

Fig. 27: Volkmann's ischemic contracture of the forearm and hand.

Reduction of fracture and holding the limb in extension may relieve arterial obstruction, but sometimes exploration of the artery may be necessary, and this must be done within six hours after the injury.

Extension Type

Reduction of the fracture is carried out by traction in flexion and pressing the lower fragment forwards over the proximal fragment while maintaining the traction. Sometimes pronation of the forearm is helpful.

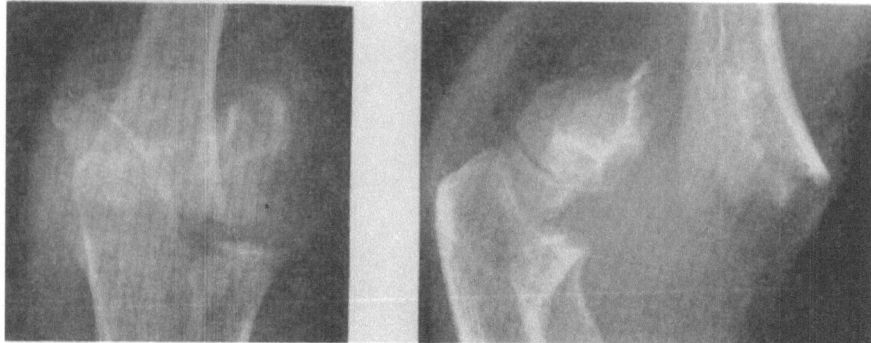

Fig. 28a: Supracondylar fracture of the humerus, with upward and backward displacement (extension) of distal fragment.

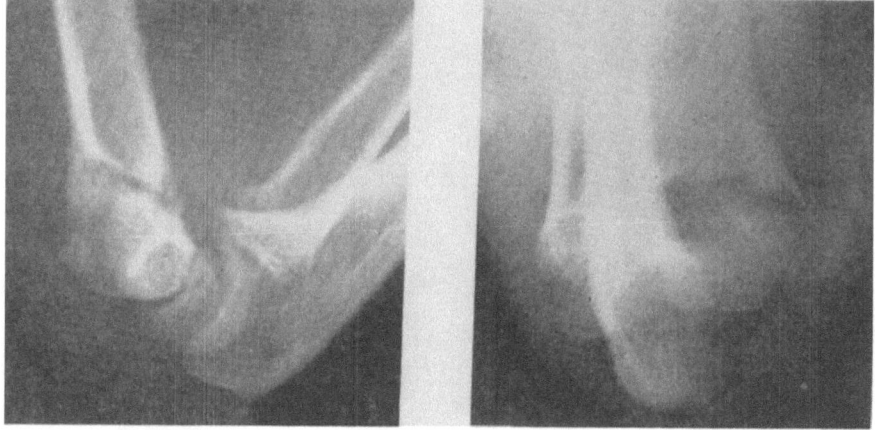

Fig. 28b: Treated by closed reduction and plaster of Paris cast.

It may be required to do two or three attempts to reduce the fracture, but it must be done at one sitting under one-time anaesthesia, not at intervals of two to three days. The carrying angle can be checked by the extension of the elbow while reduction is held. The reduction is stable in full flexion, being held by the pressure of the triceps on the back, but swelling and circulation demand slight extension of the limb. The radial pulse must always be checked after reduction.

In supracondylar fracture, in addition to posterior displacement of the fragment, there may be medial or lateral displacement of the lower fragment. This medial or lateral displacement must be corrected before reducing anteroposterior displacement.

Sometimes good apposition cannot be obtained. These fractures are easily reduced by open reduction and can be held with transfixation pins without difficulty. However, in such cases, movements return gradually.

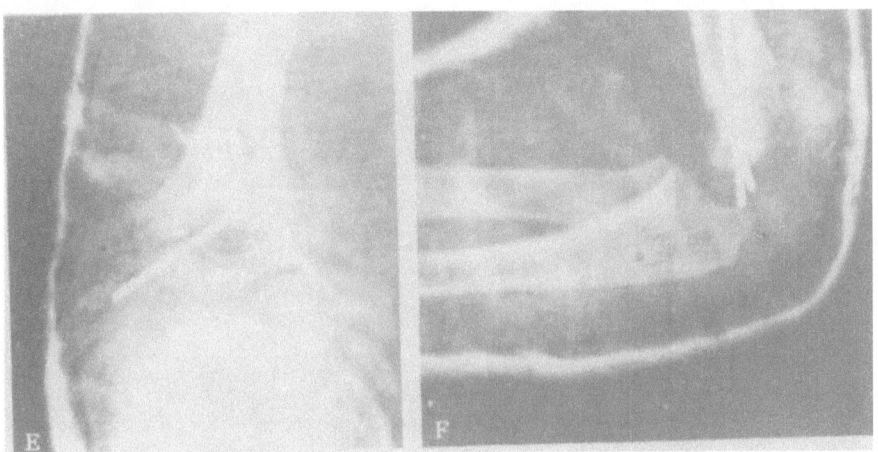

Fig. 29: Supracondylar fracture of the humours treated with reduction, pin fixation, and plaster cast.

Flexion Type

The fracture of flexion type in which the distal fragment is displaced forwards and upwards can be easily reduced by manipulation in full extension and immobilization in a plaster cast for three weeks. After that, the elbow joint should be brought to flex position and kept in plaster cast for further three weeks till complete union of the fracture takes place.

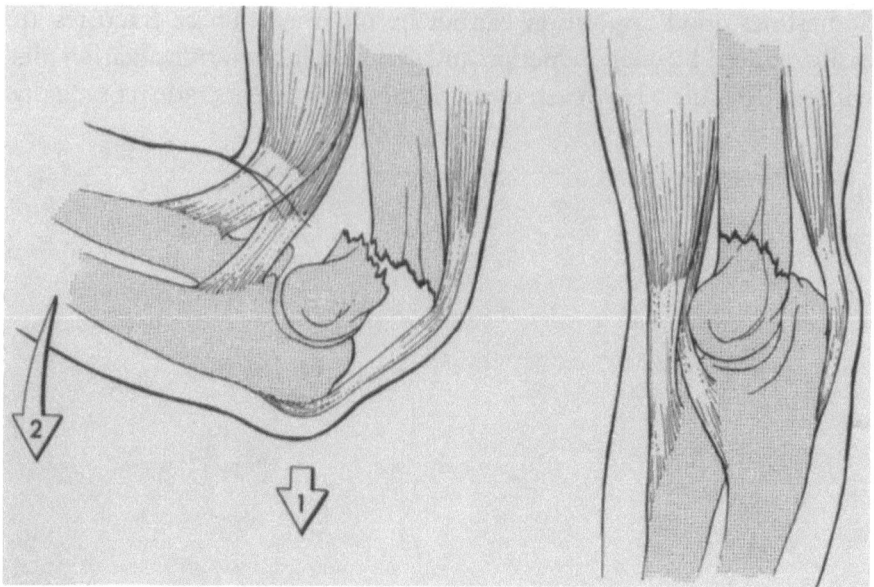

Fig. 30: Supracondylar fracture (flexion type)
is usually best held in extension.

Supracondylar fracture also occurs in elderly persons, but displacement is less. The *T-* or *Y-*shaped intercondylar fractures are more common in adults and follow a fall on the point of the elbow.

The two fragments are rotated out by the pull of the flexor and extensor muscles. Sometimes comminution of fragments occurs.

Manipulation and plaster fixation are unsatisfactory as rotational displacement of fragments recurs. Open reduction and fixation of condylar fragments give good results. Sometimes, in elderly patients, cuff-and-collar sling can be given, and active movements may be allowed gradually, but in younger patients, accurate reduction and fixation of the condylar fragments can give better result.

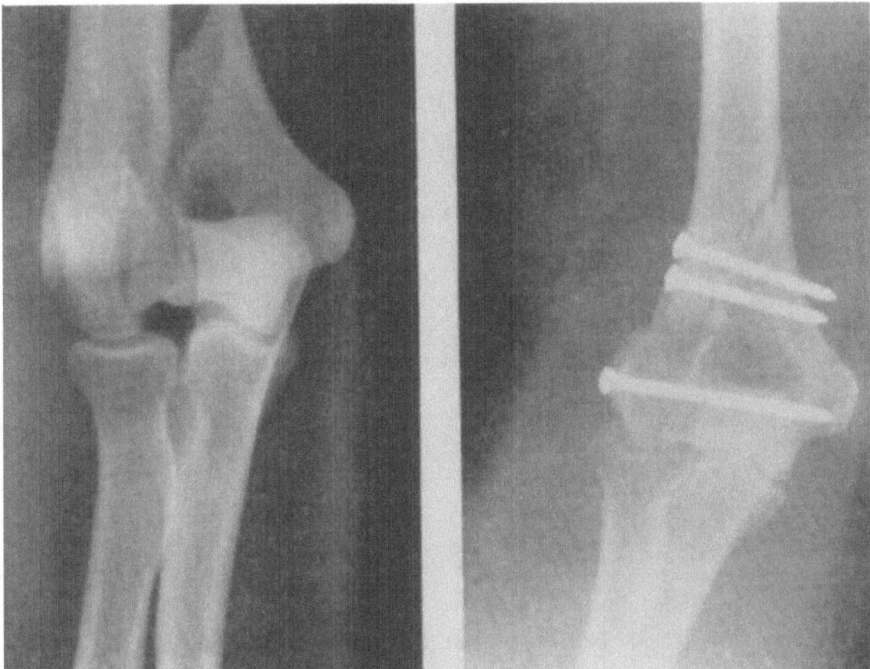

Fig. 31: Fracture of the lower end of the humerus treated with screw fixation.

Lateral Condylar Fractures

Fractures of the lateral condyle are common in children. The fragment of the fracture usually includes a small part of trochlea and a small portion of the diaphysis. The X-ray may show small portion of it because it consists largely of cartilage. The pull of the extensor may rotate the fragment so that the articular surface faces laterally. Unreduced displacement leads to non-union, disturbance of lateral growth with production of cubitus valgus, and sometimes disturbance of the trochlea growth leading to fishtail deformity of the lower end of the humerus. In such cases, closed reduction is often not successful, and open reduction is required. The fragment should be reduced and fixed with a pin. Results of this procedure are good.

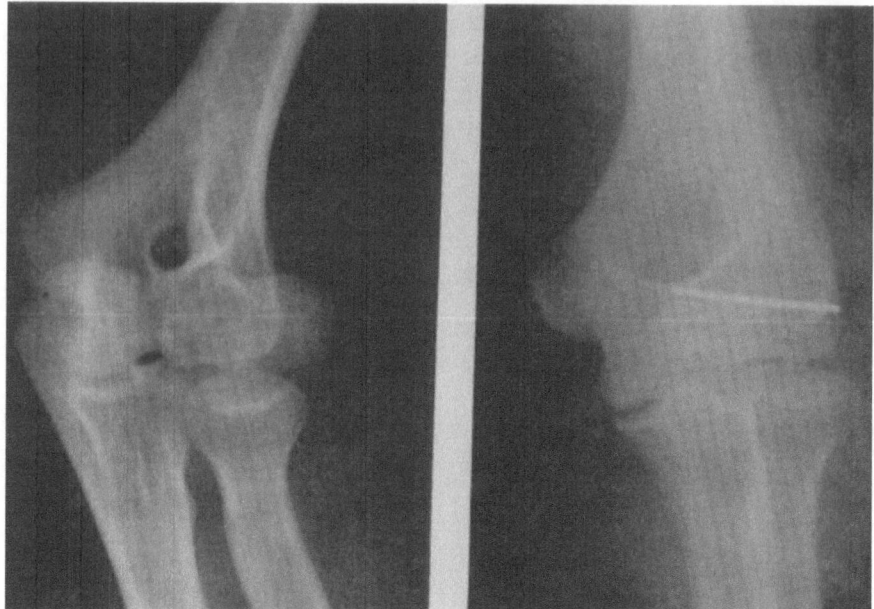

Fig. 32: Fracture of lateral condyle of humerus treated by pin fixation.

Undisplaced fracture can be treated in a plaster cast for four weeks, and no growth disturbance occurs.

Fracture of lateral condyle occurs less commonly in adults and should be treated by open reduction to prevent arthritic changes.

Capitellum Fractures

Fracture of the capitellum occurs in adults. Sometimes a small fragment is detached. Occasionally, it is associated with fracture of the head of the radius, and sometimes, the detached fragment includes a portion of the trochlea. The treatment is by operation. Small fragments are better excised, but a larger fragment must be reduced and secured in position by fixation with a pin. Results of the operative treatment are good.

Avulsion of the Medial Epicondyle

In the case of avulsion of the medial epicondyle, it is usually the epiphysis which is avulsed. The displacement may be slight, or if the medial ligament of the elbow gets ruptured, the displacement may be considerable, associated with lateral dislocation of the elbow joint. The displaced epicondyle may be trapped in the joint on the inner side. For minor displacement, conservative treatment in a plaster cast is required for four to six weeks, but if the fragment is trapped in the joint, it would require excision of the fragment and suture of medial ligament to protect the ulnar nerve from injury, or transposition of the ulnar nerve may be required.

Fracture of the Head of the Radius

Fractures of the head of the radius are common in adults. Swelling is mild, but limitation of movements, particularly rotation, and pain on movements are present. The most common type of fracture is a fissure without displacement. Conservative treatment in a plaster cast for four weeks, along with a cuff-and-collar sling, followed by gentle active movements, produces full recovery of movements and functions in two months' time.

If there is slight displacement of a small fragment, which is not touching the superior radioulnar joint, it can be treated by rest in a plaster for four to six weeks.

Comminuted and displaced fractures in adults should be treated by excision of the radial head, partial excision, or replacement by prosthesis. This produces inferior result than complete excision. The results of early excision within a week are superior to the results of delayed excision, even where fracture has been associated with dislocation of the elbow joint. After the operation, cuff-and-collar sling in flexion should be given for 14 days to allow the synovial injury to recover itself. If dislocation of the elbow joint or tearing of medial ligaments has also taken place, a plaster cast for four to six weeks is required for full recovery.

Fracture of the Neck of the Radius

In children, the neck of the radius is more commonly fractured than the head. The head is tilted to one side. Manipulation of the most prominent part of the displaced head laterally and strong pressure may reduce the tilt. When displacement is severe or manipulation is unsuccessful, open reduction is required and is usually stable without fixation. Excision will cause shortening of the radius and can lead to dislocation of the inferior radioulnar joint.

Fracture of the Olecranon

Fracture of the olecranon can occur either by a fall or blow on the point of elbow. Many fractures of the olecranon process have little or no displacement. Rest in plaster cast for four weeks is required, then active movement can be started.

Fracture in an elderly is often comminuted, and it can be treated in a plaster cast for four to six weeks, followed by active movements. It can give good result; therefore, operation is not required.

Displaced fractures of the olecranon can be treated in extension in a plaster cast for four to six weeks and will unite, but there is a risk of permanent loss of flexion movements. Therefore, this method is not advisable. Where fracture has a small fragment or comminution with the distal face of the coronoid fossa intact, excision of the fragment of the proximal portion and suture of triceps to distal fragment give good results. Transverse fractures do well with internal fixation after accurate reduction. Firm screw fixation along with plaster cast for four weeks will restore good active movements.

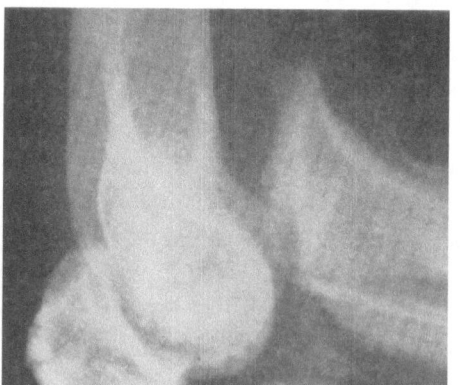
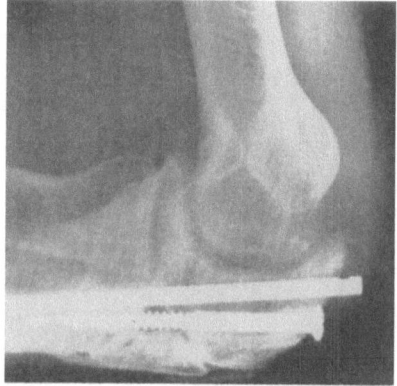

Fig 32a left – image olecranon fracture
Fig 32b right – treated by nail and screw fixation

Fracture of the Coronoid Process

Fracture of the coronoid process occurs in adults, and they are usually not displaced. It can be treated in plaster cast for four weeks with good result. Occasionally, the fragment of the coronoid is displaced into the joint and causes limitation of movements. It can be treated by excision of the fragment.

Dislocation of Elbow Joint

Dislocation of the elbow joint involves tearing of the capsule of elbow. Dislocation is of two types:

1. posterior dislocation
2. anterior dislocation.

Posterior dislocation is more common and occurs at any age. It occurs as a result of a fall or a blow with the elbow in an extended position so that the lower end of the humerus moves forwards over the coronoid process and the head of the radius, tearing the capsule of the elbow joint.

Anterior dislocation without fracture of the olecranon is rare. Lateral dislocations are less common.

The posterior dislocation can be reduced under general anaesthesia by traction in flexion, gently pushing the humerus backwards so that the coronoid and the head of the radius move forwards distal to the lower end of the humerus. Immobilization in a padded plaster cast is carried out for three weeks. The plaster cast can be changed when swelling has subsided, and further rest is given for three weeks. Then active exercises should be started and continued till function is restored.

Posterior Dislocation

Posterior dislocation of the elbow joint without fracture of the coronoid process can only occur with the elbow flexed at 45 degrees. With the elbow fixed at this position, a longitudinal force along the shaft of the radius and ulna can cause this dislocation. The olecranon process appears to stop behind in the olecranon fossa and allow the radius and ulna to slip off the joint surface of the distal end of the humerus posterior to the humerus. In the case of posterior dislocation, there is tearing of the medial and lateral collateral ligamentous structures at the elbow. In addition, some separation of the fibres must occur in the anterior and posterior capsules of the elbow joint.

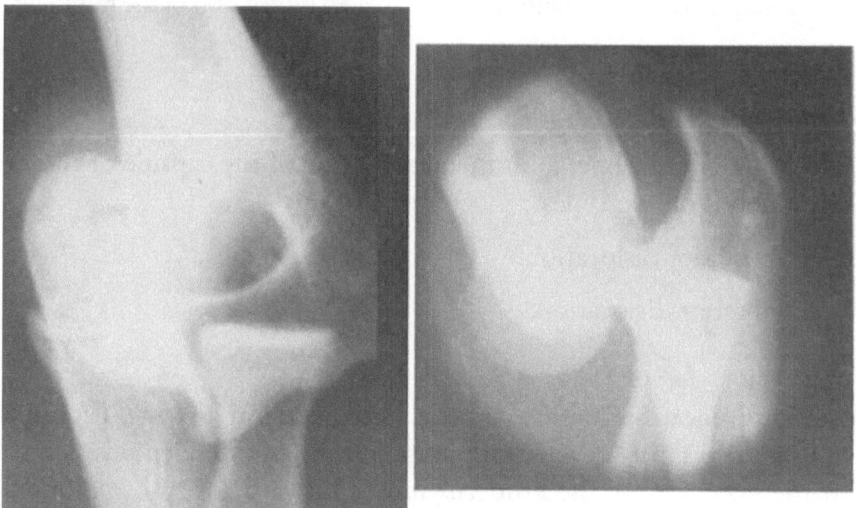

Fig. 33: Dislocation of the elbow joint. The displaced fragments can be seen.

Examination

Examination of the dislocated elbow shows the olecranon process to be posterior to its usual relationship. The elbow cannot flex and extend through its usual range of motion. Supination and pronation of the forearm are often limited.

X-ray examinations confirm the diagnosis. In anteroposterior view, the radial head and coronoid process and olecranon are superimposed directly over the joint surface of the distal humerus. In the lateral view, the X-ray film shows the radius and ulna lying directly posterior to the joint surface of the distal end of the humerus.

Treatment

The treatment of posterior dislocation of the elbow is to reduce the dislocation as soon as possible. A general anaesthesia is required.

The relocation can be accomplished with forearm supinated, the elbow flexed to 45 degrees, and a longitudinal traction applied to the forearm while counter-traction is applied to the upper arm. As soon as the radius and ulna slip back into their normal relationship with the humerus, the arm is immobilized in a long-arm plaster of Paris cast with the elbow flexed to 90 degrees. However, the reduction must be verified by X-ray before the patient is revived from the anaesthesia. For comfort, the forearm is placed in a neutral position of pronation and supination. The arm should be kept in this position for three to four weeks. The cast is then removed, the arm is placed in a cuff-and-collar sling, and gradual range of motion exercises is started.

Anterior Dislocation

Although not common, the anterior dislocation does occur, and the tearing of muscles must be accompanied by a fracture of the olecranon process. The mechanism is the use of force applied to the flexed proximal forearm from the posterior to anterior side.

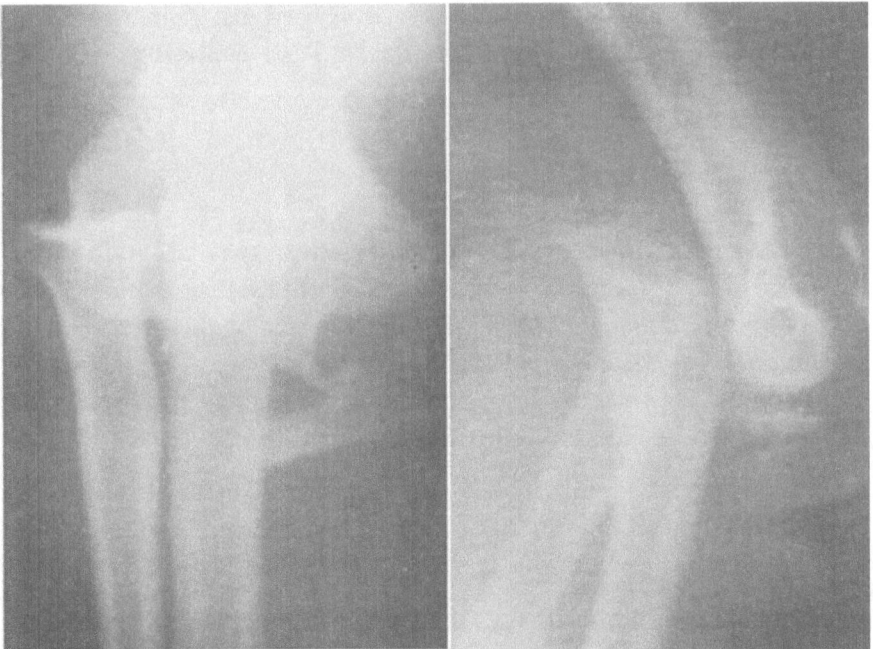

Fig. 33: Fracture–dislocation of elbow joint (anterior type).

Examination

In anteroposterior X-ray film, the proximal radius and coronoid process of the ulna are seen to overlie the distal humerus. Fracture fragments of the olecranon process are visible. In the lateral view, the distal humerus condyles are seen to lie posterior to the proximal radius and coronoid process of ulna, and there is fracture of the olecranon process.

Treatment

An anterior dislocation is unstable until reduced, and the olecranon process is fixed by open reduction. The effective method is to do open reduction of the ulna and to fix it with the figure-of-eight wire passed under the tendon of triceps and crossed at the site of the fracture on the dorsal side of olecranon. The wire is then passed through a hole drilled transversally through the ulna distal to the fracture. Tightening the wire reduces and fixes the fracture. Alternately, the fracture can be fixed by intramedullary nail or a lag screw or plate and screws.

After open reduction, the elbow should be immobilized in the plaster of Paris cast for six to eight weeks. The arm is then placed in a cuff-and-collar sling, and gentle exercises are started. Passive movements should never be given to the elbow joint.

Complications

Compression or rupture of the brachial artery may occur in elbow injuries. If reduction of displacement and slight extension of the elbow do not restore adequate circulation, exploration of the artery within six hours is necessary to avoid Volkmann's ischemic contracture. Occasionally, simple division of the bicipital fossa and release of hematoma will suffice and relieve spasm of the artery.

Neurapraxia of median or radial nerve occur in a small number of cases, but lesion of the ulnar nerve is less common. Axonotmesis is uncommon, and neurotmesis is rare.

Frictional neuritis of the ulna nerve may follow irregularity of its groove, and transposition of the nerve may be necessary.

Myositis ossificans commonly occurs and should be treated conservatively with rest in flexion until irritability has subsided. Excision of bone blocking the flexion can be attempted after a delay of several months, but it is seldom very successful.

Fracture in and around the elbow causes more complications than other injuries of the upper limb. This is due to the complex nature of the elbow joint subserving flexion, extension, and rotation movements and the large number of structures in relation to joint which are likely to be injured.

Fracture of the olecranon, supracondylar fracture of humerus, and dislocation of the elbow (with or without fracture) are likely to cause limitation of functions.

Fracture of the head of the radius and fracture of the shaft of the radius and ulna are likely to cause limitation of rotation.

The danger of passive movements to the elbow after injury is always there, and it causes stiffness, painful spasms, and myositis ossificans.

Stiff Elbow

Passive movements should never be given to the elbow joint. The patient should also be told not to do stretching of the joint on his own. Active exercises only are allowed. The patient should extend the elbow joint against resistance.

Myositis ossificans may follow dislocation, fracture–dislocations of the elbow, or forced passive movement. The development of this condition is suspected by the increasing pain in the elbow and loss of movements at the elbow joint. X-ray must be taken, and if the condition is confirmed, the elbow is rested completely in a sling until pain is gone and the X-ray film becomes negative. Subsequent mobilization should be done gradually.

Ulnar Palsy

The ulnar nerve is often damaged in elbow injuries. Complete paralysis with clawing, paralysis of the interossei and lumbricals, and sensory loss are obviously present. Slight tingling in the little and ring fingers or a little weakness in the intrinsic muscles must be examined carefully if injury to the ulnar nerve is suspected. Motor weakness may also appear slowly.

Some limitation of extension movement is inevitable after fractures of the elbow. If no improvement is seen at three weekly intervals, then further rehabilitation may not likely increase the range of movement, but time and normal use will benefit the patient up to 20 degrees of movement over a period of six months.

CHAPTER 16

FRACTURE OF THE SHAFTS OF THE RADIUS AND ULNA

Fractures of the forearm are difficult to treat because any malunion or overlap of fragments results in the loss of pronation and supination and produces disability. If only one bone is broken and fragments are angulated or overlapping, the upper or the lower radioulnar joint will be dislocated.

Non-union with closed treatment is about 6%. It is a fact that if open reduction and plating are done in the second or third week, the union rate is much improved. This differs in cases where the granulation tissue and early callus formation by closed reduction or operation may delay the healing of the fracture.

Indications for closed manipulation:
1. youthful age of the patient (a small degree of malunion is acceptable in very young patients as with growth this may disappear)
2. greenstick fractures
3. fractures with angulation of 10–15 degree but no overlap
4. transverse fractures with overlap

Indications for open reduction:
1. failure of closed reduction
2. redisplacement after successful closed manipulation
3. unstable fractures due to comminution or obliquity of the fracture line
4. unstable open fractures

When open reduction is carried out, internal fixation should be used unless the fracture line is transverse and the fragments can be locked solidly in place. Except in open fractures, cancellous bone can be packed around the bone ends in case of non-union.

Technique of Closed Reduction

It is important to ascertain the rotational position of the proximal fragment of the radius.

An anteroposterior radiograph of the forearm of the injured limb is compared with films of the normal forearm taken in neutral rotation of 30 degrees and 60 degrees of supination. By comparing the position of the bicipital tuberosity on the films, an estimate of the degree of displacement of the injured side can be made. The tuberosity is prominent on the ulnar side in full supination and becomes smaller with rotation till it appears laterally in full pronation. With patient fully anaesthetized, the elbow is flexed to right angle, and counter-traction is applied on the humerus. Traction is applied to the hand, and the forearm is rotated into the predetermined position. Steady powerful traction is maintained for three to six minutes to allow the muscle spasm to disappear, and then pressure is applied to the front and back of the forearm over the fracture site. The traction is gently relaxed. The bones are tested for telescoping, and radiograph is taken. If necessary, manipulation may be repeated. Sometimes transverse fracture can be reduced by flexing the limb at the fracture site and levering the distal fragment on to the end of the proximal fragment, but it should be done with great care.

If radiograph shows a satisfactory position, the forearm is immobilized in a padded plaster cast from the knuckles to the axilla, traction being maintained during the application of the plaster. During the setting of plaster, light pressure is applied with the hand on the front and back of the forearm at the fracture site. A cuff-and-collar sling should be given. The plaster should be changed to a lighter one after three weeks. Radiograph should also be taken to confirm the position of reduction.

Open Reduction and Internal Fixation

Fracture of the radius and ulna should be explored through two separate incisions to lessen the chances of cross-union. A rigid fixation of six-hole plate and screws is recommended. Intramedullary nails can be used, but they usually do not provide rigid fixation and may require external support of plaster cast. Sometimes an intramedullary nail may produce splinters of the bone due to its large size and narrow cavity of the ulna and radius.

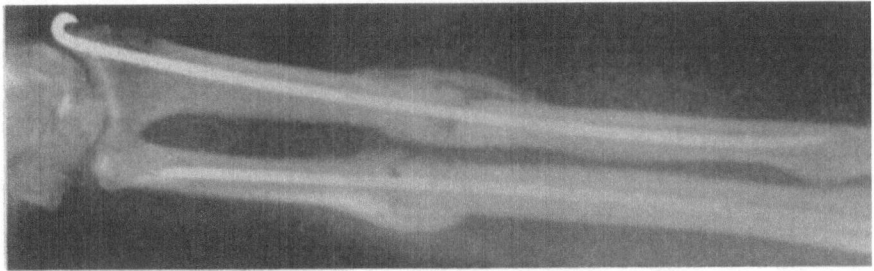

Fig. 35: Fracture of the forearm treated by rush pins.

Fractures of Both Bones Near the Lower End

A fall on outstretched hand in a child may result in a fracture of both bones of the forearm about 2 in. above the wrist joint with the distal fragments angulated backwards.

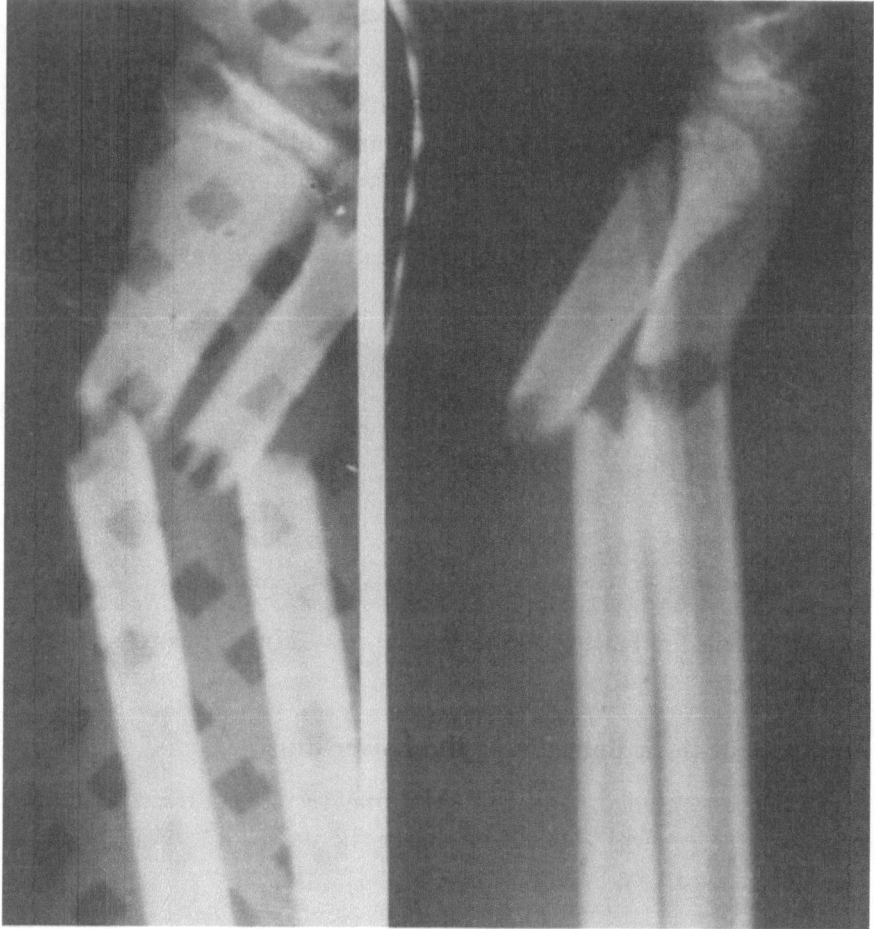

Fig. 36: Fracture of both bones of the forearm (radius and ulna) in a child.

Even when the bones are overlapped, it is possible to reduce the deformity by closed manipulation and should be immobilized in a long-arm plaster cast.

Isolated Fracture of the Lower Shaft of the Radius

Fracture of the lower shaft of the radius is usually displaced, and the fracture line is oblique or transverse. Closed reduction may not be successful; therefore, open reduction and internal fixation may be required.

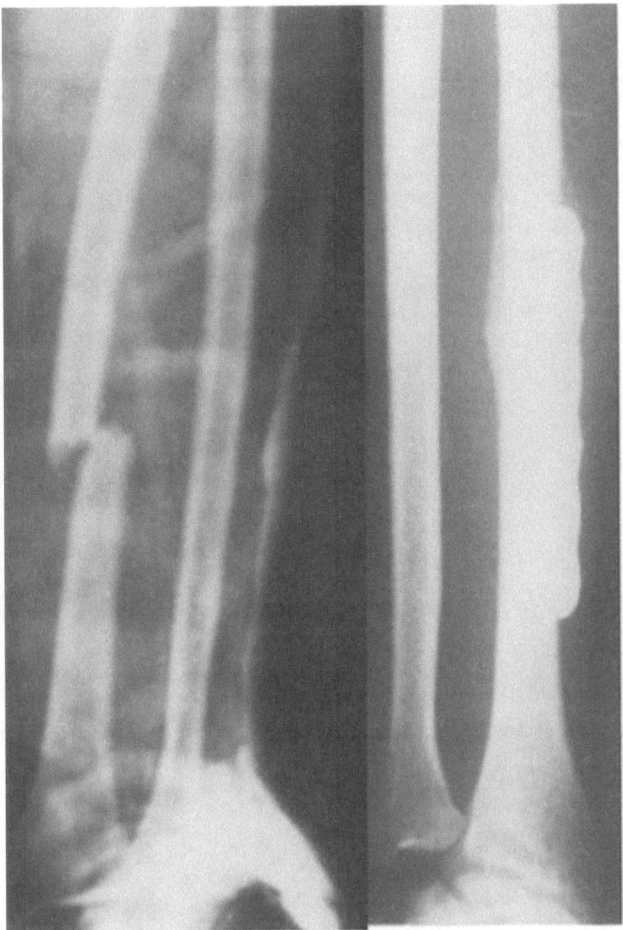

Fig. 37: Fracture of the forearm (radius) treated by fixation of plate and screws.

Fracture of the Upper Ulnar Shaft with Dislocation of the Head of the Radius (Monteggia Fracture)

The ulna is fractured near the junction of the upper and middle one-thirds and produces angulation. The radius remains parallel to the distal fragment of the ulna due to the attachment of interosseous membrane. As the ulna angulates, the radial head is thrown out of the joint at the elbow, tearing the orbicular ligament of the superior radioulnar joint.

There are two types of Monteggia fractures.

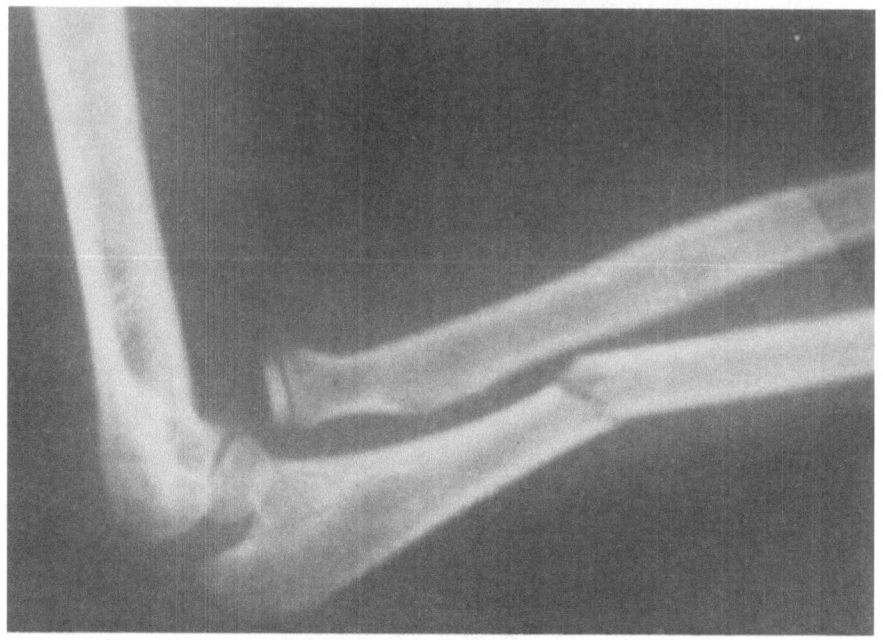

Fig. 38a: Monteggia fracture–dislocation (extension type).

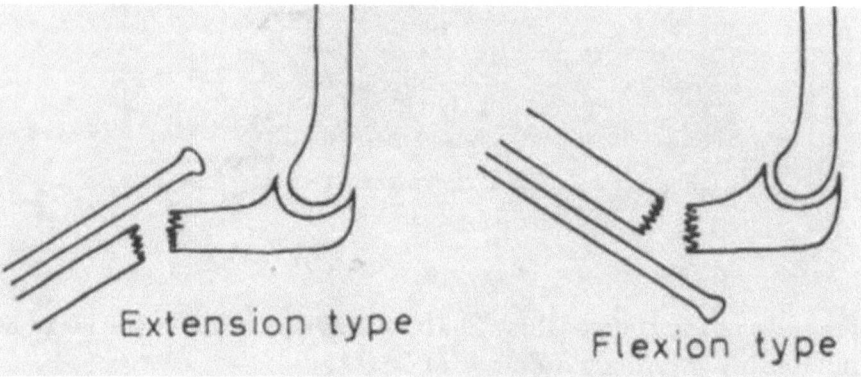

Fig. 38b: Monteggia fracture–dislocation (extension and flexion type).

Extension Type	Flexion Type
1. It occurs in 90% of the cases.	1. It occurs in 10% of the cases.
2. Ulna is angulated forwards.	2. Ulna is angulated backwards.
3. Radial head is displaced forwards.	3. Radial head is displaced backwards.
4. After reduction, it is treated in flexion position.	4. After reduction, it is treated in extension position.

Treatment

In vast majority of cases, if the alignment of the ulna is corrected, the head of the radius reduces itself.

Extension Type

Extension type can be reduced by flexion of the elbow and pressure of the hand over the front of the radial head. The reduction may not be stable and may result in incomplete reduction or redisplacement. Hence, early open reduction and internal fixation of the ulna by an intramedullary nail or plate and screws is recommended. The head of the radius may reduce itself or may require open reduction and replacement. The arm is then kept in a plaster cast for six weeks with elbow at right angle.

Flexion Type

Flexion type can usually be reduced easily by extension of the elbow, and in this position, fracture of the ulna and dislocation of the head of the radius is reduced and remains stable. A padded plaster cast can be applied from mid arm to knuckles in full extension and maintained for six weeks; however, it is better to perform open reduction. The ulna fracture can be fixed by an intramedullary nail or plate and screws. The dislocation of the head of the radius may reduce itself or may require open reduction because the orbicular ligament after rupture falls back into the cavity of the ulna and will not allow the head of the radius to be reduced. The open reduction of the head of the radius should be done through separate incision.

After surgery, the elbow should be kept at right angle in a plaster cast for six weeks.

Risk of Myositis Ossificans

New bone formation may occur around the radial head and may cause limitation of movements of the elbow joint. This will happen if the radial head is not reduced into its place and repeated manipulations are carried out for recurring displacement. In such cases, early open reduction and fixation of the ulna with reduction of the head of the radius is much safer than repeated closed manipulations.

If the mass of bone formation blocks the movements, it is better to wait for six to nine months when the bone mass becomes mature for complete excision. Early excision will allow the bone to form again and cause permanent limitation of movements of the elbow joint.

Persistent Dislocation of the Head of the Radius

If the ulna has united in malalignment and radial head remains displaced, the functional recovery may not be bad, but gross disfigurement is present. In such cases, early operation may produce greater stiffness and limitation of functions.

If after a year the patient still complains of pain or the displaced head of the radius causes limitation of movements, the head of the radius may be excised in adults, which gives good functional recovery. In children, the operation should be avoided till growth is complete; otherwise, dislocation of lower radioulnar joint will occur.

Rotation Movement

Involvement of the superior or inferior radioulnar joint and malalignment of the bone ends in radius and ulna fracture lead to restricted movements of pronation and supination. Even in fracture of the radius and ulna, stiffness does occur in prolonged mobilization longer than eight weeks and may become permanent if not treated.

Wrist

The most common fracture around the wrist is Colles fracture and fracture of the scaphoid.

Within 14 days after the removal of plaster cast, active exercises will help recover full range of movement, provided that patient has done exercises during the period of immobilization.

If the fracture involves the joint, some stiffness is inevitable. The movements to a stiff joint in osteoarthritis of the wrist joint can easily be restored. Intra-articular injection of steroid once weekly for three weeks is to be considered. A leather support can be worn for it as well. But these methods give temporary relief; permanent relief is obtained by arthrodesis of the wrist joint.

Bennett Fracture–Dislocation

The usual methods of rehabilitation are resistance exercises and games and occupational therapy. These are helpful in recovery of functions after injury, but power returns gradually.

A fibreglass splint can be worn for relieving the pain. The patient can perform most of the duties while wearing splint.

CHAPTER 17

FRACTURES OF THE WRIST AND HAND

Colles Fracture

Colles fracture occurs within 1 in. from the distal articular surface of the radius. The displacement of distal fragment is typical and is called as dinner fork deformity (fork placed on the table in inverted position). The distal fragment is displaced upwards and backwards so that the lower articular surface of the radius, which looks normally downwards, now looks upwards and forwards.

The fracture ranges from a crack, a few cracks, to a shattering, and it also includes fracture separation of the lower epiphysis of the radius.

Treatment

Treatment of Colles fracture is done in two methods:
  i. direct manipulation
  ii. closed reduction.

Direct Manipulation

The fragments are manipulated into position by direct pressure on the distal fragment in relation to the proximal fragment after applying traction and counter-traction to the forearm. Sometimes it is successful, but often it fails.

Closed Reduction

Closed reduction involves four steps:
  a. exaggeration of the deformity by pushing the distal fragment upwards
  b. disimpaction of the fragments

c. reduction of the fragments by pulling down

d. Past reduction position the wrist and hand are held in flexed position and hand is held in adduction position in plaster cast.

The plaster cast is applied in this position after padding it. The plaster cast should initially be applied above the elbow for three weeks, and it can be changed to below-elbow cast for further three weeks.

The objection to this method of treatment is that it may injure the median nerve, but in practice, it has been seen not to occur.

Badly comminuted fracture can be overcorrected. Hence, precaution is necessary not to apply too much force in such cases.

Displaced epiphyses are the easiest of all fractures to reduce, and occasional slight imperfection is corrected in the remodelling process.

General anaesthesia is most often used, but local or regional anaesthesia can be employed satisfactorily.

Splintage in the form of posterior plaster slab can be used when there is a marked swelling or a wound is present over it. However, best grip is provided by a well-padded, deeply moulded, complete plaster.

Local swelling is accommodated by the uncompressed wool at the sides. If fingers do swell, it is not enough to split the plaster; the wrist should be radiographed because one cause of swelling is displacement at the fracture site.

The wrist should be X-rayed at the end of a week of manipulation, and if the fracture is still in good position, nothing more is required to be done. A carefully applied moulded, padded plaster cast can retrain the fragments in position for three weeks. By then, fracture fragments may show some union taking place, and an unpadded plaster cast can be applied for further three weeks. Repeated manipulation should be avoided, but if displacement recurs after one week, then treatment should be started all over again.

Complications of Colles Fracture

Open fracture: This fracture occurs sometimes due to the eruption of the head of the ulna through the skin, which may have to be cut to allow the bone to return to its place. Such fracture, when treated in a routine manner, does well.

i. Malunion: When deformity is completely uncorrected, the fracture soon becomes firm. A deformed wrist is not usually much of a handicap, provided that it is not stiff. In young persons, deformity can be corrected by operation, doing osteotomy and pin fixation, added with padded plaster cast. In some cases, the head of the ulna should be removed for the sake of good appearance or if it is blocking the movement. An inch or so should be taken out with its periosteum. The operation is worthwhile, but it is often not required. It takes three to six months for functional recovery.

ii. Median nerve neuritis: Complaints of cramp, tingling sensation, numbness, and stiffness occur frequently from the compression of the median nerve, but usually, the patient recovers completely. Seldom will it require decompression for carpal tunnel syndrome.

iii. Rupture of the tendon of the extensor pollicis longus: Rupture may occur weeks or months after a fracture, which is usually a mild one or a crack near the distal tubercle of the radius. It should be sutured back, and results are good.

iv. Sudeck's atrophy: This is also called disuse atrophy. It is accompanied by painful stiffness of the wrist and fingers following the injury and is frequently accompanied by shiny redness of the skin and patchy moth-eaten rarefaction of the bones of the wrist and hand. It is a very painful condition and causes a lot of psychological suffering. It requires prolonged treatment with analgesic and support for the wrist and hand. Physiotherapy and firmness usually succeed. The patient should be encouraged to do active exercise of the whole upper limb with maximum movements of the wrist, hand, and fingers by fully flexing, extending, and spreading the joints. The success of the treatment depends on the patient's manners and expression, which may justify psychiatric treatment to achieve success.

Smith's Fracture

Smith's fracture is of three types (fig. 39):
   i. juxta-articular
   ii. trans-articular without subluxation
   iii. trans-articular with subluxation

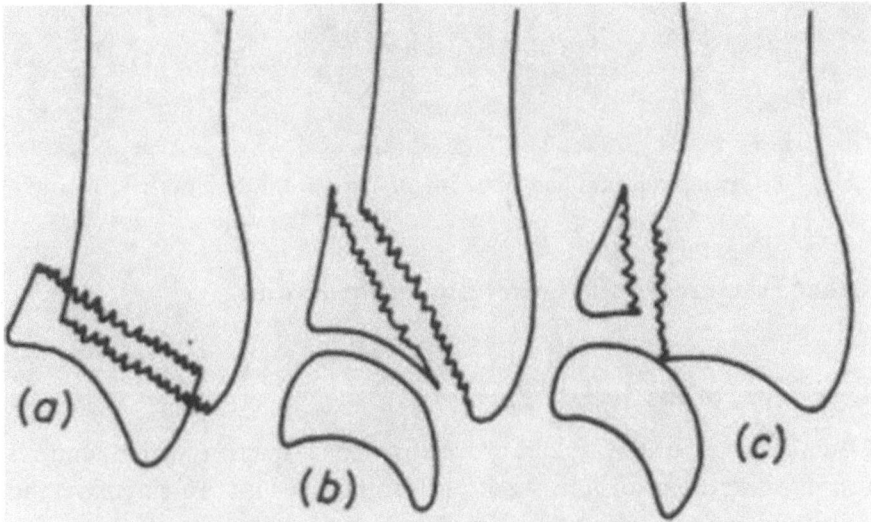

Fig. 39: Smith's fracture patterns: (a) juxta-articular, (b) trans-articular without subluxation, (c) trans-articular with subluxation.

The juxta-auricular and trans-articular fracture without subluxation can be adequately reduced and held by a padded plaster cast extending from the wrist to above-elbow position with forearm held in fully supinated position for six to eight weeks.

Trans-articular fracture with subluxation is more difficult to treat by closed reduction. It should be treated by open reduction and screw fixation (fig. 40).

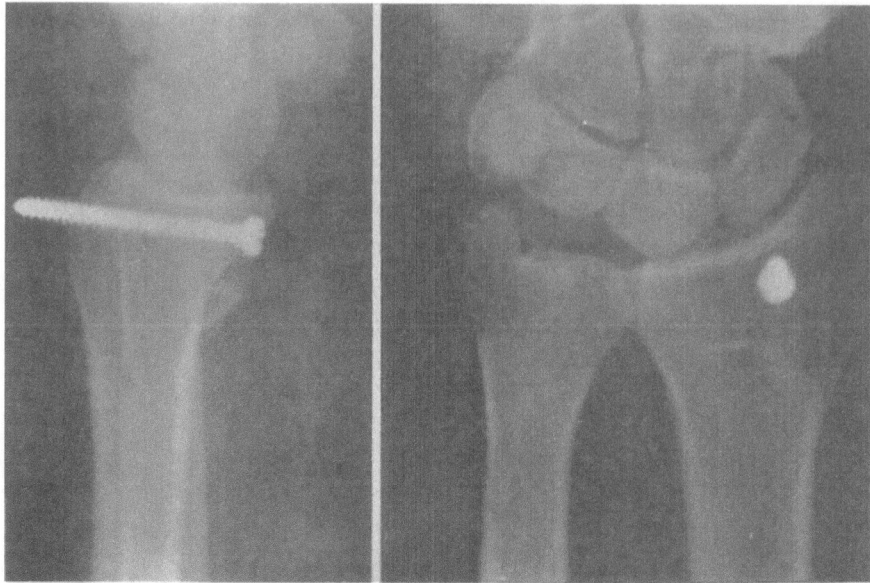

Fig. 40: Open reduction and screwing of a comminuted Smith's fracture.

Other Fractures of the Lower End of the Radius

1. Fracture of the Styloid Process

Often, fracture of the styloid process is a crack fracture which requires rest in plaster slab for four weeks, but sometimes it is an extensive and disruptive fracture which requires operative treatment to restore stability of the radiocarpal joint.

2. Fracture of the Head of the Radius

A fall on the hand may be sufficient to displace the radius upwards. This injury can cause the head of the radius to be broken into many pieces or shattered and scattered.

If there is a crack fracture of the head of the radius, rest in plaster cast for four to six weeks is required. If there is displacement of the head of the radius, it can be reduced by operation. In comminuted fracture, the head of the radius can be excised. Afterwards, the recovery of function is good.

3. Dislocation of the Lower End of the Ulna

The wrist is painful, and the hand cannot be turned due to displaced head of the ulna, which can go either backwards or forwards.

Reduction is usually easy and stable in closely fitting plaster cast, which is worn for four to six weeks. If the injury is recognized late or if it recurs after reduction, the head of the ulna should be removed.

Minor Fracture of the Carpus

The most frequent fracture is chip fracture of the marginal component of the radiocarpal joint. The distal row is less often affected.

Major Fracture of the Scaphoid

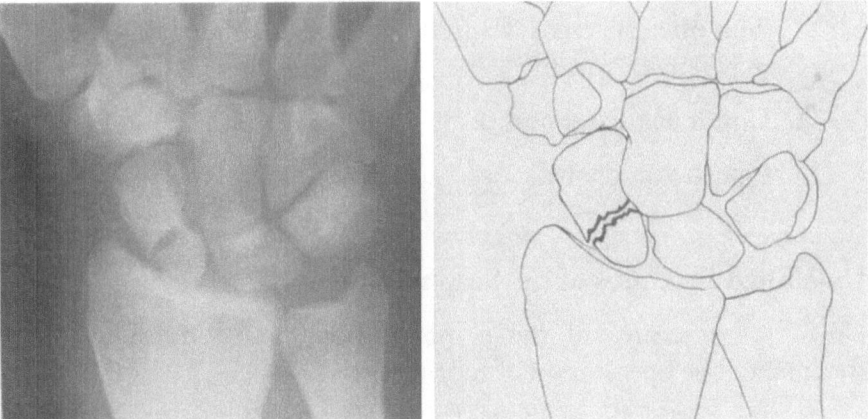

Fig. 41: Fracture of the scaphoid.

Fracture of the middle part of the scaphoid is very common. Less often, the distal position of scaphoid may show a fracture.

Majority of these fractures, if given prompt treatment, will unite. Bad result are obtained frequently due to inadequate or too much interference in the treatment.

It is necessary to apply a well-moulded padded plaster cast, which should include the bunch as well. The plaster should be kept for 8–10 weeks. After 3–4 weeks, the plaster cast can be changed to a lighter plaster cast.

Treatment

It is necessary to apply well-moulded padded plaster cast, which should include the thumb as well. The plaster should be kept for 8–10 weeks. After 3–4 weeks, the plaster cast can be changed to a lighter plaster cast. The fracture of the distal pole of the scaphoid unites quickly. This prolonged treatment is required for middle portion of the scaphoid.

Since the plaster cast immobilization will cause stiffness of wrist joint, the patient should be encouraged to actively perform exercises and movements of the wrist joint. If the wrist is stiff, weak, and painful after three to four months, one of the three courses may be applied:

i. The patient should be given assisted exercises with a bandage. This often succeeds when the fracture has united, but the wrist may remain painful.

ii. Continue the support using a removable splint.

iii. Operate on the wrist, and do arthrodesis.

Un-United Fractures of the Scaphoid Bone

Un-united fractures of the scaphoid bone will require operative treatment. The operation is of four types:

i. Removing spurs—this is worthwhile if it is blocking the movements and is painful.

Removing one or both parts of the scaphoid—this seems reasonable to do if there is local and painful arthritis. However, such operations are not often recommended.

Removing the scaphoid and lunate bones—it is carried out when there is early arthritis at the fractures site. However, success depends on removing the bones as a whole while not damaging the adjacent bones and joints.

ii. Bone grafts—these are likely to succeed when the two fragments are healthy and the wrist is weak but free from arthritis. Cancellous or cortical peg is inserted across the main body of the scaphoid bone. Sometimes a screw fixation can be carried out, and it works well. It is worth noting that sometimes spontaneous healing takes place within 6–12 months; hence, operation can be delayed.

iii. Arthrodesis of the wrist—this is indicated when there is little and painful movements of the wrist joint.

iv. Fascial arthroplasty—this is done by turning a flap of the fascia into the fracture site, giving a useful wrist for a year; however, long-term results are not successful.

Fracture of Other Carpal Bones

Fractures of the other carpal bones are uncommon. Only a degenerating condition of the lunate bone can be seen. It may require excision of the lunate bone to relieve the pain and give good movements of the wrist joint.

Dislocations of the Carpus and Related Fractures

1. Dislocation of the Lunate Bone

Usually, the lunate bone is dislocated and tilted forwards. This is best seen and visible in lateral radiograph.

The dislocated lunate bone can be reduced by prolonged traction, pushing the bone back into place while keeping the traction on the hand and gently extending the wrist from full flexion. If it does not reduce itself, operation may be required to reduce it.

2. Fracture–Dislocation of the Proximal Row of the Carpus

The typical injury separates the rest of the carpus from the lunate and half of the scaphoid which remains on the radius.

The displacement can often be reduced by pulling hard on the hand and applying pressure and counter-pressure. While doing this, the wrist can be moved medially or laterally at the same time to reduce the displacement. Operation is sometimes necessary to reduce the displacement. If there is a displacement of half of the scaphoid, it can be reduced and fixed by a screw.

3. Carpometacarpal Dislocation

Carpometacarpal dislocation is an uncommon injury. It often occurs in motorcyclists. After a fall, the carpus is driven forwards off the hand, or the hand is driven backwards off the carpus. The hand looks short, the wrist is thick from the back to front, and the fingers cannot be bent due to pain. There is overshadows of bones in the X-ray film.

Closed reduction can be done by traction, manipulation, and splintage. If closed reduction fails, open reduction with internal fixation by Kirschner wire is required to overcome the instability of the dislocated joint.

The Hand

The hand has got the necessary combination of strength and precision and delicacy of movements which can easily and permanently be upset by trivial injuries.

Classification of Fracture of the Hand

Based on the method of treatment, the fractures of the hand can be classified into three groups:

    i. where no splintage is required

    ii. where external splintage is required

    iii. where operation is required.

Signs of injury and swelling are present. The swelling may mask the injury. Radiography must always be repeated after manipulation of a fracture or dislocation.

Fractures Not Needing Splintage

Fractures that do not need splintage include nearly all the simple cracks and some fractures without deformity.

A finger that has suffered a sprain or a sprain with fracture can be protected from further injury by attaching it to its neighbour by a turn of strapping or small elastic garter. The thumb may need a light plaster cast.

Displaced fractures in the fingers need to be reduced and splinted. The brawl injuries of first and fifth metacarpal should also be corrected and splinted. However, simple crack fractures of the metacarpal need simple bandage.

Fractures Needing Closed Reduction and Splintage

Fractures that need closed reduction and splintage are mostly slightly displaced fractures of the phalanges and metacarpals. Twists, bends, and shortening can be overcome by traction in flexion, and splintage can be applied (fig. 42).

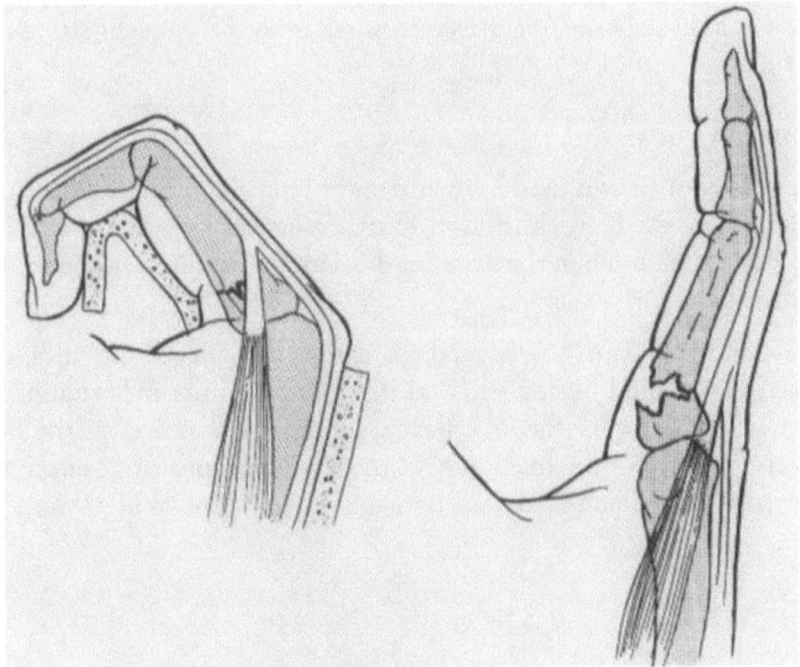

Fig. 42: Fracture of the proximal phalanx of the finger treated by closed reduction and posterior plaster slab.

Method of Splintage

As far as possible, the hand should be available for use. The splint should be easy to apply and adjust, and it should not mask radiological appearance.

Roll and strapping. The finger is manipulated and held down over a roll of bandage or held by narrow elastic strapping. This can be done without anaesthesia, but digital block or local infiltration can help the procedure to be carried out.

When only one finger is splinted, it will point towards the thenar eminence. If more than one finger is splinted, in this way, the fingers lie parallel, but if one of them does not point in the right direction, malunion will result. When more than one finger has to be kept flexed, a spherical pad should be used. An important point is to distribute the flexion evenly between the three joints and not to concentrate on the middle one. It can be done by putting a pad of the right size in the right place.

Malleable metal splints. These are available readymade with padding, as much or as little of the finger, as is required is bound down by strapping.

Plaster of Paris

The plaster of Paris is used in treatment of fractures of the metacarpals. Fractures of the first, third, and fourth metacarpals are not marked, but it is troublesome in the fifth and becomes a handicap in the second metacarpal.

The deformity can be reduced. A carefully padded and moulded plaster cast should be applied, and it does not require inclusion of the corresponding finger for its efficacy. Using the pressure on the bent finger, the head of the metacarpal can be pushed into its position, but sometimes too much force will damage the joint and skin as well (fig. 43).

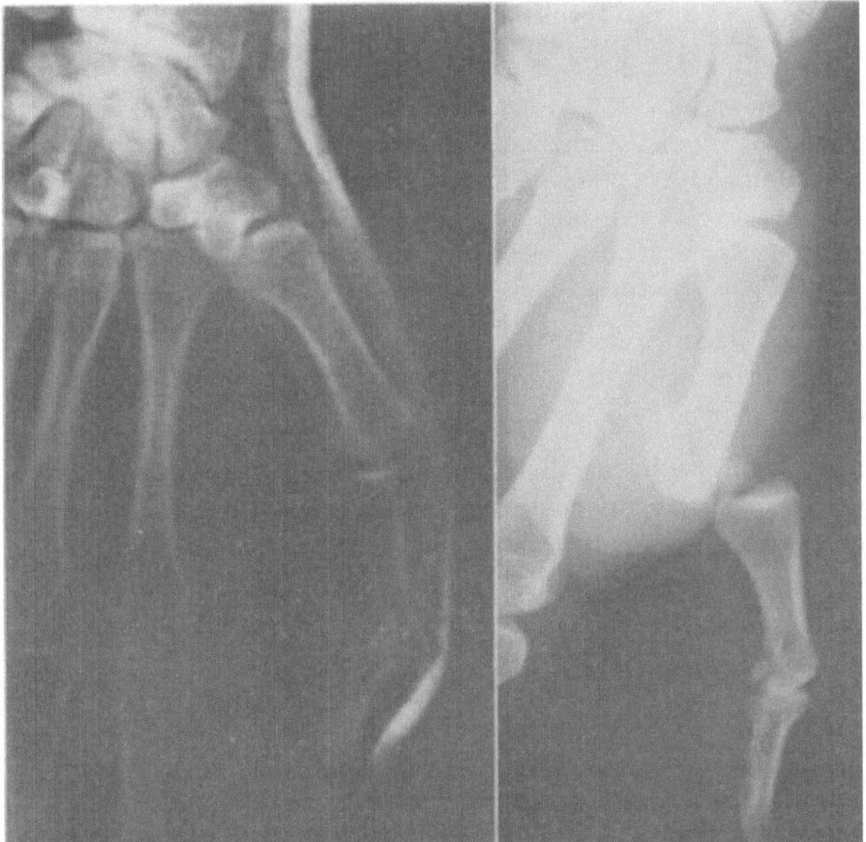

Fig. 43: Dislocation of the metacarpophalangeal joint of the thumb treated by closed reduction and plaster slab.

Fractures of the shafts require immobilization for six to eight weeks to become firm enough, and fractures of the neck of the metacarpal are united in four to six weeks. It is to be noted that pulp traction must be avoided.

Fractures Needing Operation

Open Operation

Fractures that need open operation are mostly intra-articular due to avulsion or being kept apart by soft tissue.

1. Fractures of the Terminal Phalanx

Fractures of the terminal phalanx can cause an awkward unstable fingertip, and if a large distal fragment is separated, it may not unite. Reduction by closed method may be successful, but sometimes open reduction with fixation by a Kirschner wire is required.

2. Avulsion Fractures

Avulsion fractures are best treated by operation. There is often violent injury to the ligaments. If these are repaired, they work well with no effect if the bone piece is replaced or removed.

The fracture with wide displacement and inversion of fragment at the metacarpophalangeal joint of the thumb must be corrected completely; otherwise, it will produce a disabling result.

Fractures caused by avulsion of the corresponding tendons can be repaired easily. The torn middle slip of the extensor tendon can be repaired successfully in a fresh case, but when deformity has appeared, it may not be successful. If the fragment gives trouble as a painful lump or a block to movement of fingers, it should be removed.

The mallet finger can be repaired, but on the whole, it causes less trouble if left alone. Operation is required if the flexion deformity angle is more than 45 degrees.

3. Fractures of the Condyles of the Phalanges

Fractures of the condyles of the phalanges are uncommon injuries. Communition destroys the joint, but sufficient movements can be retained with protected activity from the beginning. The simple fracture, with a small step, can be treated in the same way. If there is much displacement, the fragment should be reduced and held in place by Kirschner wire; however, it is a difficult procedure.

4. Fracture of the Head of a Metacarpal Bone

Fracture of the head of a metacarpal bone is intra-articular, and the fragment always dies and should be removed.

5. Displaced Fractures

Displaced fractures of the shafts of the metacarpal or phalanges can be reduced by operation and fixed with a Kirschner wire (fig. 44).

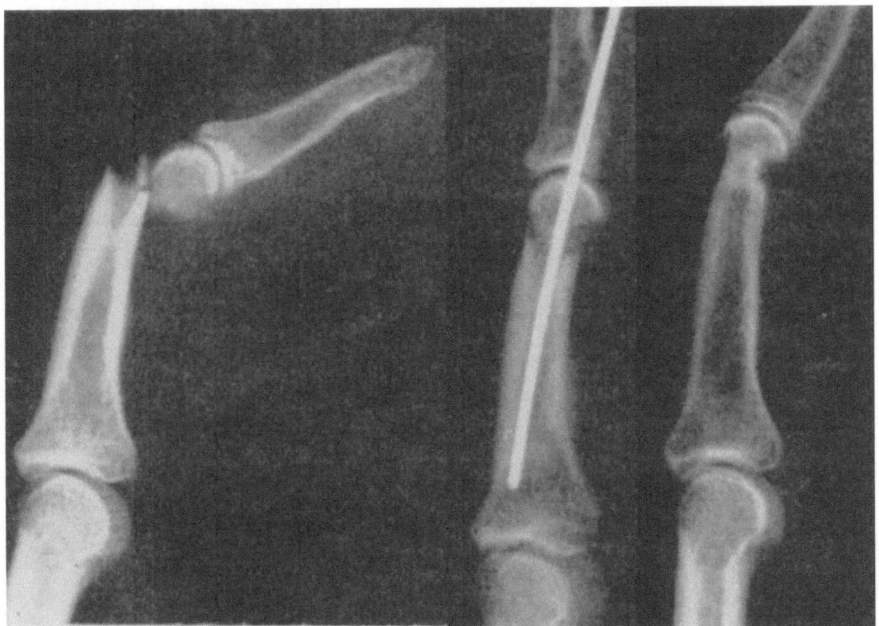

Fig. 44: Fracture of the phalanx treated by Kirschner wire fixation.

6. Bennett Fracture–Dislocation

Bennett fracture–dislocation should be treated by open reduction, and fragment can be screwed from the dorsal aspect.

The screw can be passed from the larger fragment, and it can hold the small fragment as well. If there is a small fragment or comminution, it can be fixed in a reduced position by a Kirschner wire.

7. Open Fractures

The relationship between the skin and bone in the hand is so close that fixation of fractures usually allows the skin to heal with simple sutures or by means of a skin graft.

The shattered joint. This is often treated by formal excision and arthrodesis. Sometimes shortage of skin can be overcome by removing the bone.

Open fracture of the tip. This is usually either a comminuted fracture or a crush injury and may be accompanied by avulsion of the base of the nail.

When it is necessary to amputate a crushed finger, it is always better to save as much as possible, especially all attached bony fragments. The simple fracture is treated by a Kirschner wire. The nail acts as a splint and should be retained even if the rest of the tissue is required to be removed due to sepsis.

CHAPTER 18

FRACTURES AND DISLOCATION OF THE SPINE

The spine has a characteristic feature. Apart from the first two cervical vertebrae and five fused sacral vertebrae, the rest of the vertebrae have got the same pattern, like a body, two transverse processes, and a spinous process with strong muscles and ligaments attachments. In addition to it, there is anterior and posterior synovial joint system. These facts allow a lot of mobility to the spinal column and also influence the type of injury (e.g. the junction of the fixed thoracic spine with the mobile lumbar spine is a common site for injury).

Mechanism of the Injury

The spinal ligaments, like ligaments elsewhere, are constructed to withstand tension and stress. However, a torsional stress placed on the ligament produces a different result, and all ruptured ligaments are caused by a twisting force.

There are many variations in magnitude and direction in which a force can act on a spinal column. However, every spinal injury can be classified into one of the five groups, according to direction in which force acted on the column and subsequently tended to displace the column. The five groups are:

1. flexion
2. extension
3. rotation
4. longitudinal pressure
5. shear.

Besides those, there is a sixth group of injuries which are produced by strong muscle contraction. These injuries are fracture of the bony vertebral processes, such as spinous process and transverse process, which are commonly avulsed by the large muscle attachment to them. They are unimportant injuries and require symptomatic treatment. Although the fractured processes often fail to unite by the bone, the stability of the spine is unimpaired, and the function is also not affected.

Pathological Anatomy

Each injury has a different pattern to present itself. They are discussed as below:

Flexion Injuries

In a flexion injury, the anterior portion of the body of the vertebra is compressed together, and the spinous processes are separated. Since no ligament is ruptured, and the posterior ligament remains intact, the force is spent on the front of vertebral body, which is crushed and forced into the shape of a wedge (see fig. 45).

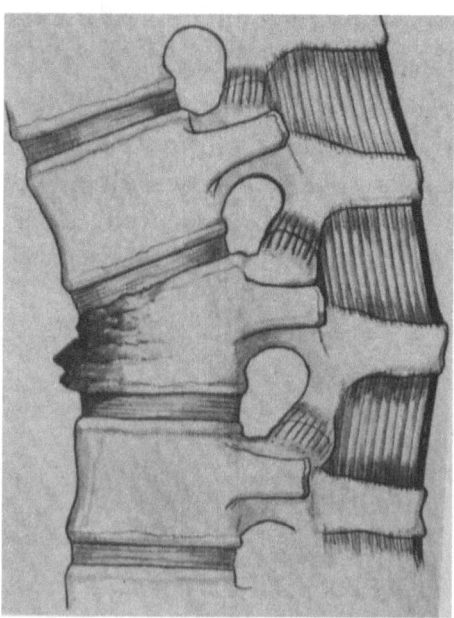

Fig. 45: Wedge fracture of the vertebra.

Extension Injuries

Extension injuries occur most commonly in the cervical region. In this injury, the vertebral arch, particularly the facets and pedicles, is compressed and sometimes fractured in older persons. A mild extension may not cause fracture but may damage the spinal cord. The cord damage is due to infolding of the ligamentum flavum or the posterior longitudinal ligament. Such injuries are undisplaced and stable.

Rotation

A rotational force of sufficient strength applied to the spine will rupture the spinal ligaments. If combined with flexion, the posterior ligaments will rupture, and if combined with extension, anterior ligaments will rupture. By far, the most common is the flexion–rotation injury (fig. 46).

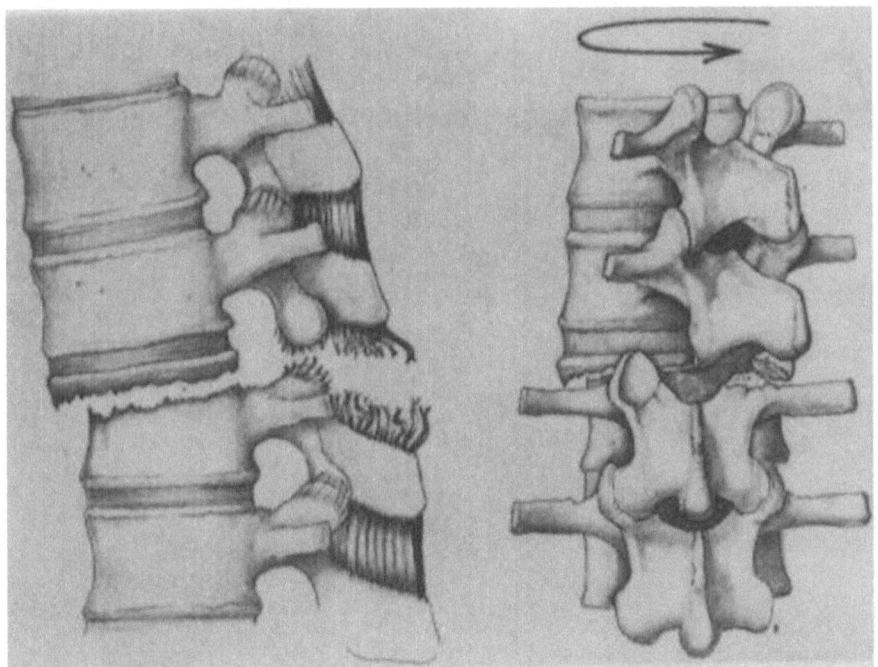

Fig. 46: Flexion–rotation type of fracture–dislocation at the dorso-lumbar junction.

The result of flexion–rotation injury depends on the level of the spine affected. In the cervical spine, it will cause simple dislocation as the upper vertebra moves forwards and sidewards. In lumbar and dorso-lumbar junction, it results to a fracture of one or both pairs. At times, the associated flexion force may result in fracture–dislocation. Both these rotational injuries are grossly unstable and very commonly produce damage to the spinal cord and nerve roots.

Longitudinal Violence

Longitudinal force can act only on those regions of the spine which can be held straight—that is, the cervical and lumbar spines.

Both cervical and lumbar spines become straight when the normal lordotic curves are slightly flexed. The longitudinal pressure, at first, forces out the blood from the cancellous vertebral body, but if the pressure is great enough, the end plate fractures and the vertebral body is disrupted. This is called burst fracture. Since ligaments are not broken, the fracture is a stable one (fig. 47).

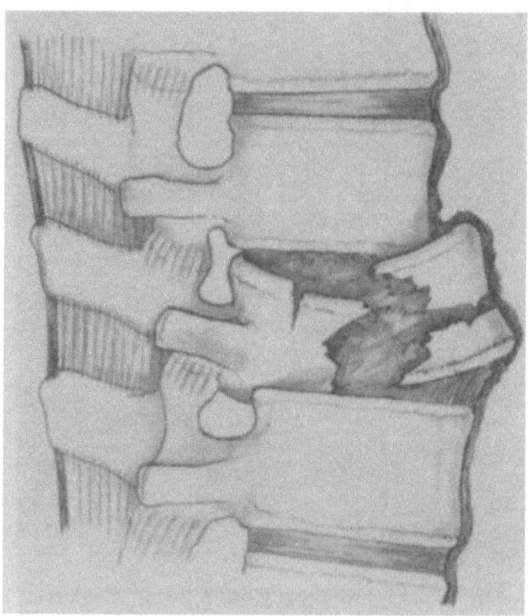

Fig. 47: The burst fracture.

These fractures are associated with spinal cord damage (in the cervical spine) or root damage (in the lumbar spine) as the fragments of the vertebral body are thrust backwards into the spinal canal.

Shearing Violence

Shearing violence is most often seen in the dorsal spine. The ribcage holds this area rather rigidly, and a force is applied directly to one area of the dorsal spine, shears of the upper segment of the dorsal spine of the lower. Not only is one vertebral body sheared forwards off the one below, but the posterior bony elements are also fractured (fig. 48).

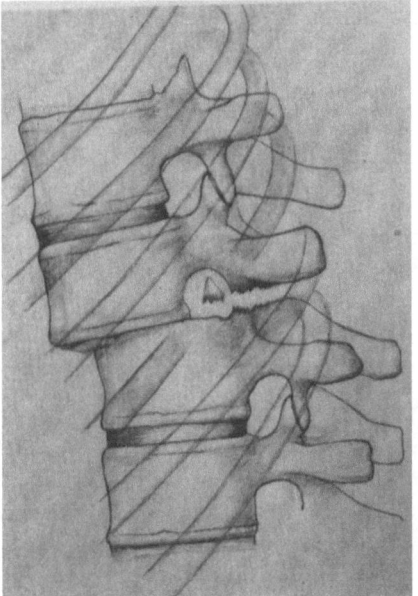

Fig. 48: Thoracic shearing fracture.

Such fracture–dislocations are frequently associated with complete paraplegia, although theoretically unstable, in that anterior and posterior spinal pillars are disrupted; in practice, the ribcage holds the displaced vertebrae firmly in position, and further displacement will not occur.

It must be noted that posterior group of ligaments are key factors in the various injuries. The supraspinous and interspinous ligaments are the only spinal ligaments directly palpable. They are torn, like ligaments elsewhere, by torsion violence, and the gap produced by their rupture is easily felt. If rupture of these ligaments is associated with fracture or dislocation of the vertebral bodies, then the injury is a unstable one.

Spinal injuries can be classified into two groups, the stable and the unstable. In general, a stable injury has got intact posterior ligaments; hence, it only requires symptomatic treatment. An unstable injury has got ruptured posterior ligaments; therefore, it first requires reduction (if displacement is present) and then immobilization.

Classification

Fracture	Force	Area of Spine
A. Stable		
Force	Fracture	Area of Spine
wedge	flexion	thoracic
burst	vertical compression	cervical, lumbar
fracture–dislocation	shearing	thoracic (stabilized by ribcage)
B. Unstable		
Force	Fracture	Area of Spine
Flexion-rotation	Dislocation	Cervical (rarely lumbar)
fracture–dislocation	flexion–rotation	dorso-lumbar junction and lumbar spine
extension–rotation	fracture–dislocation	Dosso-lumbar junction and lumbar spine
Extension-rotation	fracture–dislocation	Cervical

Clinical Diagnosis

1. Inspection

Inspection of the back and head may reveal abrasion or bruising, indicating the site of the application of force. The mechanism of the spinal injury can then be deducted. For example, abrasions on the top of the head are often associated with fractures of the cervical spine. Abrasion over one scapula suggests a twisting force on the trunk and is common in rotational fracture–dislocation of dorso-lumbar junction.

2. Palpation

Palpation of the spine is of utmost importance. The gap left by the rupture of ligaments can be easily felt and is certain evidence of an unstable injury. If the displacement of the bodies of the vertebrae is gross, a marked step may be palpable between one spinous process and the next.

3. Radiological Diagnosis

Good-quality anteroposterior and lateral X-rays are the minimal requirement. In addition, the right and left oblique views in the cervical region are essential for accurate assessment of the position of the posterior articulations. Oblique views often provide help in dorso-lumbar injuries.

The lower cervical and upper dorsal vertebrae are difficult to X-ray. The lower cervical spine may be X-rayed while the head is steadied. Traction is made on the arms to pull the shoulder downwards. In the upper dorsal injuries, lateral views may be clearer if the 'crawl' swimming position is adopted—one arm elevated above the head and the other placed along the body.

Indications for Treatment

The aim of the treatment of fractures and dislocations of the vertebrae is to produce a stable painless spine. It is a fact that ultimate stability is more important than restoration of the anatomical position. Reduction of uncomplicated spinal injuries is only necessary if it will produce stability between damaged fragments. There is not the slightest need to reduce stable, uncomplicated fractures. If the bony injury is complicated by the damage to the spinal cord and the nerve root and clinical examination suggests that recovery is possible (that is, the nerve damage is not complete and irreparable), reduction is indicated to relieve pressure on these structures.

If the cord injury is complete and irrecoverable, reduction is necessary only if the displacement of the bones is gross and likely to interfere with subsequent rehabilitation.

Indications for Immobilization

Immobilization is not always necessary. However, immobilization may be required to control pain. This rule applies even to stable fractures.

In unstable fractures, immobilization is necessary. It is necessary to do so if the injury has caused fracture of the bodies of the vertebrae. In fracture–dislocation, immobilization is very necessary, and sometimes internal fixation may be required to produce stability of spine.

Treatment of Individual Injuries
1. Stable Injuries

Wedge Fracture

Wedge fractures are stable fractures and require neither reduction nor immobilization because they are usually uncomplicated. Symptomatic treatment by bed rest until pain subsides is all that is required. However, the fracture can be reduced if necessary or desired to do so. The method of reduction is known as two-table method.

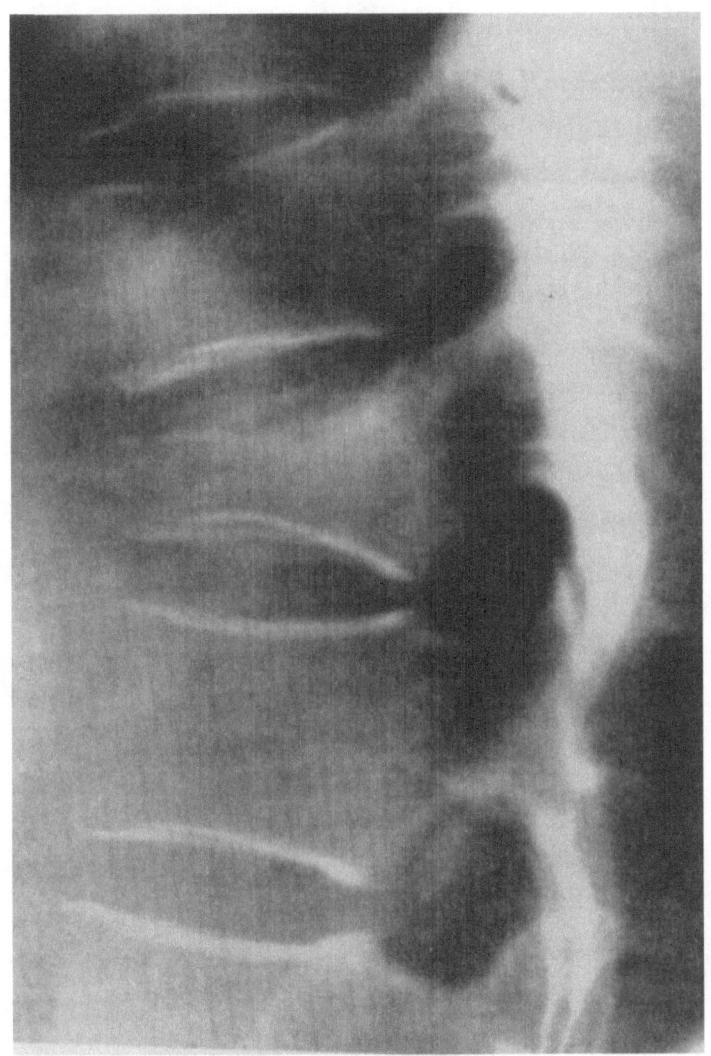

Fig. 49: Wedge fracture.

Two-Table Method

Two operation tables are used for it. One table is 18 in. high, and the second is 12 in. high. The patient lies down on it with face down. The head, neck, and arms of the patient rest on the higher 18 in. table while the thighs and legs rest on the lower 12 in. table.

The body of the patient hangs free between the two tables. By this method, the wedge of the fractures of body of vertebra is corrected. Since the ligaments of the spinal column remain intact, sometimes little pressure can be applied over the prominent spinous process of the vertebral body to reduce and correct the deformity. This method is often successful to reduce the fracture. Afterwards, a plaster of Paris jacket can be applied for immobilization, which remains for 10–12 weeks. The patient is allowed to move about after four days' rest, when the pain has subsided (see fig. 50).

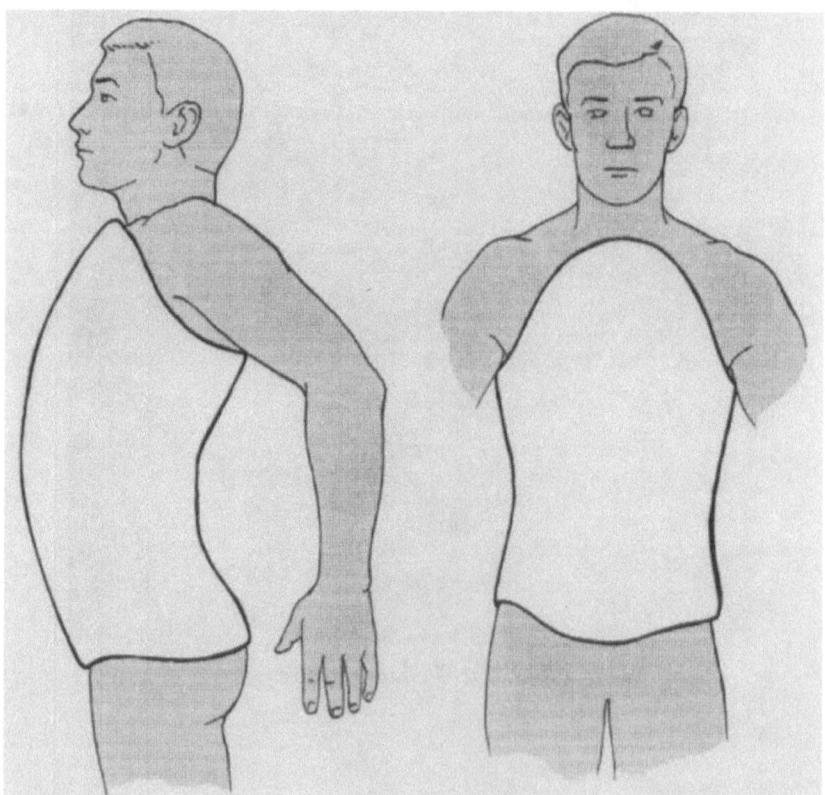

Fig. 50: Plaster jacket applied for spinal fracture for immobilization.

Vertebral Burst Fractures

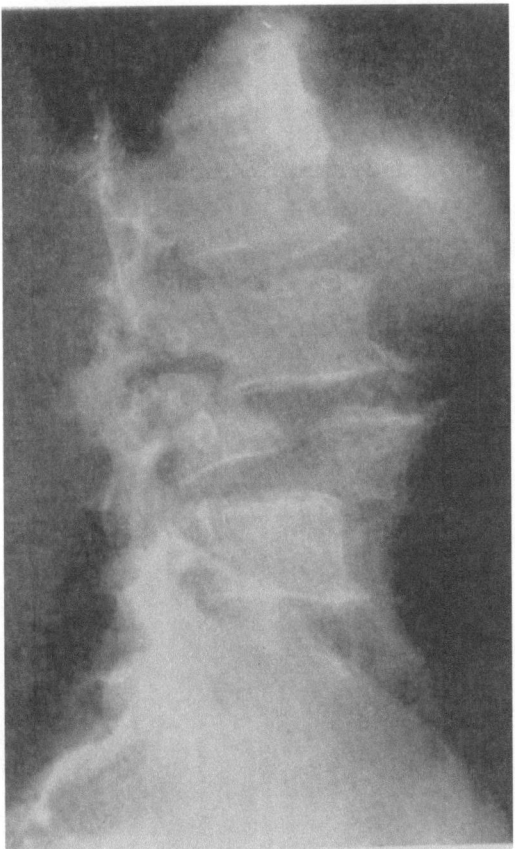

Fig. 51: Burst fracture of the lumbar spine.

The comminution of vertebral body causes great pain, and immobilization of the fracture is necessary. In lumbar spine, a plaster of Paris jacket is given, which remains for three months, when the fracture is completely united.

In the cervical spine, traction through skull callipers is the simplest way of relieving the discomfort. This will also decrease spreading of bony fragments.

It is worth remembering that the plaster cast (Minerva jacket) for cervical injury is a very cumbersome method because it extends from the head, neck, both shoulders, and spine to rest on the hip bones. It is a fact that not many patients can tolerate it, and they do not like to have it. The cervical traction results to a bony union and stable painless spine.

Thoracic Shearing Fractures

In thoracic shearing fractures, the displacement of the fragments occurs, but the ribcage firmly holds these fracture–dislocations in the displaced position; therefore, no treatment, whether closed or open reduction, is required. A plaster of Paris jacket for 10 to 12 weeks is to be given to help relieve the pain and allow the fracture–dislocation to unite in its position.

2. Unstable Injuries

Pure Dislocation

Pure dislocation commonly occurs in the cervical spine (fig. 52).

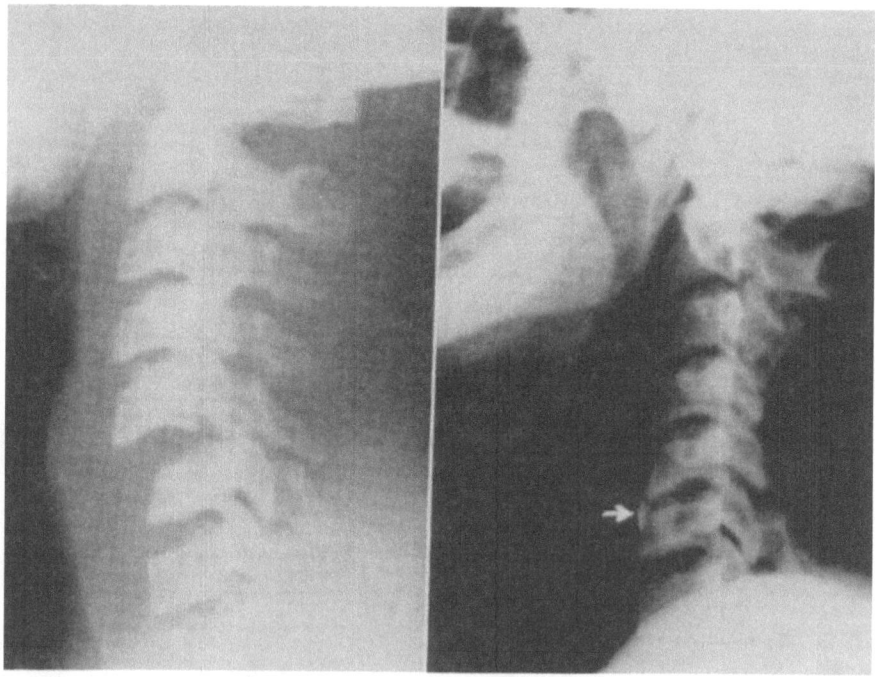

Fig. 52: Cervical dislocation of C5 on C6 is treated by traction with skull callipers.

It is not accompanied with neurological damage. They must be reduced, and it is most easily accomplished by gentle manipulation under general anaesthesia. It is immobilized by traction through skull callipers. The traction is maintained for three weeks. At the end of this period, sometimes bone formation is visible. If it happens, then traction is continued for further three weeks and is then replaced by polythene collar, which is worn for further two to three months until the vertebral body fusion takes place and dislocation becomes stable.

Rarely, dislocation may occur in the lumbar spine. This dislocation needs open reduction. Reduction, immobilization by using a metal clamp or plates across the spinous processes, and ultimately, a cancellous bone grafting may be required to produce stability of the spine.

Fracture–Dislocation (Flexion–Rotation)

This injury commonly occurs at the dorso-lumbar junction (fig. 53).

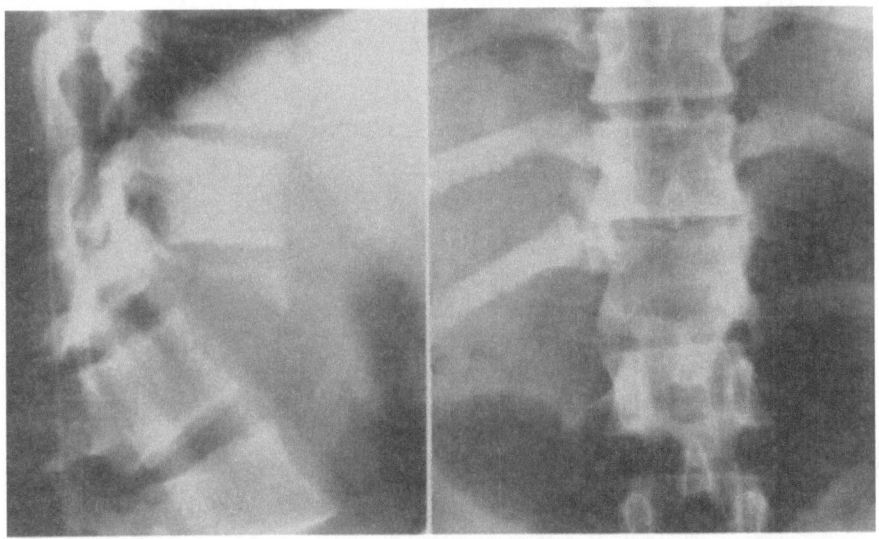

Fig. 53: Fracture–dislocation and dorso-lumbar junction of the spine.

The vast majority of this injury is associated with paraplegia and treatment is dictated by it. Since there is danger of movements at this site and during the nursing care further damage to the spinal cord and nerve roots may occur, the best treatment is open reduction of the dislocation, and fixation by internal metal splints should be carried out. This will help the subsequent nursing and mobilization easy.

If there is no neurological damage, the fracture–dislocation can be reduced by closed method, and the spine is immobilized by plaster jacket for three months until sound healing has taken place.

Fracture–Dislocation (Extension–Rotation)

Extentions–rotation injuries are rare. If they occur, they can be treated by manipulation under anaesthesia and immobilization by traction through skull calliper.

Laminectomy for the Spinal Injuries

Formal decompression by laminectomy is indicated only in partial cord lesion, which shows a worsening of the neurological picture in the first 48 hours.

In partial lesions, an increase in the paralysis may occur after laminectomy. If improvement does occur, it may have taken place without laminectomy because there is no evidence that it has resulted from decompression. However, if there is complete loss of motor and sensory functions below the lesion and if it persists for more than 12 hours after the injury, it is sure evidence that the spinal cord damage is complete and irrecoverable. Decompression in these cases is valueless and should not be done.

CHAPTER 19

FRACTURE OF THE PELVIS

Fractures of the pelvis may be divided into three main groups:
1. disruption of the pelvic ring
2. intra-articular fracture
3. solitary fracture of a pelvic bone.

Disruption of the Pelvic Ring

The commonest fracture is that when the pelvic ring is broken in two places. Often, the ramus of pubis and ramus of ischium are broken on the same side (fig. 54). But as far as the pelvis is concerned, the ring is broken only in one place, so it cannot be called as two fractures of the pelvis.

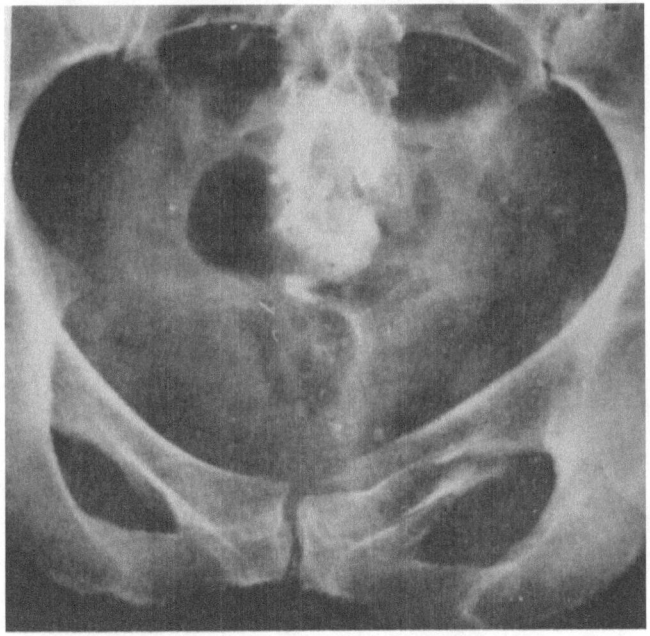

Fig. 54: Fracture of the rami of pubis
and ischium of the pelvis.

A disruption of the pelvic ring implies that there are two breaks with an intervening detached fragment (fig. 54). The detached fragment is displaced by the force of blow, and in the process, the structures within pelvis may be injured. These internal injuries are serious in nature.

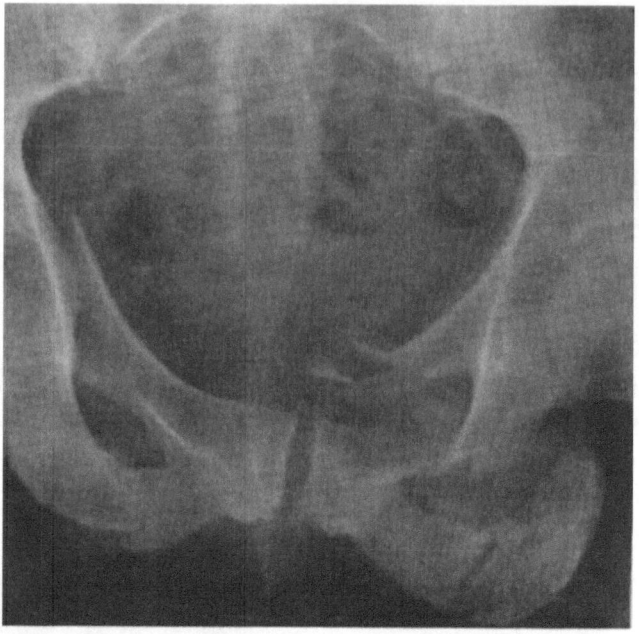

Fig. 55: Disruption of the pelvic ring showing the detached ligament.

Intrapelvic Injuries

Three structures are likely to be injured:

a. a large vessel

b. the urethra

c. the sciatic nerve.

Torn Vessels

Massive haemorrhage is common and accounts for profound shock. Blood transfusion can be given to maintain the blood pressure and overcome the shock. Sometimes a large subperitoneal haematoma may occur which may cause paralytic ileus. It is to be noted that gut is never injured in closed fracture of the pelvis, and in closed fracture of the pelvis, the sacrum is never fractured or displaced.

Rupture of the Urethra

Rupture of the urethra is the most important type of injury which occurs in crush type of disruption and not in the others. Usually, the urethra is torn above the urogenital triangle.

The presence of blood at the meatus is a diagnostic sign, but it may be absent. Precise information can be obtained by a soft catheter. If the catheter passes easily and clear urine is withdrawn, injury to the urethra and bladder can be excluded. When no urine is obtained or when the urine is bloodstained, operation should be done as soon as possible.

Sciatic Nerve Palsy

Sciatic nerve palsy happens only when there is a deep type of disruption of the pelvic ring. The palsy is incomplete and usually recovers.

Skeletal Pelvic Injury

Skeletal pelvic injury occurs due to anteroposterior compression of the pelvis, such as having rolled on by a horse or wheel of a car or having fallen from height.

The fractures are the following:

 i. compression fracture
 ii. hinge separation of the symphysis
 iii. vertical fracture.

Diagnosis

Clinical features are common in all injuries. The patient cannot stand. The patient is in profound shock. There is pain in and around the pelvis, which is aggravated by movements. The patient feels that he is falling to pieces. He cannot lift his legs, but passive gentle movements at the hips are possible. Exact diagnosis can be made only after radiographs have been taken.

Compression Fracture

Compression fracture occurs when the pelvis is squeezed from before backwards as when a person is trapped between the tail end of a vehicles and the wall. The weaker anterior half of the pelvis gives way. Fracture line runs through the ramus of the pubis and through the ramus of the ischium on both sides (a butterfly-type fracture).

Diagnosis

There is no shortening of the limbs, and movements of the limbs are the same on both sides. A radiographic examination confirms the diagnosis.

Treatment

Although the detached fragment is displaced, it needs not to be corrected (fig. 56). The fracture is stable and can be treated by plaster of Paris application of necker type, incorporating the whole pelvis and both hip joints up to the mid thigh on both sides. The period of immobilization is ten to twelve weeks. The patient is allowed to walk with crutches as soon as the pain has subsided.

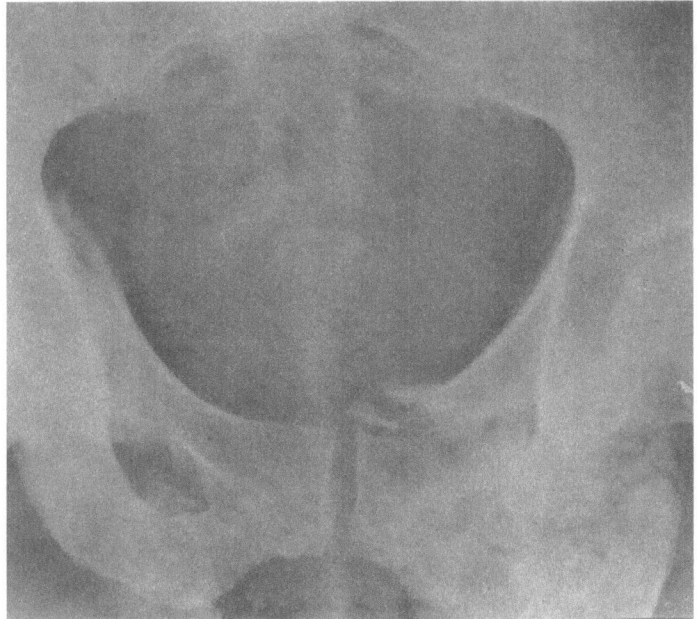

Fig. 56: Disruption of the pelvic ring showing healing of the fracture three months after the accident.

Often, urethra is injured with this type of injury and needs to be treated. A stricture of urethra is likely to develop unless it is prevented by repeated dilatation by sounds. The skeletal injury recovers completely and leaves behind no after-effects.

Hinge Separation of Symphysis

Hinge separation is a result of a rolling injury. Either the patient is run over by the wheel of a car or he is rolled on by a falling horse. Due to the force of injury, the symphysis pubis is separated, and one sacroiliac joint is hinged open.

Diagnosis

Often, a gap can be felt at the symphysis. A look at the feet shows that there is no shortening but the leg or the damaged side is rotated out. Radiograph examination is distinctive. At the symphysis, there is a gap and downward displacement of one ileum which shows the side of the pelvis that has been damaged (fig. 57).

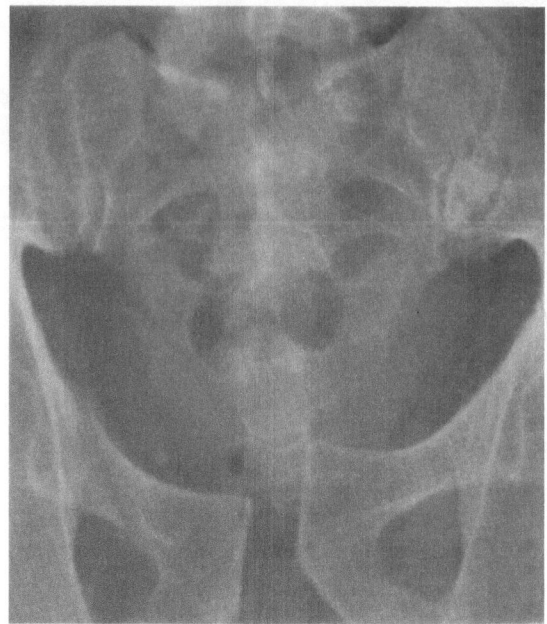

Fig. 57: Hinge separation of the symphysis showing downward displacement of the damaged side.

Widening of the sacroiliac joint is present in such injury. The way this injury is caused and the way it is treated are both unique and should not be confused with any other injury. With this type of injury, the intrapelvic injuries are minimal, and internal haemorrhage may be severe. The urethra is occasionally torn, but sciatic nerve is not injured.

Treatment

Reduction of displaced fragment can be done under general anaesthesia. The patient should lie on the uninjured side. The damaged half of the pelvis is firmly rotated forwards by applying pressure on the back and side of the injured part (fig. 58).

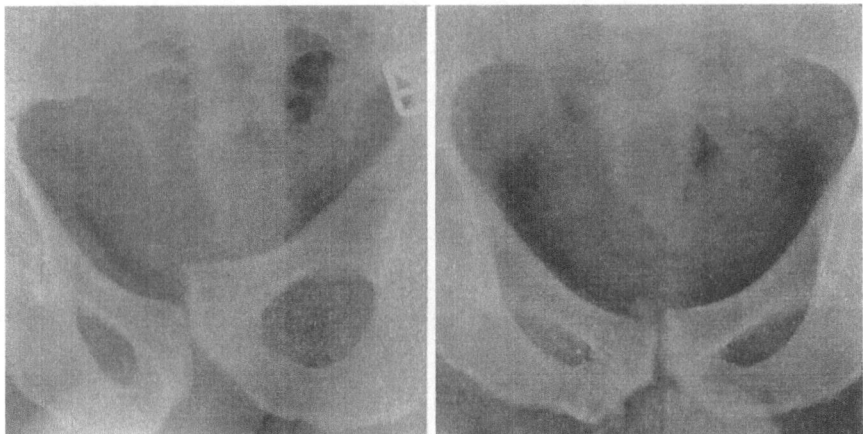

Fig. 58: (A) Hinge-separation injury. (B) The injury after six weeks' treatment.

A plaster of Paris cast is applied around the pelvis while the patient remains in this position, lying on the uninjured side. When the plaster cast is dry, the patient is allowed to lie in bed on his back. The plaster cast remains for 8 to 10 weeks, and weight-bearing is not allowed during this period. After this, the patient is allowed to walk with a stick, which can be discarded after three to four weeks. Prognosis is good. Apart from the pain felt at the sacroiliac joint for some time, full recovery is expected.

Vertical Fracture

The damaging force is usually a result of a fall from a height, such as a tree or upper-storey window. There are vertical fractures through the pubis and ischium on one side, and on the same side, a vertical split through the ilium, lateral to sacroiliac joint, is present (fig. 59). The fracture fragments are displaced upwards as much as 1 in.

Diagnosis is based on the nature of the injury. A look on the feet reveals shortening of the limb on the injured side, but rotation movements of the legs are not affected.

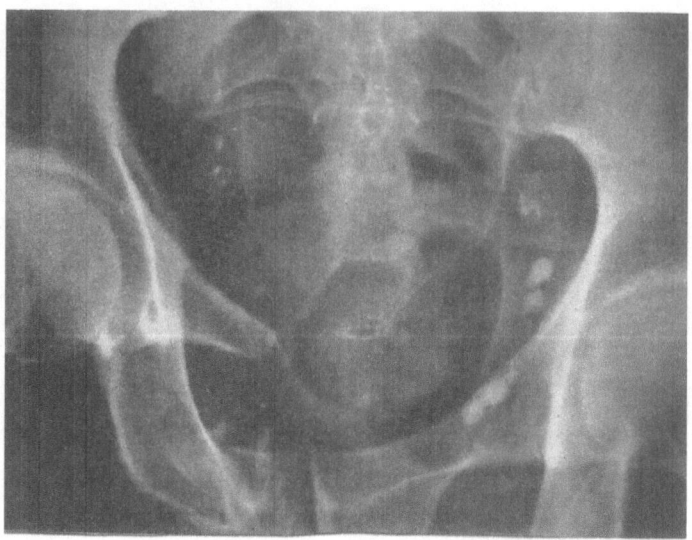

Fig. 59: Vertical fracture of the pelvis.

Intrapelvic Injuries

As with other injuries of the pelvis, internal haemorrhage is severe. Urethra is not injured, but the branches of the sciatic plexus are usually damaged.

Treatment

A strong pull on the affected leg reduces the upward shift, and reduction is maintained by skeletal traction through the tibia for six weeks, a short hip spica can be given for further six weeks. Weight-bearing is not allowed for three months, but the patient can get up and walk with the help of crutches.

Prognosis is good when the upward displacement has been corrected. The partial lesion of the sciatic nerve takes a few months to recover.

Intra-Articular Fracture

This group contains two fractures—one is trivial, and the other is serious:
 1. fracture of the posterior rim of the acetabulum
 2. fracture of the sidewall of the pelvis.

Fracture of the Posterior Rim of Acetabulum

This type of fracture happens to a passenger in a motorcar accident when he is thrown forwards and the front of his knee strikes the dashboard. The force is transmitted, and it breaks the posterior rim of the acetabulum and pushes it backwards. The head of the femur usually remains in the socket, but it may follow the fragment. Diagnosis is not easy because no clinical signs are present. There is no shortening. The degree of rotational movements is the same. Sciatic nerve is not injured. Movements of the knee and ankle are possible.

Radiographic examination shows the detached fragment which presents itself like the segment of a circle and is lying separately (fig. 60). There is no intrapelvic injury, but sometimes the detached fragment may strike and damage the sciatic nerve.

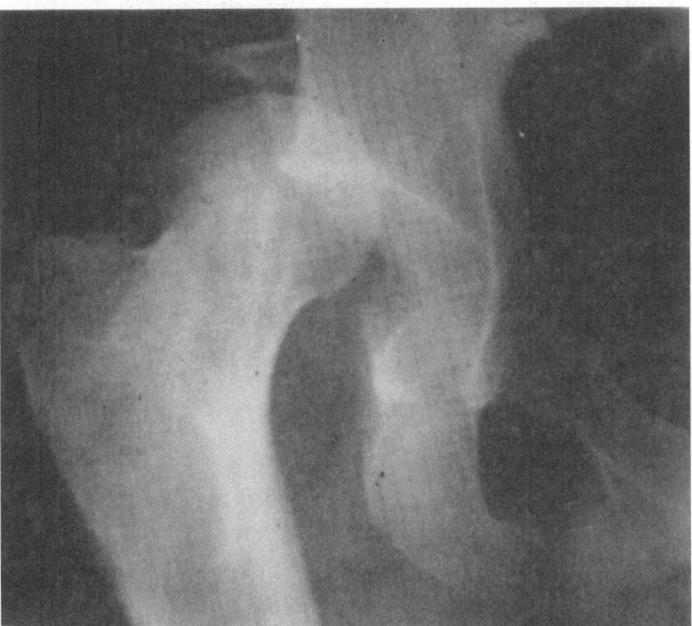

Fig. 60: Fracture of the acetabulum with posterior displacement of the femur. The detached fragment can be seen like a segment of circle.

Treatment

The detached fragment can be replaced only by open reduction. It can be held in place by two screws. The patient should rest in bed for 8–10 weeks. However, after two weeks, the patient is allowed to walk with the help of crutches without putting weight on the injured and operated side. Recovery is usually complete, and functional results are good after this treatment. However, two skeletal injuries may demand more active treatment:

1. A small piece of bone may have been clipped off the head of the femur; if so, the loose fragment trapped inside the joint must be removed.

2. The head of the femur may leave the socket and follow the displaced fragment backwards. It rises up when the leg is straightened. X-ray film shows that the head of the femur is displaced. It should be treated by applying skeletal traction to the leg through the tibia for six weeks. Thereafter, the patient is treated by routine manner as if the complication were not there.

Prognosis

Aseptic necrosis is a possible delayed complication. This may not be visible in X-ray film for a year. However, it should be kept in mind if patient complains of pain three months after the injury, for by then, he should have recovered completely.

Fracture of the Sidewall of the Pelvis

Fracture of the sidewall of the pelvis is a serious injury because it is both a disruption of the pelvic ring and also an intra-articular fracture (fig. 61).

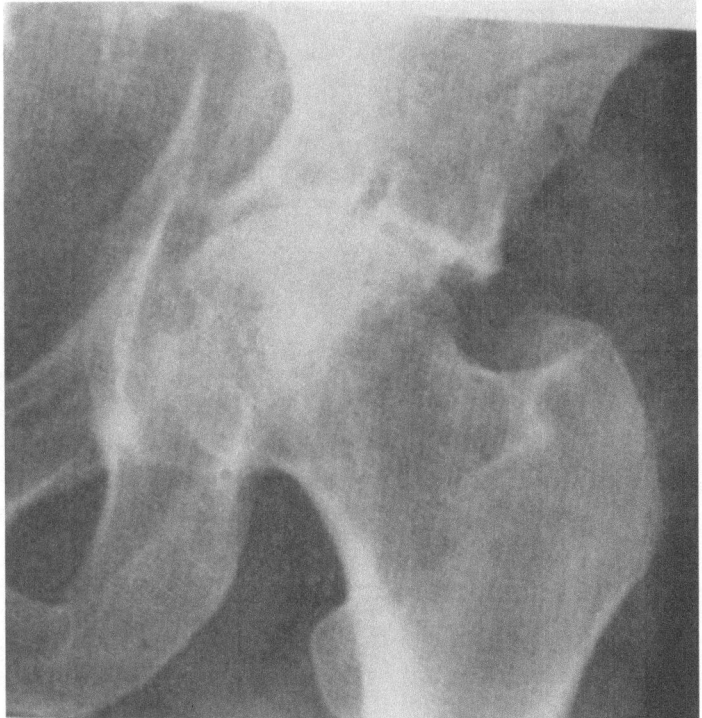

Fig. 61: Injury to the sidewall of the pelvis showing fracture into the roof of the acetabulum.

The commonest cause is car accident. It may also occur due to a fall from height if the patient lands on his side on the ground. The strong force strikes the sidewall of the pelvis and breaks the pelvis. A segment of the sidewall of the pelvis which includes part of acetabulum is displaced inwards or upwards as well. The head of the femur is also displaced in a similar manner. Diagnosis is not difficult. History of the patient is meaningful. The patient is in great pain. The hip on the injured side is immobile, and any movement of it increases the pain.

Radiograph shows that the fracture line is not often clearly defined, but the commonest fracture is that in which one fracture line is just below the acetabulum and the other line runs through the roof of the acetabulum. However, the following variations may occur:

1. The upper fracture may run above the acetabulum instead of through the roof.

2. The lower fracture may be invisible, and the only indication of another ring fracture is that the head of the femur is displaced either inwards or inwards and upwards.

3. Sometimes the two fractures in the ring of the pelvis may be close that the head of the femur appears to have been driven through the floor of acetabulum. This injury is often called central dislocation of the hip joint.

4. Sometimes the upper fracture runs through the roof of the acetabulum, but the lower fracture is below the acetabulum on the other side of the pelvis.

5. Often the fracture lines are not visible, but the doubt is resolved by looking at the roof of the acetabulum and the head of the femur. If they are not congruous, it is certain that there are two breaks in the pelvic ring.

6. Sometimes the head of the femur is displaced to such an extent that it appears to have been dislocated. This, in fact, is a fracture where part of the roof of the acetabulum has been displaced up and has dragged with it the head of the femur (fig. 62).

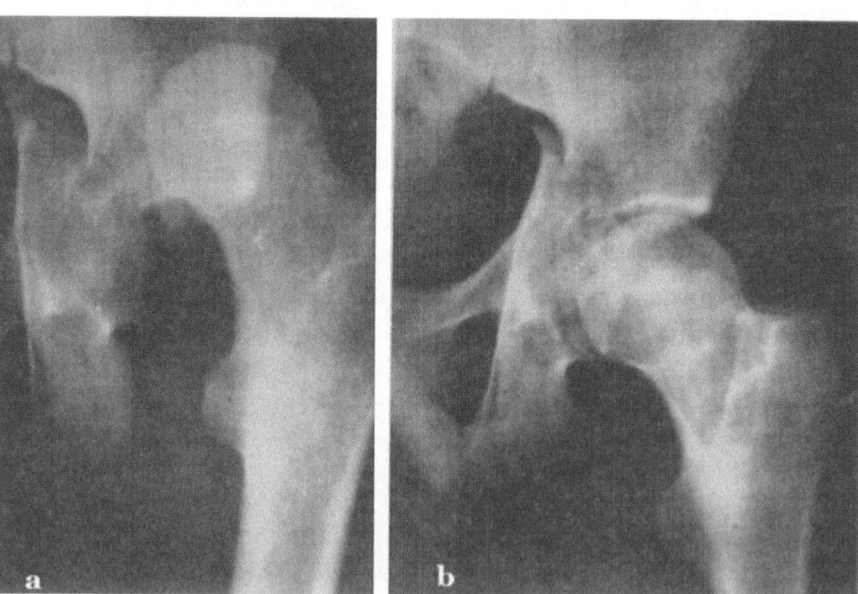

Fig. 62: (A) Fracture of the roof of the acetabulum with displacement of the head of the femur. (B) The head of the femur has returned to its normal position after treatment with skeletal traction for ten days.

Intra-Pelvic Injuries

Severe internal haemorrhage does occur, and shock is always there. The urethra is not torn, but a bony fragment may penetrate the bladder. However, usually the bladder also escapes the injury. The sciatic nerve is not injured.

Treatment

Traction reduces all the upward displacement and part of the inward displacement. If closed treatment is not successful, operation and internal fixation may be carried out. However, even after the surgery, exact anatomical reposition may not be obtained. This fracture is unstable, and early weight-bearing is not recommended. A reasonable procedure is to continue skeletal traction for six weeks, and if X-ray film confirms good union, then non-weight-bearing movements should be allowed with the help of crutches for four weeks. At the end of 10–12 weeks, weight-bearing may be allowed. However, the patient must use the sticks for six months from the date of accident. Prognosis immediately after the injury is good, and movements at the hip gradually increase. However, threat of aseptic necrosis in one year and osteoarthritis in five years should be remembered.

Solitary Fractures of the Pelvic Bones

These solitary fractures of the pelvic ones are fractures which do not disrupt the pelvic ring and do not involve the hip joint.

They include unilateral fracture of the rami of the pubis and the ischium, fracture of the ilium, traction–separation of the pelvic apophyses, fracture of the sacrum, injuries to the coccyx.

In these fractures, intrapelvic structures are not damaged, and shock is mild. They do not require treatment. Bed rest for a few weeks is beneficial, and no splintage is required. Weight-bearing may be allowed on crutches. Even with mild displacement, results of treatment are good, and there are not any delayed consequences.

CHAPTER 20

INJURIES OF THE LOWER LIMB

Injuries of the lower limb are divided into two:
  i. common
  ii. less common.

Common injuries are:
  1. dislocation of the hip joint
  2. fracture–dislocation of the hip joint
  3. fracture of the neck of the femur
  4. trochanteric fracture of the femur
  5. subtrochanteric fracture of the femur
  6. fracture of the shaft of the femur
  7. fracture of the lower end of the femur
  8. fracture of the upper end of the tibia
  9. fracture of the shaft of the tibia
  10. fracture of the ankle joint
     a. single malleolar
     b. both malleolar
  11. fracture of the calcaneus
  12. fracture of the metatarsals and phalanges.

Less common injuries are:
  1. fracture of the acetabulum
  2. fracture of the head of the femur

3. fracture of lesser trochanter
4. fracture of the medial or lateral condoyle of the femur (unilateral)
5. fracture of the condoyle of the tibia (unilateral or bilateral)
6. fracture–dislocation of the ankle joint
7. fracture of the third malleolar of the tibia (lower end of posterior portion of the tibia)
8. fracture of the neck of the talus
9. fracture of the small bones of the foot.

CHAPTER 21

FRACTURE AND DISLOCATIONS OF THE HIP JOINT

Mechanism

The dislocation of the hip joint commonly occurs due to car accidents. The victim is usually a passenger in the front seat, sitting with the hips flexed and knees crossed, and in this position, a powerful thrust against the dashboard with his flexed knee and adducted thigh will force the head of the femur out of the acetabulum and cause dislocation of the hip joint, usually posteriorly. This injury is often associated with fractures of the upper end of the tibia. If similar violence is applied with the leg in an abducted and externally rotated position, the head of the femur is displaced forwards and comes to lie in the obturator foramen or even on the pubic crest. This is usually known as anterior dislocation.

Types

The dislocations of the hip joint are of two types:

1. anterior
2. posterior.

Anterior dislocation is uncommon and occurs in 10% of the cases (figs 63a and 63b). Posterior dislocation is common and occurs in 90% of the cases. Posterior dislocation with fracture of acetabulum rim occurs in nearly 30% of the cases. The sciatic nerve is injured in 5% of the cases.

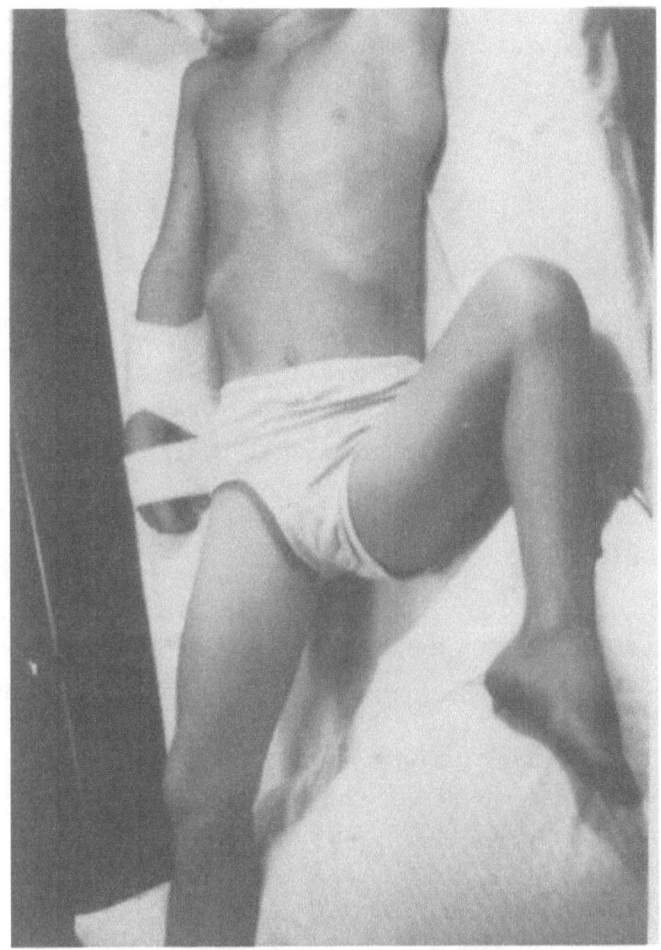

Fig. 63a: Position of the limb in anterior dislocation of the hip joint.

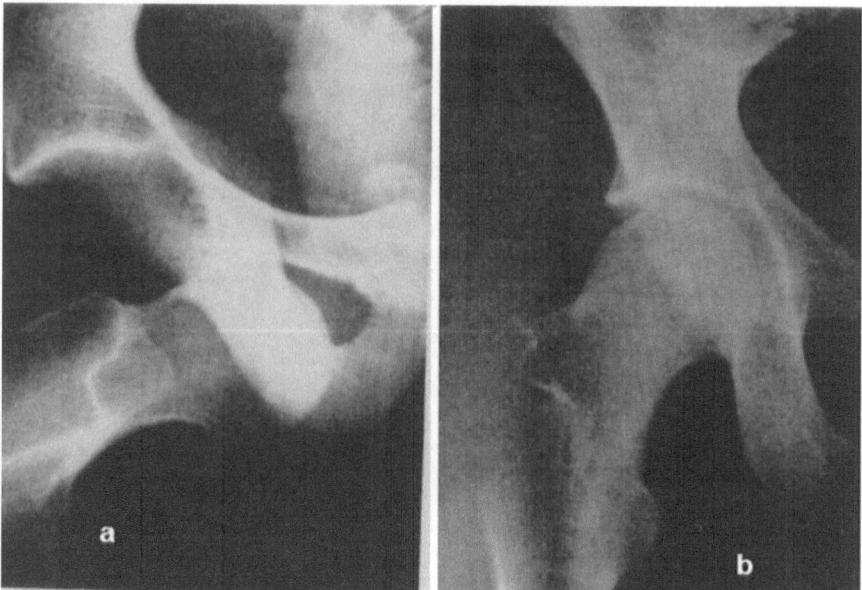

Fig. 63b: (A) Anterior dislocation the femoral head lies in front of the obturator foramen. (B) After reduction.

Method of Reduction

Dislocation of the hip joint is the only injury of the skeletal system which is reduced and treated on the floor. The patient is fully anaesthetized, and reduction is performed with the patient in a supine position on the floor. The pelvis is steadied by an assistant by kneeling by the side of the patient and placing his both hands on both anterior and superior iliac spines. The hip is flexed, and the knee is placed into a right-angle neutral position. In this position, upward and forward traction is applied to the limb with strong force, and the head of the femur will slip back into the acetabular cavity (figs 64a and 64b). It is necessary to avoid sudden forced vigorous movements, but the position of the flexion movements may be changed to varying degrees to help the head to reduce in acetabulum. Occasionally, closed reduction fails due to buttonholing of the femoral head through anterior capsule and psoas major muscle. Such cases require open reduction.

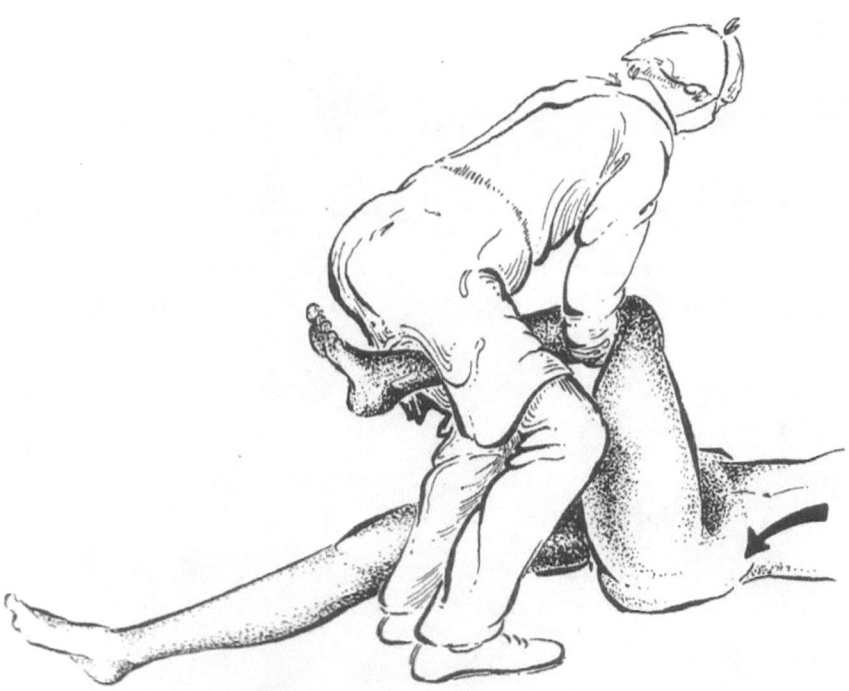

Fig. 64a: The method of reduction of posterior dislocation of the hip joint.

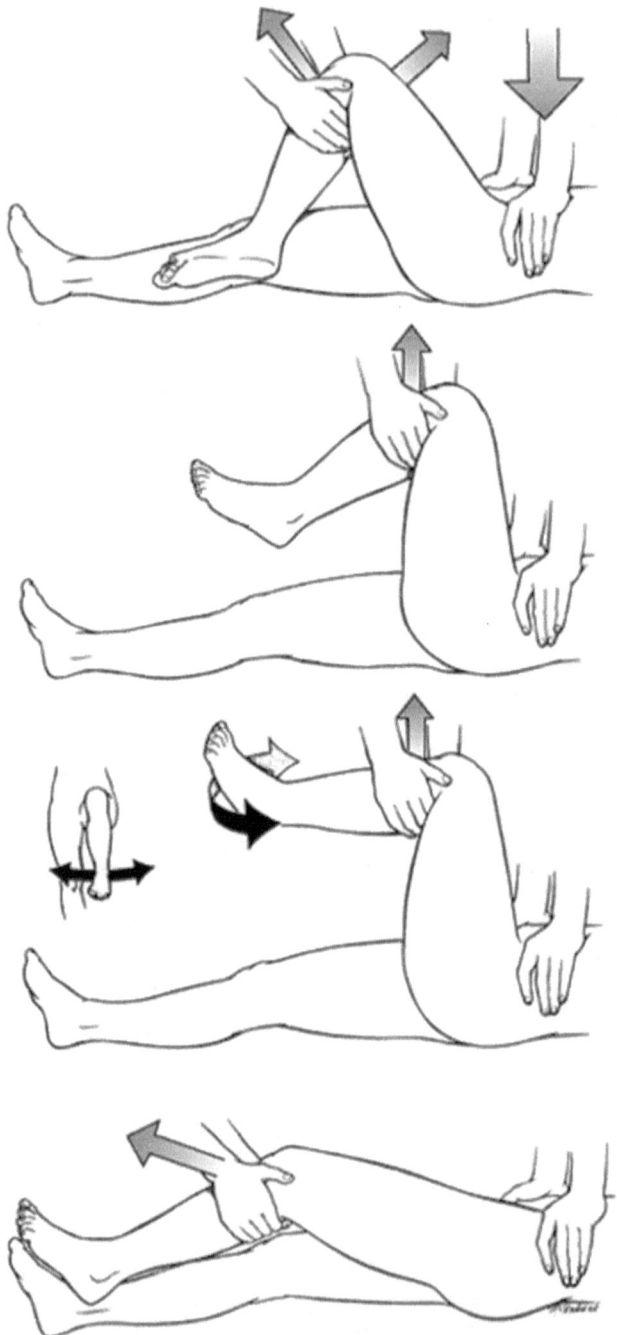

Fig. 64b: The steps of reduction of posterior dislocation of the hip joint.

Grades of Dislocations

There are four grades of dislocation, depending upon the severity of the injury.

Grade 1: Simple dislocation without fracture or a minimal chip fracture of the acetabulum.

Grade 2: Dislocation with one or more large rim fragments but with sufficient socket to ensure stability after reduction.

Grade 3: Explosive or blast fractures with disintegration of the rim of the acetabulum producing gross instability.

Grade 4: Dislocation with fracture of the head or neck of the femur.

Fracture–Dislocation of the Hip Joint

When a dislocation is associated with fracture of the posterior margin of the acetabulum, sometimes the fragment may lie within the acetabulum, and reduction of the femoral head into the acetabulum may trap it. In a good anteroposterior X-ray film, widening of the joint space or disturbance of the Shenton's line after reduction means that the loose fragment is still present in the acetabulum. It is always better to remove such fragment by early operation to avoid future disintegration of the hip joint.

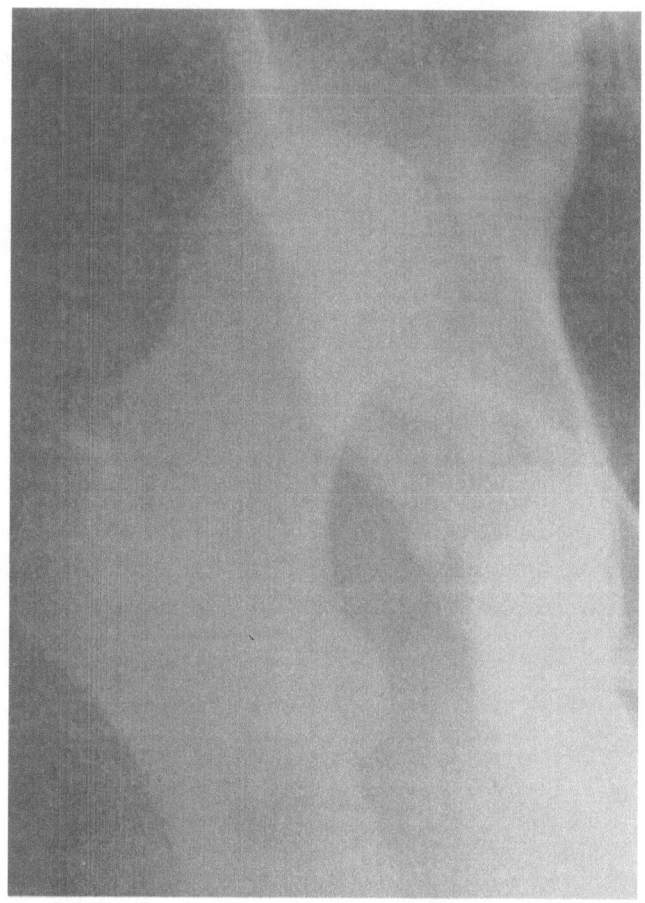

Fig. 65a: Posterior dislocation of the hip joint with fracture of the posterior lip of the acetabulum.

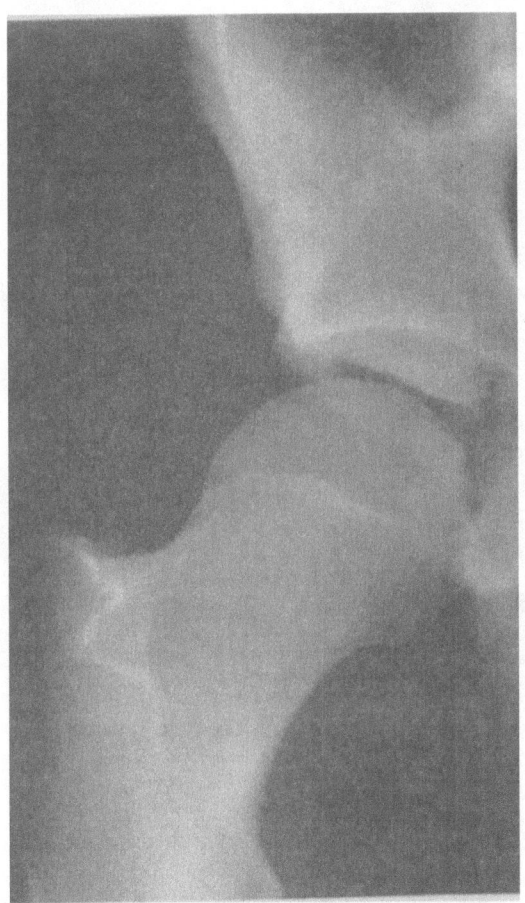

Fig. 65b: After reduction, two loose fragments remain trapped in the joint, displacing the femoral head away from the acetabulum.

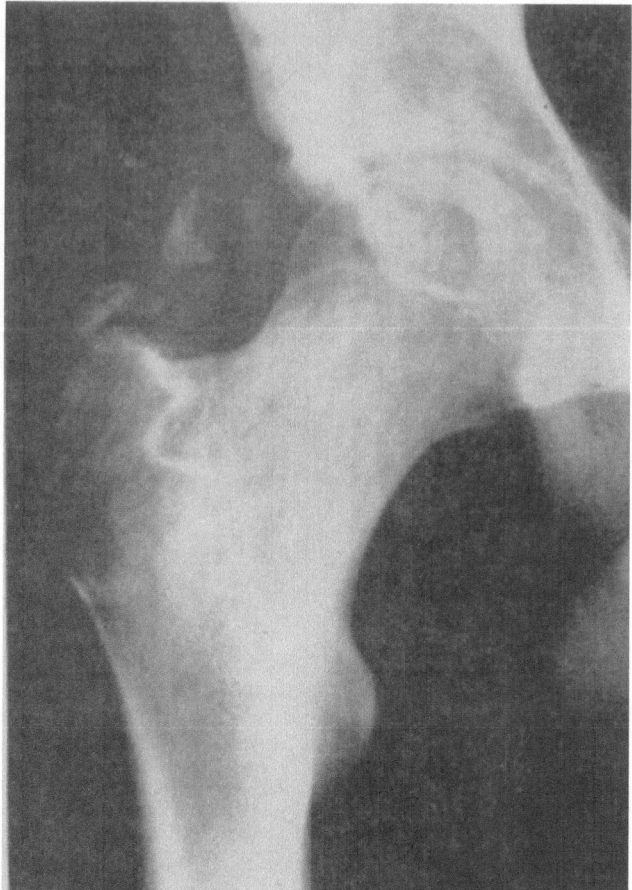

Fig. 65c: Full reduction after arthrotomy and replacement of acetabular fragments.

If early open reduction is not required, the dislocation should be reduced by closed manipulation. However, if a fragment of posteriors margin of acetabulum is lying separate, it should be fixed in its place by one or two screws, before reduction of dislocation of hip joint (figs 66a and 66b). Exploration of the joint should not be delayed for more than 7–10 days, as fibrosis of the periarticular structures can make the operation very difficult.

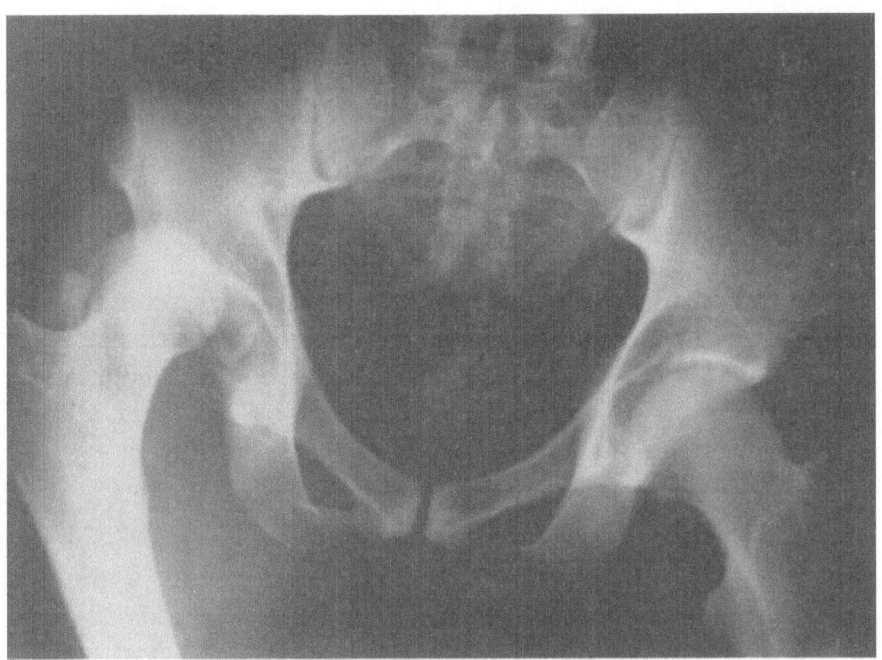
Fig. 66a: Fracture–dislocation of the hip joint.

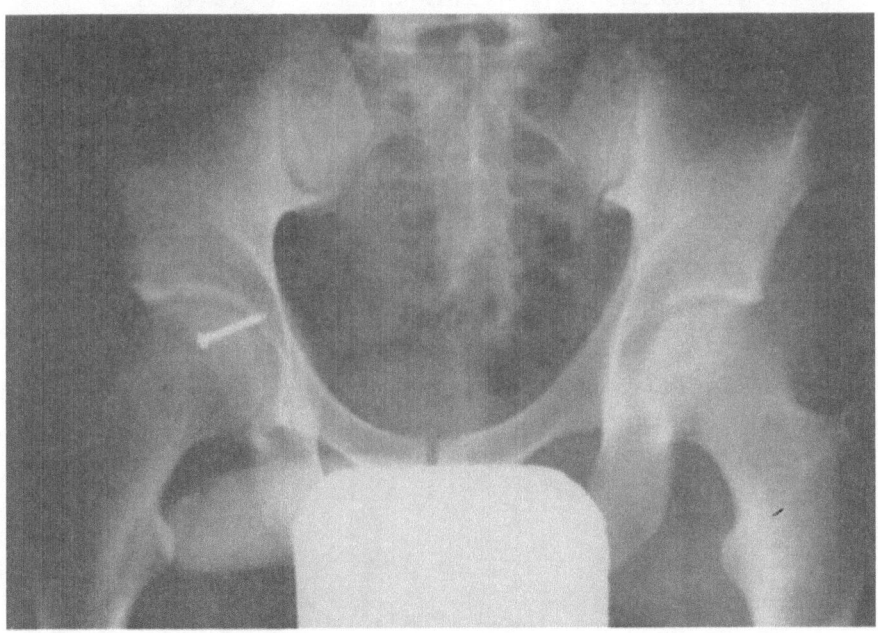
Fig. 66b: After reduction of dislocation acetabular fragment has been fixed by a screw.

Complications

i. Sciatic nerve palsy is three times more common after fracture–dislocation than after simple dislocation.

Any case in which there is evidence of sciatic nerve palsy persisting for two weeks which is associated with a displaced acetabular fragment posteriorly should be explored.

ii. Avascular necrosis: The incidence of avascular necrosis is about 10% in such injuries though post-traumatic arthritis may not appear for several years. The damage to the blood supply at the time of injury occurs, but it is further increased by the delay in reduction of fracture–dislocation.

iii. Myositis ossificans: Dislocations and fracture–dislocations are severe injuries with considerable degree of disruption of periosteal attachment of muscles and capsule. There is a great deal of haemorrhage in the periarticular tissues, and calcification and ossification may occur. These are usually small localized deposits of no clinical significance and are seen after open reduction of a fracture–dislocation (see fig. 65c). These deposits do not cause any trouble. But sometimes massive bone formation occurs in the periarticular tissues and muscles. If it causes trouble or limitation of function, it has to be removed. However, if the dislocation is reduced within a few hours of the injury and the leg rested for three or four weeks, such complication can be avoided.

Operative Approach

The best approach is a posterior one. The muscle is detached, and sciatic nerve is identified and separated. Hip joint is exposed. Small loose fragments are excised, but a large fragment should be replaced and fixed with two screws.

Aftercare

It is better to use a short hip spica, or boots and bar should be applied to the foot and leg to prevent movement at the hip joint because often the patient cannot have sufficient rest in bed and there is likelihood of displacement of the fragment. The hip spica or boots and bar should be retained for six to eight weeks to provide stability to the joint.

Treatment of Unreduced Fracture–Dislocation

Fracture–dislocation of the hip is often missed in the presence of severe multiple injuries. In some cases, a marginal fracture of the acetabulum is overlooked, and the hip joint gradually subluxates. In other cases, the posterior rim of the acetabulum is so shattered that it is impossible to reduce or fix it. In such cases, traction is applied for six to eight weeks, and the fracture will unite with gradual moulding process. No surgery proves beneficial in such cases. Many patients regain some degrees of movements. If pain persists, arthrodesis of the joint or a total hip replacement may be considered.

Dislocation of the Hip Joint Associated with Fracture of the Upper End of the Femur

Dislocation of the hip joint that is associated with fracture of the upper end of the femur is a rare complication, but occasionally, it occurs. It may be a marginal fracture of the head of the femur, and if it lies within the hip joint, it should be removed. Dislocation associated with fracture of the neck of the femur is a difficult problem, and it leads to avascular necrosis of the head of the femur. The treatment is to excise the head of the femur and replace it with prosthesis. Occasionally, dislocation may be associated with fracture of the shaft of the femur. In such cases, the fracture of the shaft of the femur should be treated first by internal fixation, and dislocation of the hip joint may be reduced afterwards.

Traumatic Dislocation of the Hip in Children

Dislocation occurs more frequently than fracture of the neck of the femur. Sometimes it may be associated with other severe injuries which should be treated first. The dislocation of the hip joint should be treated by closed reduction. It usually is successful and gives a good result.

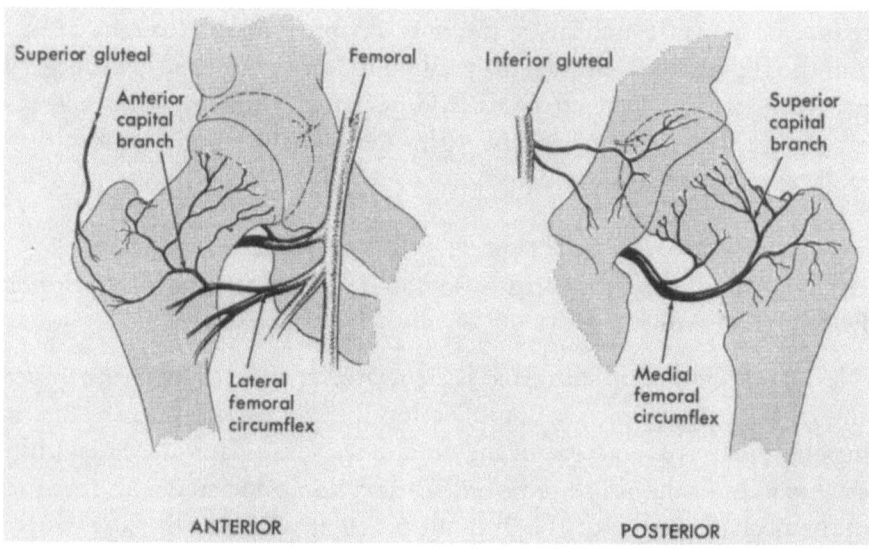

Fig. 67: The blood supply to the head and neck of the femur. This shows that the fracture of the neck of the femur may heal slowly or may fail to heal at all while fractures in the trochanteric region heal readily.

CHAPTER 22

FRACTURE OF THE NECK OF THE FEMUR

The strength of the upper end of the femur depends on calcar femorale with trabeculae spreading out in a fan-shaped direction to the articular surface. These trabeculae known as compression group are the main weight-bearing system.

Bone fragility increases sharply with age, and it is more common in women than men. This accounts for greater occurrence of the fracture of the neck of the femur in women.

Blood supply of the neck of the femur is important, and the main sources are (fig. 67):

1. the artery in the ligamentum teres, which remains patent in the aged
2. the inferior metaphyseal vessels lying along the anteroinferior aspect of the femoral neck
3. the lateral epiphyseal vessels which are responsible for the blood supply of practically the whole of the capital epiphysis in young children and probably at least the outer two-thirds of the femoral head in adult life.

In their course, these arteries are all intra-articular, covered by folds of synovial membrane, and are liable to be torn at the time of fracture or during manipulation, leaving the head dependent on the supply from the ligamentum teres. It is this precarious blood supply of the femoral head which accounts for the very different behaviour of the fracture of the neck of the femur.

The fracture commonly occurs in persons above 60 years of age and in females. It is twice more common in females than in males.

Mechanism of the Fracture

Many cases of this fracture occur as a result of a trivial twist, such as tripping over a mat or missing a step.

Clinical Features

The classical picture is of an elderly female lying with the injured leg shortened and externally rotated, extremely painful on the slightest movements, and unable to raise the leg from the bed. Occasionally, the initial injury results in a fracture of the neck of the femur with no displacement, and the patient may be able to move the hip with some extent and even walk a little. Complete displacement may not occur until some days or weeks later. It must be remembered that any elderly person who complains of pain in or around the hip following trivial injury must be considered to have sustained fracture of the neck of the femur until a good anteroposterior and lateral X-rays have excluded the injury.

Types of Fracture of the Neck of the Femur

Fracture of the neck of the femur may be divided into:

a. subcapital

b. transcervical

c. basal

d. intertrochanteric.

There are three main problems associated with the treatment of this injury:

1. A satisfactory reduction is often difficult to achieve.
2. In high fractures, it is difficult to provide rigid fixation which will endure until the fracture unites.
3. A proportion of cases will inevitably go on to avascular necrosis.

Classification of the Fracture

The classification of fracture of the neck of the femur is as follows:

Type A

1. abduction
2. adduction

Type B

1. intracapsular
2. extracapsular

Type C

1. subcapital   ⎫
2. transcervical   ⎬ intracapsular
3. basal   ⎫
4. intertrochanteric ⎪
5. comminuted intertrochanteric ⎬ extracapsular
6. subcervical   ⎪
7. subtrochanteric   ⎭

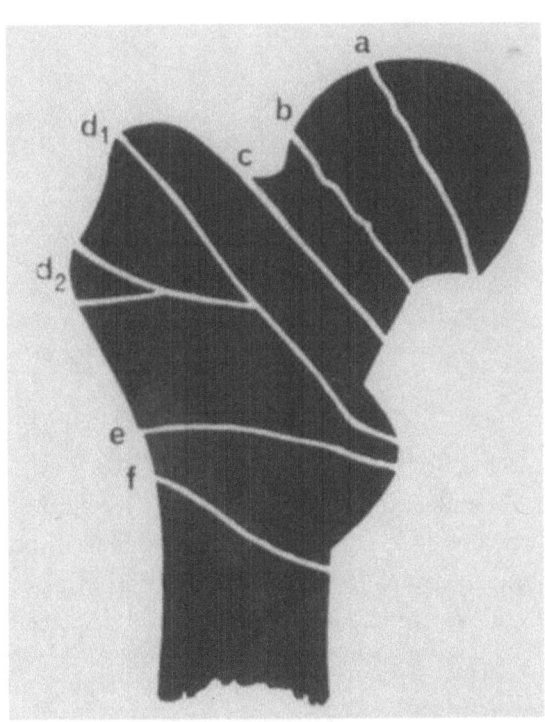

Fig. 68: Common fracture sites at the upper end of the femur.

A recent classification is based on the trabeculae pattern of the head and neck of the femur, which are directed upwards. The classification is shown in figure 69.

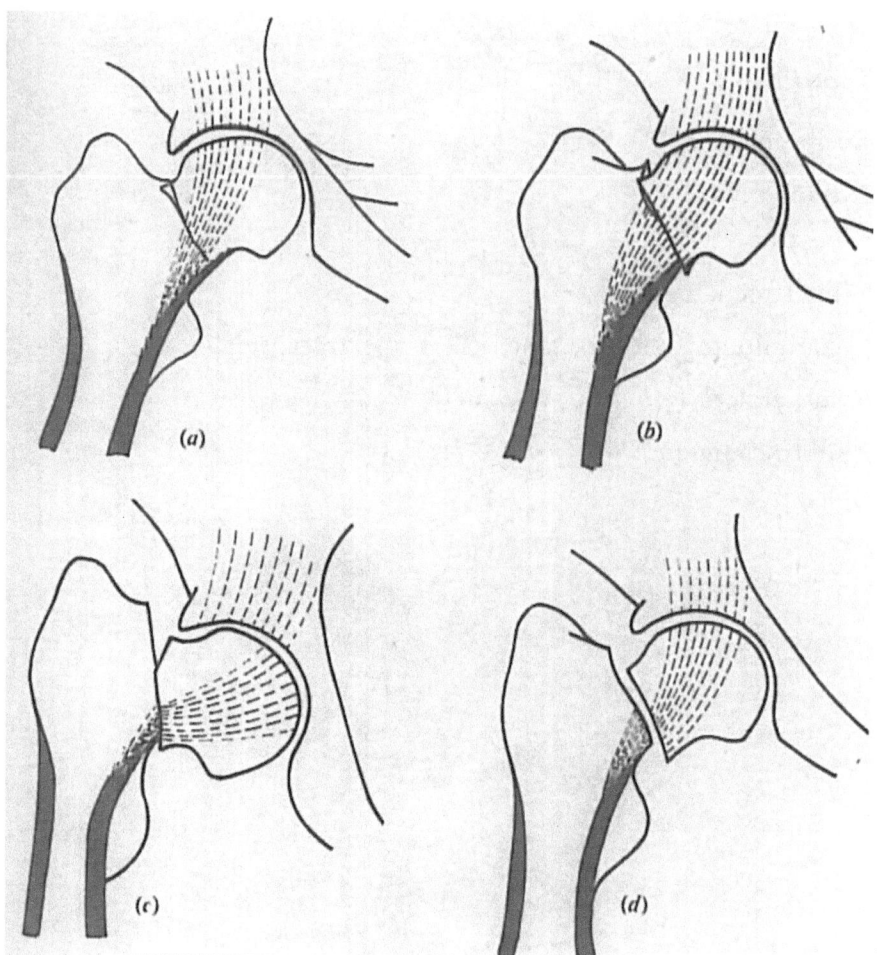

Fig. 69: (A) Grade 1: incomplete greenstick fracture in a valgus position. (B) Grade 2: complete fracture without displacement. (C) Grade 3: complete fracture with partial displacement. (D) Grade 4: complete fracture with full displacement.

Besides it, the following points need consideration.

1. Level of fracture line:
    i. subcapital
    ii. transcervical
    iii. basilar

2. Relationship of the fracture fragments:
    i. varus type of fracture
    ii. valgus type of fracture

3. Direction of the fracture line:
    i. fracture line nearly horizontal
    ii. fracture line nearly vertical

4. Displacement of the fragments:
    i. impacted
    ii. unimpacted or displaced

The significance of the consideration of these points is that they contribute certain important factors in the prognosis. Fractures near the base of the neck of the femur have a better prognosis than subcapital fracture. Fractures that are impacted have a better prognosis than those that are not impacted. Fractures whose line of division is nearer the horizontal than the vertical will have better prognosis. Fracture in some valgus position will have a better prognosis than in varus.

Reduction of the Fracture

There are two reasons why perfect anatomical reduction is important:

1. Full reduction, particularly in slight valgus with the cortex on both sides of the fracture interlocking, provides a degree of stability which can be retained by a well-placed internal device.
2. It is not possible to insert any type of nail or screw through the neck of the femur into the head without tilting the capital fragment unless the reduction is accurate.

It must be remembered that nothing is more dangerous to complete the damage to the vascular supply of the head of the femur than allowing the patient to lie in bed for days without applying leg traction. It may not only immobilize the fracture but may also reduce it in good position (fig. 70).

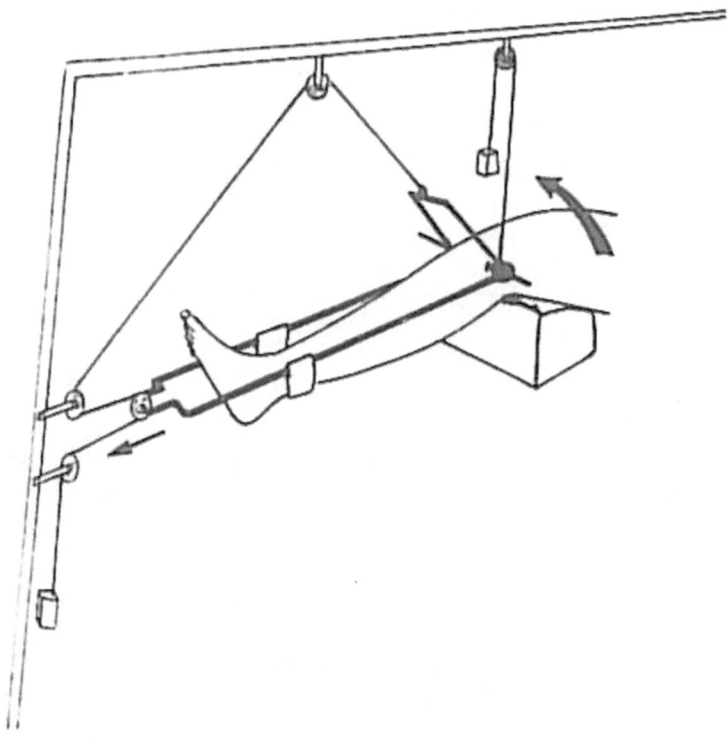

Fig. 70: Apparatus used for the reduction of the fracture of the neck of the femur.

Method of Reduction of the Fracture

If displacement is present, the fracture can be reduced by this method. Traction is exerted in the line of the femur with the hip flexed to 90 degree before rotating the leg internally and slowly extending it in about 30 degrees of abduction. The shortening of the limb disappears, and external rotation of the limb also disappears when the foot is held in the palm of the hand after reduction.

Treatment

1. Hip spica: It is an outdated method of treatment of fractured neck of the femur. It is likely to produce more complications of the chest, abdomen, urinary tract, and skin, and it may also develop bedsore.

2. Boots and bar: In this method, after reduction, plaster of Paris boot and bar is applied with a wooden bar placed underneath and fixed with plaster. It prevents rotation of the limb, and the patient is allowed to prop up or sit in bed after the pain is relieved. It is recommended for patients where internal fixation is not possible due to the absence of facilities or due to intercurrent problems of cardiovascular disease or diabetes.

3. Smith-Petersen nailing (fig. 71): It provides adequate fixation for incomplete or undisplaced fracture, but it has disadvantages as well, like the following:

    a. It has only two points of bony contact, the outer shell of the shaft and the cancellous bone of the head of the femur.

    b. Any form of fixation has to contend with the tendency for the limb to rotate externally. Hence, there is a tendency for a horizontally placed nail to cut out, owing to a relatively poor fixation in the cancellous bone of the femoral head. However, a more stable fixation can be achieved by inserting the nail in a low-angle position.

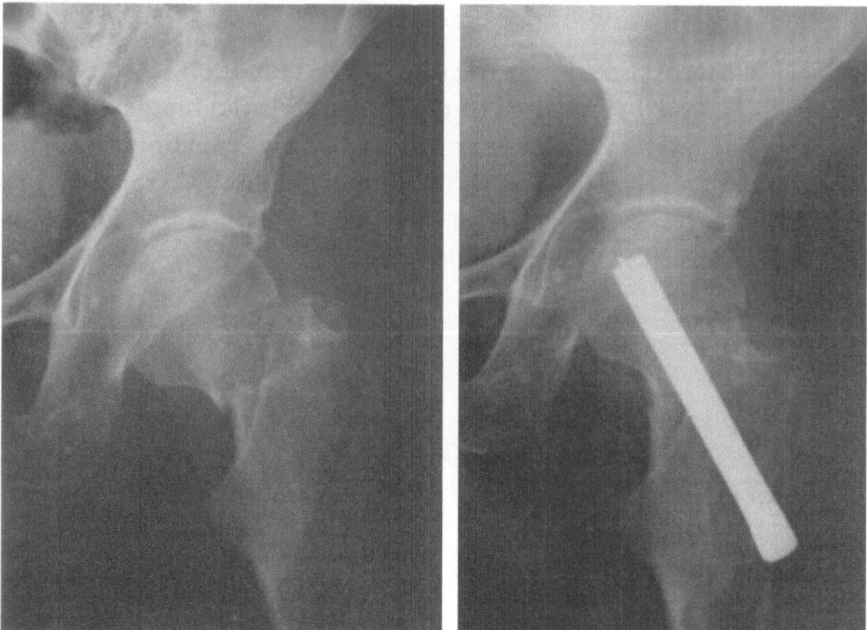

Fig. 71: Fracture of the neck of the femur treated by SP nailing.

Abduction Type of Fractures

In abduction type of fracture, there is some degree of coxa valga with impaction of the upper part of the femoral neck with no angulation or displacement. This can be confirmed by anteroposterior and lateral X-ray examination. The fracture usually heals without nailing. Although fracture is stable, in some cases, displacement may occur later on. In such cases, protected weight-bearing is required, or internal fixation with nailing must be considered.

Vascular Factor in the Healing of Fractures

Accurate reductions with rigid fixation are essential for healing of fracture, which depends on the maintenance of adequate blood supply. Since the fracture is widely displaced and the lower fragment is externally rotated, the vessels are likely to be torn completely. Therefore, avascular necrosis is likely to develop, which will be demonstrated in X-ray films taken repeatedly at one-month interval (fig. 72). Later on, the head of the femur may crumble and become fragmented.

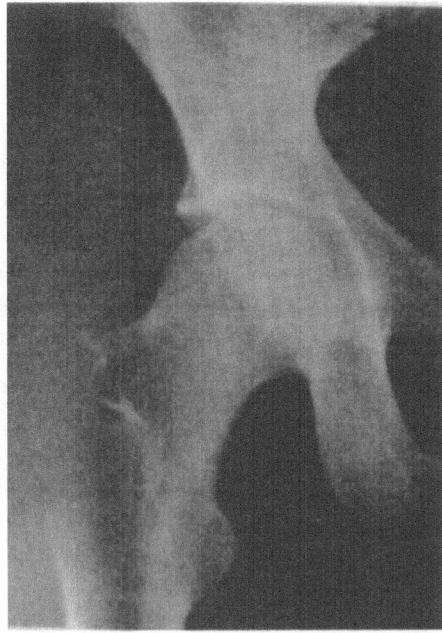

Fig. 72: Early avascular necrosis of the head of the femur.

When studying the effect of fractures on the blood supply of the femoral head, the questions which one has to answer are:

1. Is the vascular state of the head determined at the time of fracture?
2. Does the method, traction or manipulation, or the timing of reduction affect the incidence of avascular necrosis?
3. Does the type of fixation device used have any effect on the degree of necrosis?

It is very difficult to give the answers to these questions, but it is a fact that good results are likely to be achieved through accurate reduction by gradual traction, followed by internal fixation, which will allow impaction and avoid distraction. But it is a fact that whatever method is used, nearly 30% of the patients have failure rate and need to be considered for prosthetic replacement. In some cases and in view of the high failure rate, prosthetic replacement may be the treatment of choice immediately after the fracture to avoid the complications of general nature. As a rule, the use of prosthesis is indicated in grade 3 or 4 fracture, more particularly in elderly patients with an age of over 70 years.

The results of prosthetic replacement in fresh fractures are significantly better than those cases done later on, treated by other methods.

Treatment of missed or un-united fracture occurs where the original fracture was trivial and was accompanied by mild pain. Increasing pain and limp and gradual increasing limitation of the function will compel to do X-ray examination, which may show commonly a mid-cervical fracture with displacement. At this stage, accurate reduction is impossible. Therefore, such fracture should be treated with internal fixation using nails and plates, which gives good results.

Intertrochanteric Fractures

Fractures occurring between the base of the neck and the subtrochanteric region are known as intertrochanteric or pertrochanteric fractures. Basal and subcervical fractures, which lie below lesser trochanter, are included in this group.

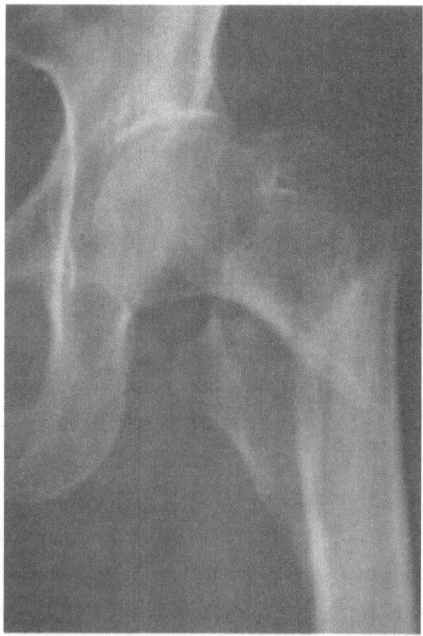

Fig. 73: Intertrochanteric fracture of the femur.

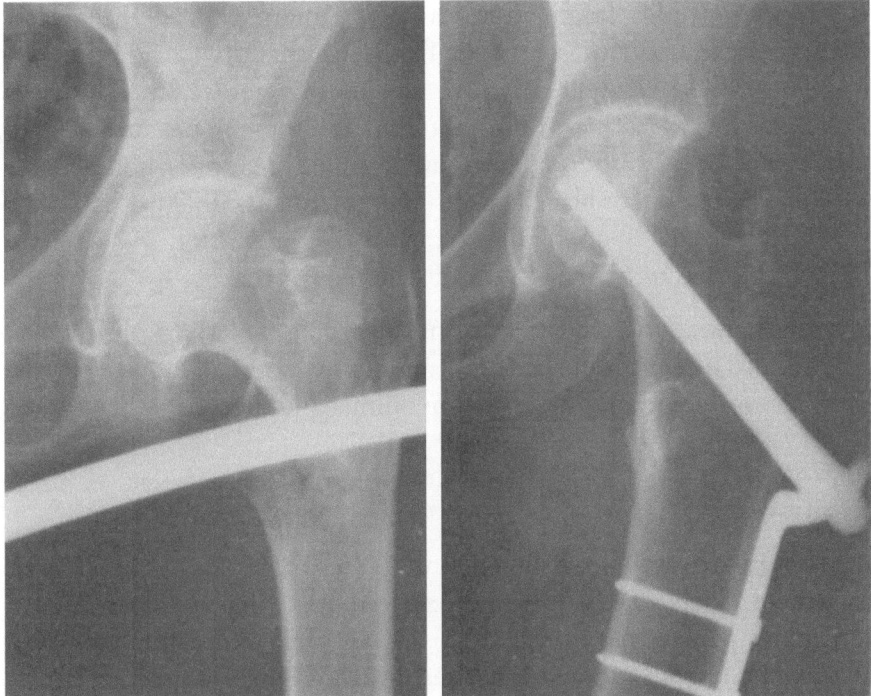

Fig. 74: Intertrochanteric fracture reduced and held with a nail and plate.

Classification:
1. basal fractures
2. intertrochanteric
    a. non-comminuted
    b. comminuted
3. subcervical or reversed intertrochantesic fractures

Pattern of Fracture

Majority of intertrochanteric fractures are comminuted with three main fragments:
1. A proximal fragment which comprises the head and neck of the femur and the line of fracture running almost parallel to the intertrochanteric line.

2. A posterior fragment forming the main part of the greater trochanter and separated from the shaft by a fracture line running at right angle to the main fracture line. It has a powerful abductor and external rotator muscles attached to it, and it is often comminuted, providing a poor hold on any fixation pin or blade plate used in treating the fracture. Accurate reduction is often difficult, and nail migration may lead to external rotational deformity and coxa vara.

3. A distal fragment consisting of a detached shaft which may also be comminuted. This fragment is externally rotated by the unopposed pull of gluteus maximus and iliopsoas when intact.

Treatment

Conservative treatment: Although union can be obtained by conservative treatment, such as traction and external splinting and rest in bed, not many people now consider this as an ideal treatment. However, shattered and comminuted fractures, in which there is great difficulty of maintaining rigid internal fixation, should be treated by skeletal traction with an internal rotation pull. This traction is to be maintained for 12–16 weeks, and satisfactory union takes place in most cases with good functional results. However, most of these frail elderly patients are unsuitable for the time-consuming procedure of reduction and traction method of treatment. These patients are better off treated by operation and internal fixation procedure, which can be easily carried out in the operation theatre under X-ray control (see fig. 74).

Various fixation devices are available and can be used for internal fixation. Results are generally good (fig. 75).

The patient should be watched for post-operative complications, such as pneumonia and urinary retention. Deep vein thrombosis can occur if the patient is confined to bed longer. Hence, early mobilization is recommended. If the internal fixation is stable and the general condition is good, the patient should be made to sit in bed and allowed to be out sitting a chair 48 hours after the operation. Gentle and passive exercises of all the limbs should be started the day after the operation.

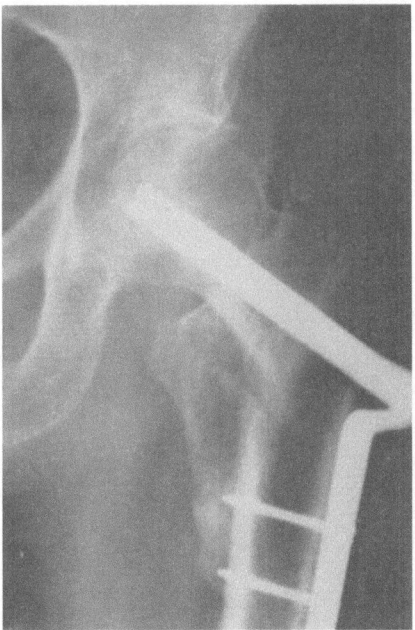

Fig. 75: Intertrochanteric fracture of the femur treated by nail and plate.

It must be noted that most of the benefits of internal fixation are lost if the patient is kept in bed for several weeks or months. It is always better to help the patient on his feet or into a chair by the bedside as the initial discomfort has settled.

If the reduction is complete, fixation is rigid, early protected weight-bearing appears to have no harmful effect, and the patient may be allowed to walk with crutches or walking aid within a few days after the operation (at least after 48 hours).

Fracture of the Neck of the Femur in Children

Fracture of the neck of the femur occurs in children due to severe violence. It is rare, but when it occurs, it causes separation of normal epiphysis or fracture of the neck through the middle of the neck or the basal or intertrochanteric regions.

In children, the blood of the femoral head is small, and special care is taken not to damage the blood supply by injudicious treatment.

The treatment is best carried out by strong skeletal traction for accurate reduction of the fracture, and then it should be maintained by the use of Knowles pin (fig. 76), which always gives good result. Delayed union with coxa vara should be treated by subtrochanteric wedge osteotomy.

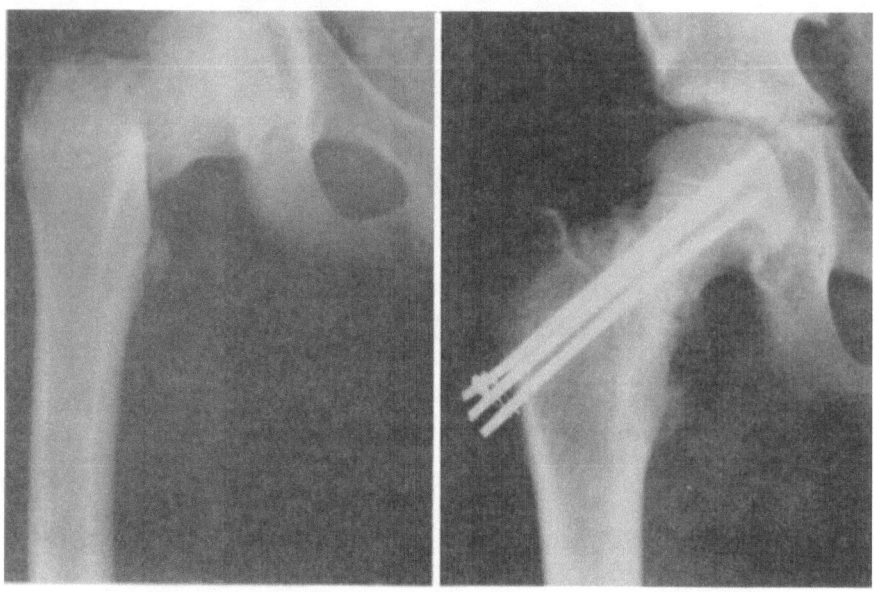

Fig. 76: Fracture of the neck of the femur in a boy of 12 years, immobilized by Knowles pins after accurate reduction.

CHAPTER 23

FRACTURE OF THE SHAFT OF THE FEMUR

Fractures of the Middle Portion

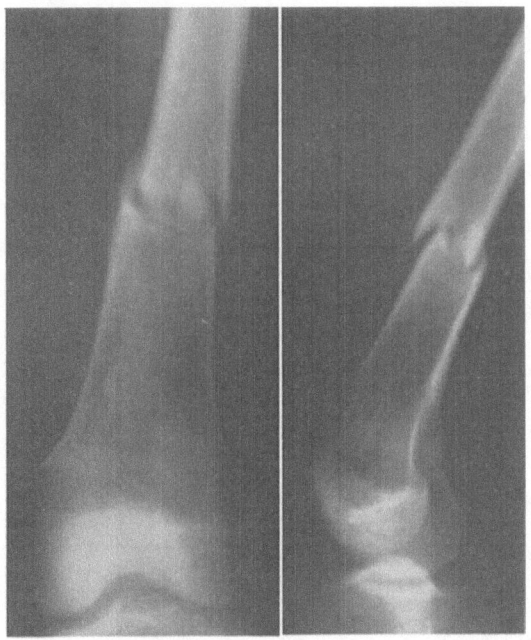

Fig. 77: Fracture of the femur (middle portion) is reduced, and position is satisfactory.

Conservative Treatment

When the fracture of the femur is an isolated injury and occurs as oblique or comminuted fracture, conservative treatment is the treatment of choice. A Thomas splint with a split ring suspended with weights gives good support and helps the patient in toilet requirements. Traction is required to prevent undue shortening. Skin traction with adhesive strapping is applied for traction, but if the patient is well built, skeletal traction with a Steinmann pin is applied through the upper end of the tibia.

In adhesive skin traction, the patient may be sensitive to adhesive strapping, or if more than 12 lb of weight is applied, it will come off and cause damage to superficial layers of the skin. In skeletal traction, the pin should be applied in aseptic conditions and at right angle to the line of pull. However, pin track infection is very common, and pin may become loose or come off.

Reduction under Anaesthesia

Unless the overriding is minimal, it is better to undertake reduction of the fracture under anaesthesia. Simple traction for a few days may reduce a gross displacement, but sometimes even weight of 25 lb or 30 lb may be required for the first week. Even then, the position may be unsatisfactory. The manipulation should aim at the following:

1. Clinical correction of the alignment with particular attention to the rotational deformity if present.
2. Correction of shortening. The length of the femur should be measured from anterior superior iliac spine to the upper pole of the patella and should be compared with the sound side, held in an identical position. When limb appears satisfactory clinically, radiographs are taken to see the exact position of the limb.

Standard of Reduction

It is of no significance if the fragments are not in accurate position. Anatomical reduction may delay the union by bringing the two bone ends together. Separation of fragments by the full diameter of the shaft is of no consequence, and in the femur, few degrees of angular deformity is of little significance.

Maintenance of Reduction

Once the fracture has been reduced, the position is maintained by traction on Thomas splint with 15 lb of weight applied. Radiographs are taken at weekly intervals for the first month to check the alignment and leg length. The rotational deformity must be examined clinically as well as with radiograph. Minor degree of posterior displacement should be corrected by suitable pads beneath the fracture site or towards the lower end of the femur by flexing the knee. The anterior displacement is corrected by extending the knee and elevating the whole leg. The varus deformity can be corrected by wide abduction of the leg.

Mobilization

From the beginning, static quadriceps contractions and foot exercises are practised. The time taken for healing is 10–12 weeks. Knee exercises can be started after six to eight weeks when the callus is firm. At the end of 12 weeks' time, mobilization is allowed with the help of crutches.

If this traction method is not desirable, then a full hip spica can be applied for three months, in which the patient can get up and walk after six weeks. In average case, partial weight-bearing is started in four months' time, but this can be delayed by a few months if callus formation is not sufficient.

Internal Fixation

For internal fixation, a Küntscher intramedullary nailing or plate-and-screw fixation can be carried out. With successful internal fixation, the patient can start walking in three to four weeks' time, though bed rest is desirable till the soft tissue has healed. With internal fixation, the leg length and alignment can be easily achieved, and knee flexion is regained quickly.

Indication for Internal Fixation

The operation is indicated in the fracture of the shaft only.

1. pathological fracture
2. wide separation of fragments with possible interposition of soft parts

3. complicated fracture of the femur with dislocation of the hip joint, fracture of the femur and tibia on the same side, or fracture of the tibia on the opposite side
4. fracture of the femur complicated with the injury to the femoral artery

Choice of internal fixation is done on the basis of economic and social factors, but it must be considered seriously because the chances of technical failure and infection are present. Mechanical success of the nailing or plating does not exclude the non-union of the fracture.

Infected Internal Fixation

If the internal fixation by nail or plate gets infected, it is a serious complication and may need several drainage operations. Whether internal fixation should be removed or not is debatable. Perhaps it is better to leave the nail until the fracture is united as long as adequate drainage is provided.

The Stiff Knee

Whether treated by conservative method or operation, some stiffness of the knee joint is inevitable. In most cases, this recovers with active exercises, but sometimes the adhesions are so formed in the joint or between the quadriceps and fracture site that it causes limitation of movements at the knee joint. Once the fracture has consolidated, the patient should start active knee flexion and quadriceps contraction for three to five minutes every hour of the day. If after a month, the flexion range is not improved, the joint should be gently manipulated under anaesthesia, giving another 30–40 degrees of motion. Too much manipulation at one time will cause painful reaction in the knee, and joint will become stiff again. The manipulation of the joint can be repeated two to three times at an interval of two to three weeks.

If the joint remains stiff despite exercises and manipulation under general anaesthesia, the question of quadriceps palsy should be considered.

Subtrochanteric Fracture of the Femur

Displaced subtrochanteric fractures (fig. 78) are difficult to treat by conservative method because the proximal fragment is pulled into acute flexion and abduction. In such cases, it is better to do open reduction and internal fixation by long plate and screws.

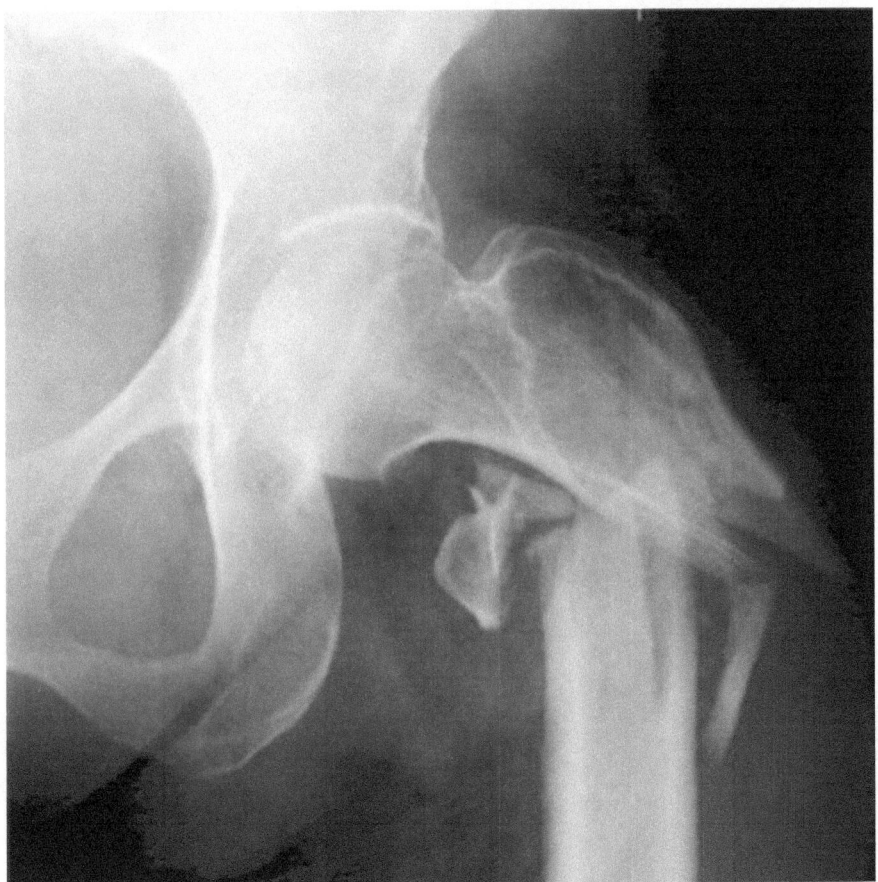

Fig. 78: Subtrochanteric fracture of the femur.

Supracondylar Fracture of the Femur

In supracondylar fracture of the femur (fig. 79), gross deformity occurs due to strong pull of gastrocnemius, and the distal small fragment is placed into acute flexion at the knee. Manipulation and reduction may be successful, but the fracture position will be maintained with knee in flexed position. As this position is difficult to maintain, it is better to do open reduction, and internal fixation by *L*-shaped plate should be carried out. For a *T*-shaped fracture, reduction and fixation by two rush nail inserted through each femoral condyle will work better, or ultimately, an *L*-shaped plate can be used. However, before applying this, it is better to fix the two condyles together by two screws. The results are usually satisfactory by this method of treatment.

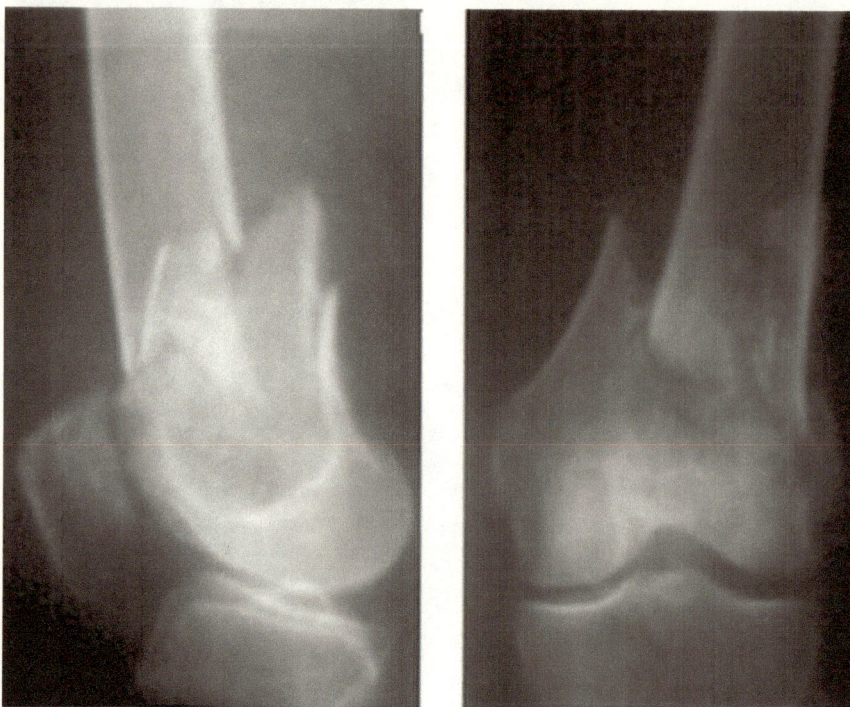

Fig. 79: Supracondylar fracture of the femur with displacement.

Shaft Fracture in Children

Bryant's traction (fig. 80) is a good method for treatment of this fracture in children. Both legs are suspended by strapping, with sufficient weight to keep the buttock just clear off the bed cloths. This method is not recommended for children older than 3 years of age, and circulation of feet must be carefully watched.

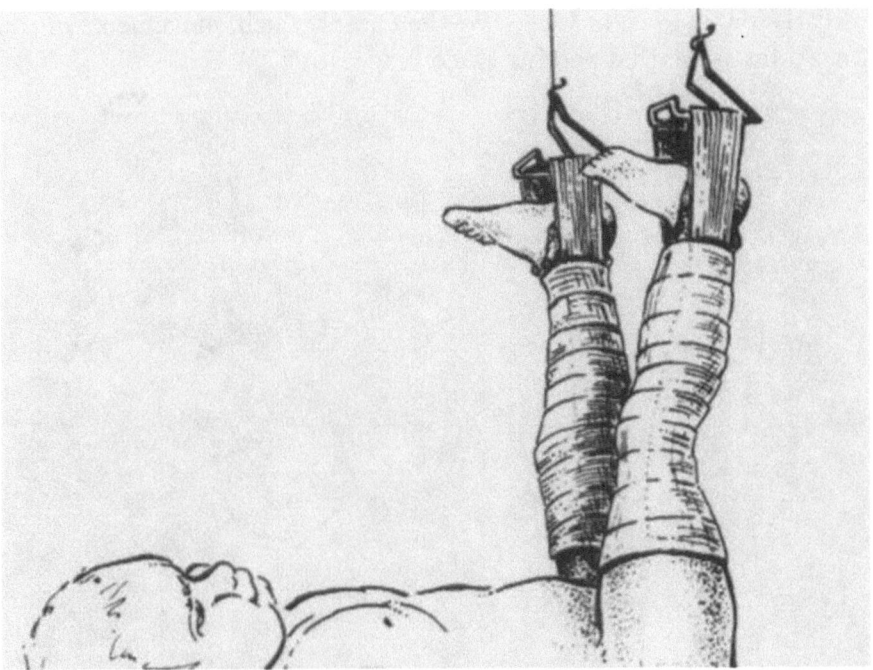

Fig. 80: Bryant's traction for fracture of the femur in children.

Malunion with a minor degree of angulations improves during the growth, but rotational deformity will need correction. If it is present, open reduction and fixation by plate and screws are recommended. In children, the intramedullary nail should be avoided as it will cause damage to the superior epiphysis of the femur, resulting to deformity or stunting of growth.

Dislocation of the Knee

Knee dislocation (fig. 81) is a severe injury, but it is rare and is always the result of severe violence. The tibia may be displaced anteriorly, posteriorly, medially, or laterally. All of the supporting tissues are completely torn, and when the knee is reduced, any stability remaining is due to the bone structures. Injury to the popliteus muscles is a common accompaniment, and treatment is carried out with this fact in mind. The dislocation is easily reduced under general anaesthesia if the patient is seen early after the injury. The limb is immobilized in a long plaster of Paris for six to eight weeks. At the end of which, movements of the knee joint are started and increased gradually.

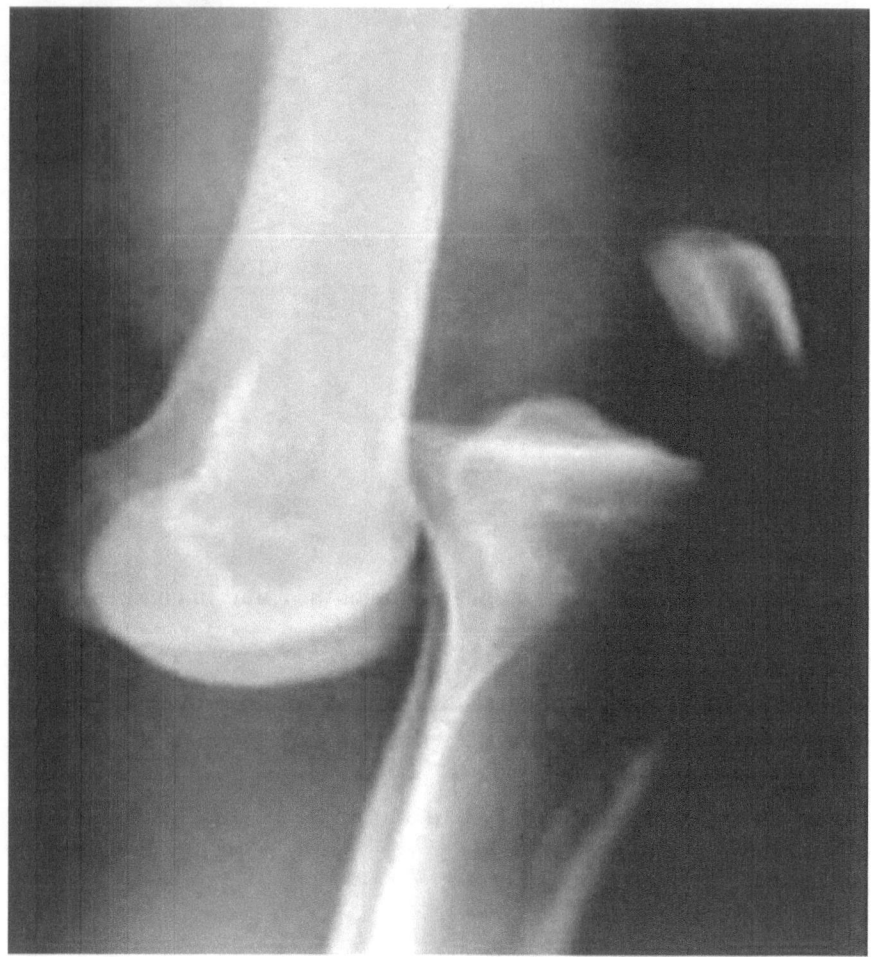

Fig. 81: Dislocation of the knee joint.

Fracture of the Patella

Fracture of the patella may be classified according to the type of injury. Those that are due to direct violence show a multiple irregular fracture lines in the patella with little separation of fragments. Those that are due to indirect injury with strong muscle pull, forced flexion of the knee is an important cause in the production of a transverse fracture line. All degrees of severity may be incomplete. The fracture line may extend completely across the patella with no displacement of the fracture fragments. The fracture line may extend medially and rate really as a tear into the quadriceps retinaculum, and the fracture fragments may be then widely separated. A combination of the two types of fractures is frequently seen with one separated fragment crushed by a direct injury.

Diagnosis

A history of indirect and direct injuries to the knee joint is typical of fracture. Examination will show swelling of the knee joint. If the patellar fragments are separated, an indentation is easily palpable. X-ray examination will show the extent of bone injury, and physical examination will reveal the extent of soft-tissue injury.

Treatment

The aim of the treatment in patellar fracture (fig. 82) is always the restoration of extensor apparatus of the knee, of which patella is an important part.

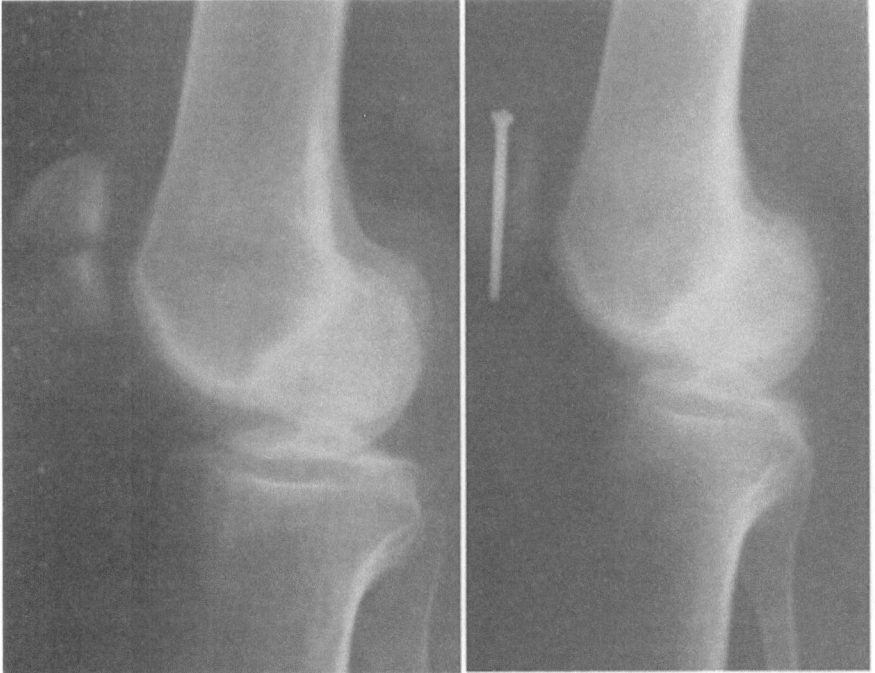

Fig. 82: Fractured patella treated by screw fixation.

Fractures that show no displacement and are associated with no tear of the retinaculum require rest for four to six weeks. After that, progressive flexion and extension exercises are started, and return to normal activity is promoted. With the separation of the patellar fragments and the associated tear of the quadriceps retinaculum, open reduction and fixation of fragments, together with the repair of the soft-tissue tear, are indicated, and fixation of the patellar fragments after reduction may be obtained by catgut, silk, fascia lata, or wire suture. The soft tissue is repaired as part of the procedure. If the patellar fragments are severely comminuted, excision may be preferable to leaving an irregular joint surface. External support in the form of a plaster of Paris cast is maintained for four to six weeks. Weight-bearing may be encouraged. After the removal of the plaster cast, exercises and movements are encouraged, and often, full functional recovery occurs.

CHAPTER 24

FRACTURES OF THE SHAFT OF THE TIBIA & FIBULA

Fibula

An isolated fracture of the shaft of the fibula occurs from direct violence to the leg (fig. 83). The bone damage is not significant, but often, there is damage to the soft tissue, which causes pain and swelling and bruising. Elevation of the leg may be required for a few days to help the swelling to subside. No splintage is required. A supporting bandage is applied, and the patient is allowed to walk with full weight-bearing. When pain is marked, a plaster of Paris cast may be applied.

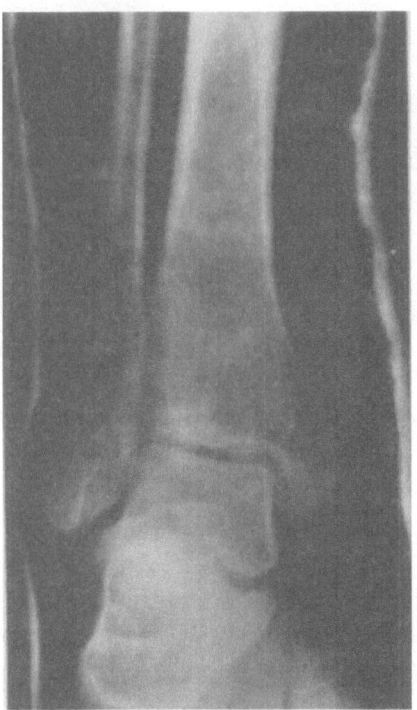

Fig. 83: Solitary fracture of the fibula treated by a plaster cast.

Undisplaced Fracture of the Tibia

These injuries are fairly common, especially in children. The leg is immobilized in a padded plaster cast from the toes to the upper part of the thigh, with the knee slightly bent. Weight-bearing in plaster is allowed after about three weeks while fracture gets united in 10 weeks.

Displaced Fracture

The fracture is reduced by manipulation under general anaesthesia, and a padded plaster cast is applied up to the mid thigh (fig. 84). Sometimes inserting of a pin through the calcaneus during manipulation and plastering help to control the position.

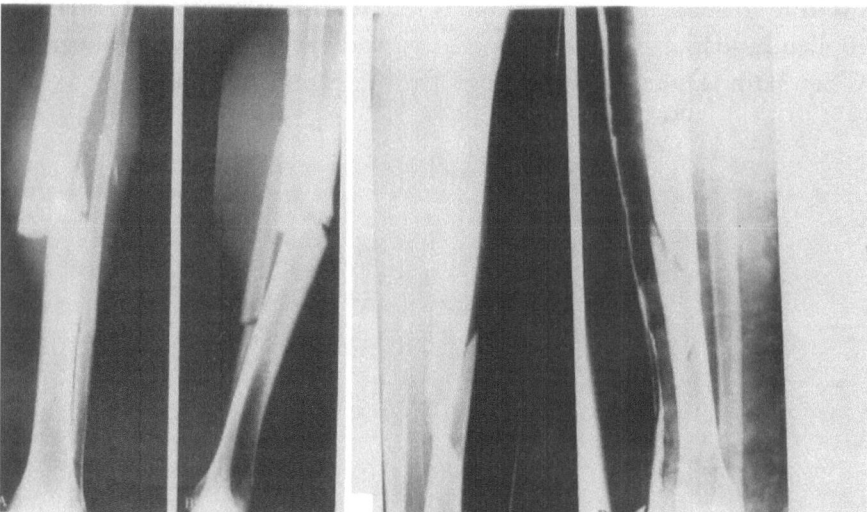

Fig. 84: Fracture of the tibia and fibula treated by closed reduction and plaster cast.

When radiograph shows good position, a padded plaster cast from the toes to the tibial tuberosity is applied, and as it sets, the tibial fragments are moulded together. When this part of the plaster has consolidated, the plaster is extended up to the upper part of thigh, with the knee kept in 30 degrees of flexion (fig. 85).

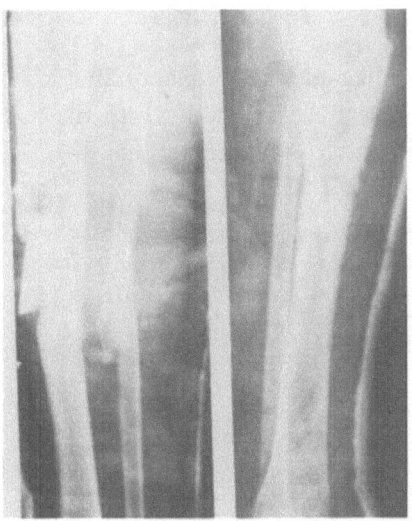 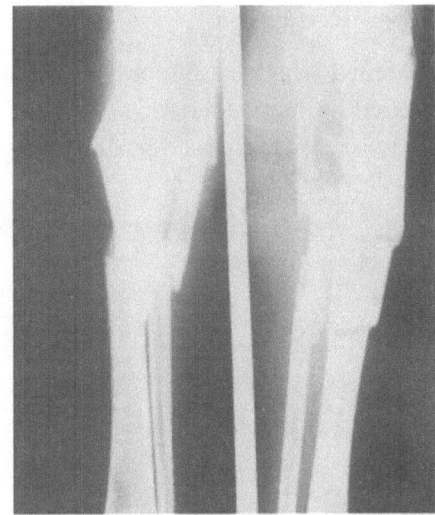

Fig. 85: (A) Fracture of the tibia and fibula in plaster cast. (B) The fracture after healing.

Care is taken that at no stage should the plaster be pressed into the skin. The limb is elevated for a few days to allow the swelling to subside. If the plaster cast becomes loose in two to three weeks' time as oedema subsides, it must be changed. Minor degree of angulation at the fracture site can be corrected by wedging the plaster, but rotational deformity should not be allowed to remain. Weight-bearing should be allowed, but at the end of two to three weeks, the patient can start non-weight-bearing walking with the help of crutches. Weight-bearing may be allowed when clinical union has taken place.

The application of continuous traction will delay the union, or if too much weight is applied, it will produce non-union. However, if swelling is present, traction can be applied to the limb through the calcaneus, with the limb placed on a pillow for two weeks. During this period, the swelling disappears, and reduction becomes easy. The limb can be immobilized in full-length plaster cast, and the pin can be removed.

Open Reduction

Fractures which cannot be reduced or are unstable after reduction should be treated by open reduction and internal fixation. In a spiral fracture, fixation by two screws in different directions will hold them together (fig. 86).

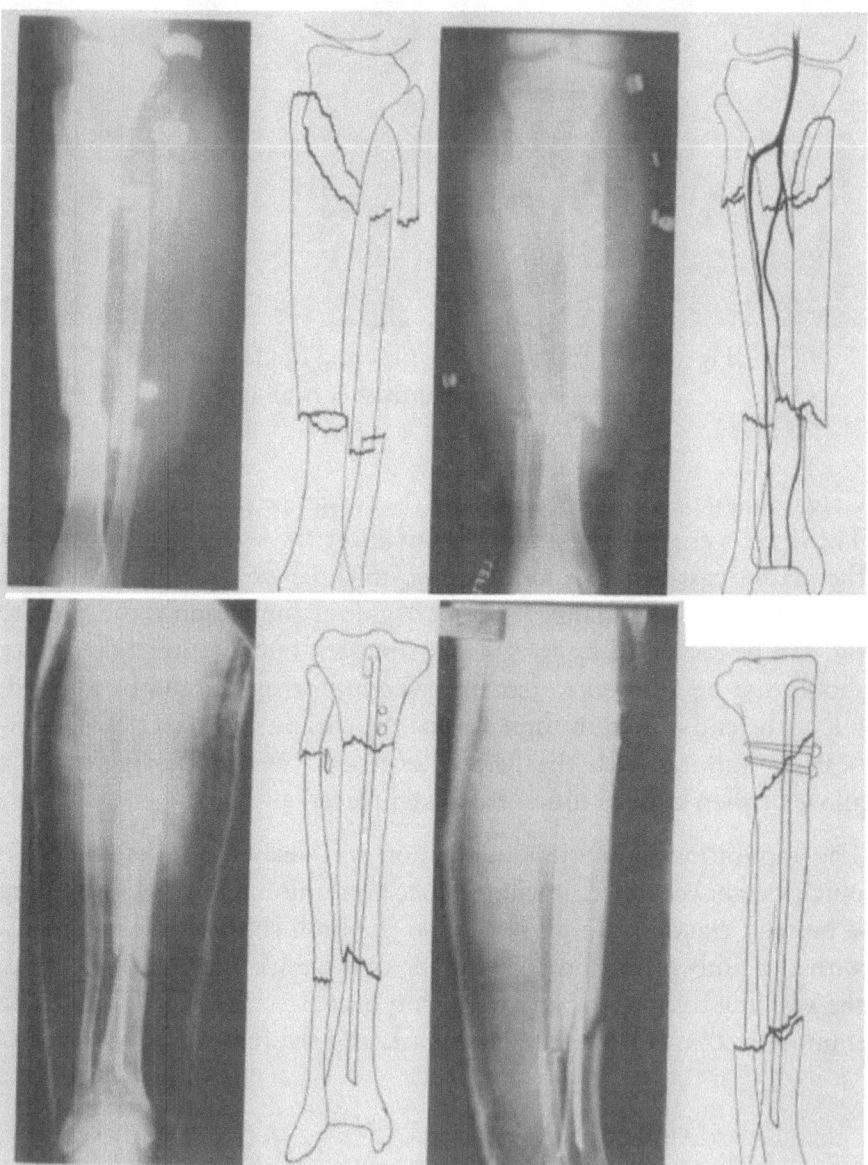

Fig. 86: Fracture of the tibia and fibula treated by (a) intramedullary nailing and (b) nail-and-screw fixation.

Comminuted and transverse fractures are better fixed by plating. Following the operation, it is better to apply a long leg plaster cast. But if the patient can rest and does not place weight on the limb, the plaster cast may not be applied, and the patient may be allowed to walk with non-weight-bearing on crutches. This way, stiffness of the knee and ankle does not occur. However, exercises of the toes, ankle joint, and knee joint must be performed daily.

In case of open reduction, the complication of the wound infection may develop. Great care must be taken to prevent it from taking place.

Delayed Union

If at the end of six months the fracture is not united clinically, immobilization is prolonged for further three to four months for it to unite. But it is advisable to do bone grafting in such cases of delayed union. However, in some cases, rigid internal fixation may help complete the union. Sometimes when the plaster cast is removed for two to three weeks for skin toilet, the fracture rapidly unites before any operation. Hence, decision must be taken in individual cases.

Compound Fracture and Skin Loss

The subcutaneous position of the tibia exposes it more often to compound fracture. The routine of early wound-cleaning must be followed, but skin loss may be present. Cortical bone exposed to air will soon necrose, and many months will pass before sufficient granulation tissue develops to allow split-skin grafting, and perhaps after sequestrectomy. Delay in union does occur. Every effort must be made to cover the fracture site with healthy skin, and for it, skin-relaxing incision on both sides of fracture site may be given. Sometimes cover may be obtained by a local skin flap, but it may slough down due to trauma of the accident.

If immediate cover is not possible, it may be proper to apply rigid internal fixation so that no external splintage is needed and bone is covered with saline dressing. For such procedure, external fixation is the best method to be used. If applied properly, it helps the bone to heal. Also, skin loss can be corrected by using a planned skin graft. By such procedure, the infection is also controlled, and results are good.

CHAPTER 25

INJURIES OF THE ANKLE

The ankle joint is a complex joint which can be labelled as hinge, saddle, or mortise joint at the same time. But if considered as part of a joint complex which includes the subtalar and midtarsal articulations, it allows a wide range of movements in all directions.

Ankle Injuries

The ligament injury without fracture is of two types:

1. sprain
2. avulsion.

Sprains

A sprain is a strain of a ligament not amounting to a complete rupture and not resulting in any permanent stretching of the ligament. The common sprain of the ankle joint is of lateral side, which results from an inversion injury to the foot and involves the anterior portion of the fibular collateral ligament. The diagnosis is easy by the presence of pain and tenderness in the front and below the lateral malleolus, accompanied by swelling and sometimes bruising.

Avulsion

Avulsion occurs from a severe injury. It is a complete rupture (fibular collateral) of the lateral ligament over the ankle joint, which occurs with more extreme degree of inversion injury. The avulsion occurs at the fibular attachment of the ligaments, and a small fragment of the bone may be avulsed from the tip of the malleolus. Pain and tenderness are present over the tip and front of the malleolus, and swelling and bruising are usually marked. In an acute stage, the instability cannot be demonstrated because of the pain, spasm, and swelling, but if

X-rays are taken with forced inversion of the foot under local or general anaesthesia, tilting of the talus between 10 and 30 degrees can be seen, and a lateral film taken in plantar flexion may show subluxation of the talus touching the inner side of the fibula and lateral malleolus of the ankle joint (fig. 87).

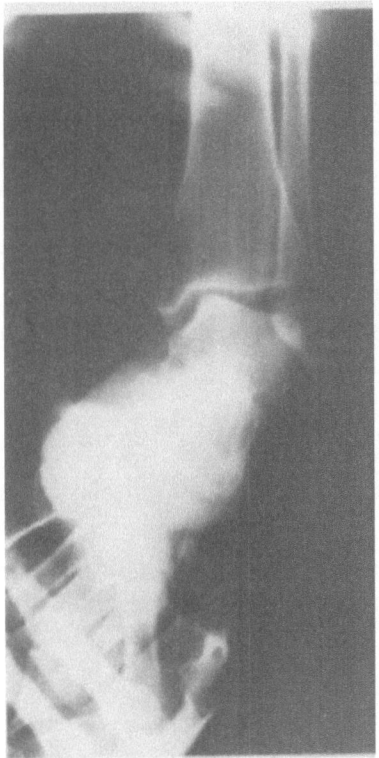

Fig. 87: Avulsion injury of the ankle joint with tear of the lateral collateral ligament. The talus is touching the inner side of the fibula and lateral malleolus.

Hypermobile Ankle

Recurrent sprain or recurrent giving way of the ankle occurs in persons, usually young women, without history of injury or complete avulsion of ligaments. These cases are due to laxity of the fibular collateral ligament, which may be congenital in origin or may be due to an old forgotten inversion injury of the ankle joint.

Other Sprains of the Ankle

Footballer's ankle. This results from forcible plantar flexion of the foot, usually caused by receiving an oncoming ball on the dorsum of foot, which forces the foot into plantar flexion. The essential lesion is an avulsion of the anterior capsule of the joint. There is pain, swelling, and bruising. The foot is held in plantar-flexed position, and movements are limited.

Injuries of Deltoid Ligament of the Ankle Joint

Injuries of the deltoid ligament of the ankle joint are uncommon injuries, owing to its greater strength and limited range of eversion movement of the foot. More severe injuries occur with complete rupture of deltoid ligament and a fracture of the fibula. If rupture of deltoid ligament does not occur, then fracture of the medial malleolus may occur.

Strain of the Anterior Tibiofibular Ligament

An isolated injury of the anterior tibiofibular ligament may occur due to external rotation injury of the foot. The signs are tenderness and swelling over anterior aspect of this joint. An X-ray film may show widening of the syndesmosis. In this case, the whole length of the fibula must be X-rayed to exclude the possibility of high fracture of the fibula.

Treatment of Ligamentous Injuries

Simple sprain. The treatment depends upon the degree of pain and swelling that occurs. Minor sprain responds rapidly to strapping of the ankle in eversion. In some cases, a plaster of Paris for two to three weeks provides better results and complete healing of the sprain. However, severe sprains are best treated by local infiltration of 2% xylocaine along with hyaluronidase (to reduce pain and swelling), pressure bandaging, and elevation for 48–72 hours, followed by gradual walking with the help of supporting strapping or plaster of Paris cast. Similar measures may be employed for simple sprains of deltoid and anterior tibiofibular ligaments.

Complete avulsion. When diagnosis in an acute stage is made, this injury must be treated by immobilization in walking plaster for six weeks.

But often, the diagnosis is not made until later when recurrent attacks of giving way of the ankle joint occur, requiring reconstruction of the fibular collateral ligament by ronaoviot tenodesis of the peroneus brevis tendon along with immobilization in walking plaster for six weeks. The results are quite satisfactory.

Complete rupture of deltoid ligament usually responds well to immobilization in a walking plaster for six weeks.

The hypermobile ankle. Exercises to strengthen the peroneal muscles and 'floating out' the heel of the shoe on the outer side are usually sufficient, but occasionally, reconstruction of the external ligament may be required.

Avulsion Fractures

When a ligament is avulsed from its attachment, it often pulls off a fragment of bone with it. In the ankle, such injuries occur in the following sites:

    i. the tip of either malleolus with injuries to the collateral ligaments

    ii. the superior aspect of the talus in a footballer's ankle

    iii. the anterior tubercle of the tibia with injuries of the anterior tibiofibular ligament.

These injuries do not require special treatment but should be treated as a severe ligamentous avulsion fracture in a walking plaster of Paris cast for six to eight weeks.

Fracture–Dislocation of the Ankle

Fracture–dislocation of the ankle is classified as follows:

1. external rotation injuries
2. abduction injuries
3. adduction injuries
4. vertical compression injuries
5. shearing or sideswipe injuries.

External Rotation Injuries

Forcible outward rotation of the foot or forcible inward rotation of the leg produces pressure on the outer aspect of the lateral malleolus, and it twists off the lateral malleolus and causes fracture, with the fracture line being oblique and running upwards and backwards from the level of the ankle joint. In pure external injuries, the obliquity of the fracture line is more marked. The fracture line may be as high as the fibular notch of the tibia. If it is the sole lesion, there is seldom any displacement. However, if the rotation strain is severe, a fracture of the medial malleolus will also occur, and the foot is rotated externally and displaced laterally. Further force will cause fracture of the posterior margin of the tibia, and the foot is usually displaced backwards as well as laterally (fig. 88).

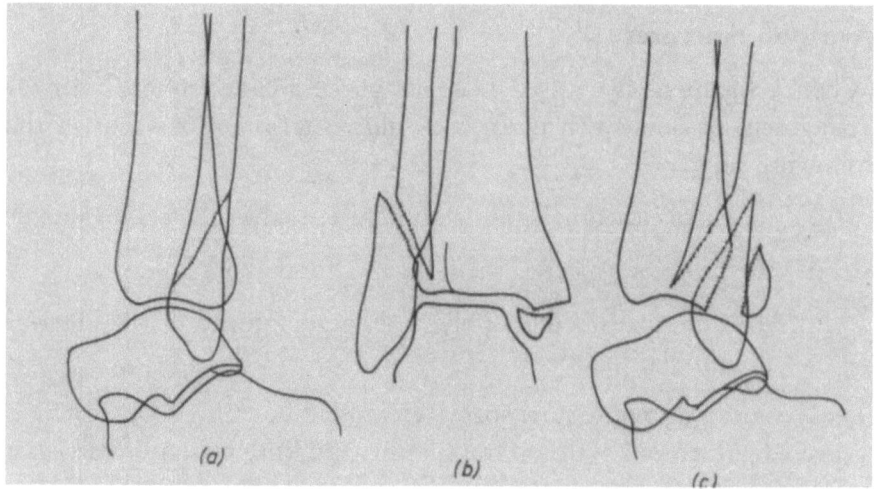

Fig. 88: External rotation injuries: (A) long oblique fracture of the fibula running upwards and backwards from the joint line. (B) Fractured fibula with fracture of the medial malleolus and lateral displacement of the talus. (C) Fractured fibula with fracture of the posterior malleolus of the tibia and posterior displacement of the talus.

Treatment without Displacement

No reduction of fracture is required. The patient can best be treated in a padded below-knee plaster cast for six to eight weeks. When initial pain and swelling have subsided, weight-bearing may be allowed.

In case plaster cast is not applied, infiltration of the fracture site with xylocaine and hyaluronidase will relieve the pain and swelling. It may be followed by pressure bandaging and elevation of the foot for a few days, followed by an elastic bandage strapping. Then the patient may start walking with weight-bearing. However, some tenderness and swelling are likely to persist for two or three months, which should not be the cause of any worry. No notice should be taken of it.

Fractures with Displacement

In fractures with displacement, proper reduction must be carried out under general anaesthesia with correction of any lateral or posterior displacement of the foot. The main criterion of reduction in all ankle fractures is the accurate replacement of the talus in the ankle mortise. In external rotation injuries, reduction can be achieved by forcible internal rotation of the foot since rotational deformity cannot be easily controlled by simple below-knee plaster and displacement is also marked. Fixation can be achieved by above-knee plaster cast with the knee flexed by 15 degrees or by a below-knee plaster cast incorporating a Steinmann pin through the upper end of the tibia. The plaster should be removed after three weeks, and if the X-ray film shows satisfactory position, below-knee plaster cast may be applied, and the Steinmann pin also may be removed. Light weight-bearing may be allowed.

Immobilization in plaster cast continues for 8–10 weeks. After the removal of the plaster cast, a crepe bandage must be applied, and exercises to the ankle joints must be given to restore the movements of the ankle and foot. Usually, it takes the same time as the period spent being immobilized in a plaster cast. It is important to accurately restore the displaced medial malleolus and the large posterior marginal fracture of the tibia by operative procedure and screw fixation to avoid any irregularity and early degeneration of the tibial articular surface and ankle joint (fig. 89).

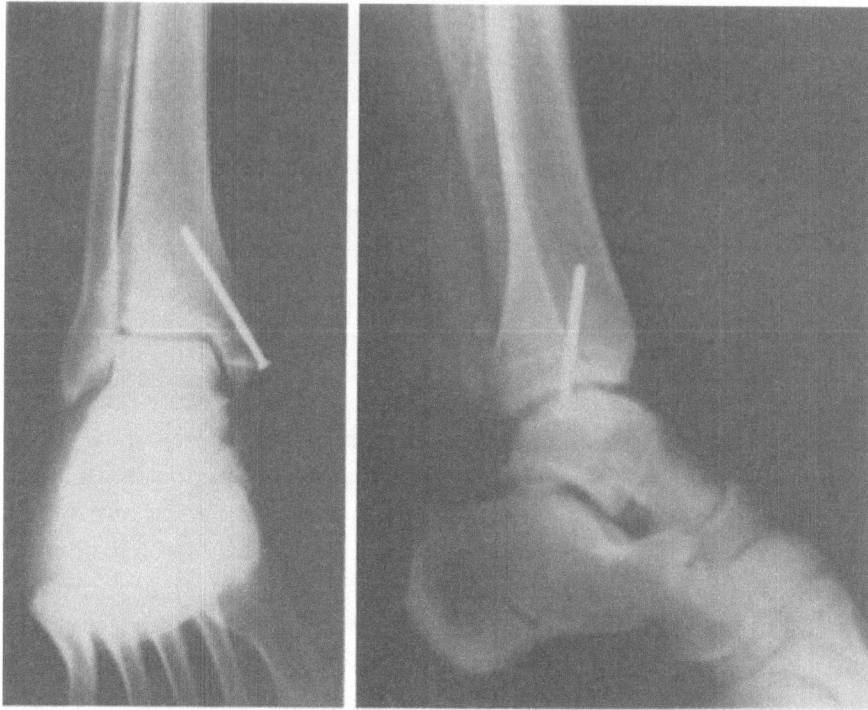

Fig. 89: Fracture of the medial malleolus treated by a single-screw fixation.

Fracture of the Fibula with Diastasis of the Ankle Joint

Fracture of the fibula with diastasis of the ankle joint is an uncommon injury and results from severe external rotation injury. In this injury, the inferior tibiofibular ligaments rupture, freeing the fibula from its tibial attachment, and the fibula is fractured in its upper third. This is also accompanied by diastasis of the inferior tibiofibular syndesmosis. As pain and swelling are mainly located at the ankle joint, the X-ray film shows diastasis of the syndesmosis, but X-rays of the upper part of the fibula shows an oblique or spiral-type fracture.

It may be possible to reduce the diastasis by closed manipulative reduction and plaster application, but it usually recurs as swelling subsides and plaster gets loosened. Hence, it is advisable to do screw fixation of the syndesmosis and immobilization by below-knee plaster cast for two months (fig. 90).

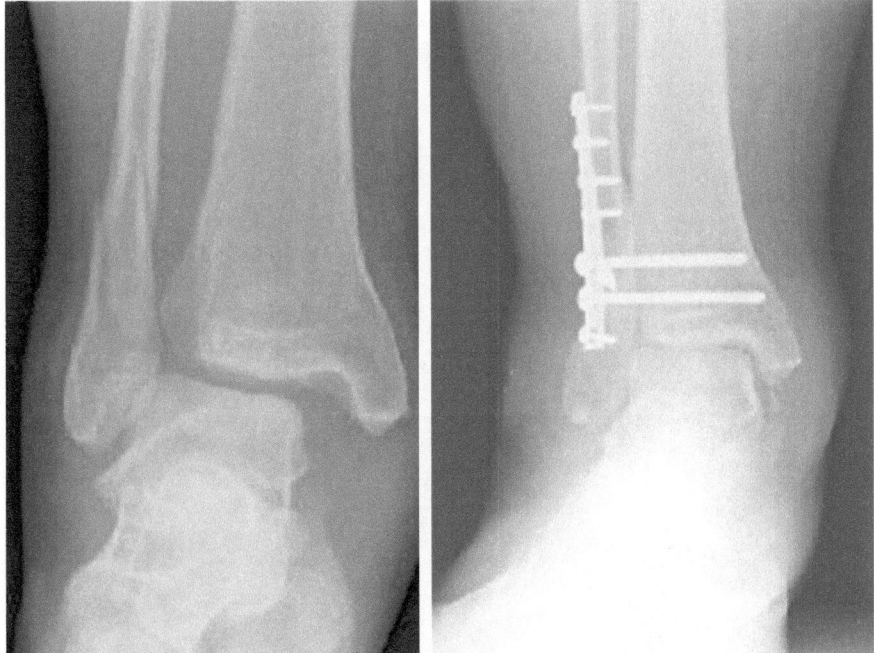

Fig. 90: Rupture of the syndesmosis with displacement treated by open reduction and plate fixation.

Abduction Injuries

Abduction injuries occur in about 20% of the cases but are markedly less common than external rotation injuries. However, certain amount of external rotation accompanies them, and pure abduction injuries are uncommon.

Abduction strain along with weight-bearing is an essential factor in the production of this fracture. The injury takes place in the manner that abduction strain causes first a fracture of the medial malleolus, usually transverse and near the tip, or rupture of the deltoid ligament. If the force continues, it will make the talus to impinge upon the lateral malleolus and result in:

1. rupture of the ligaments of the tibiofibular syndesmosis, diastasis, and fracture of the fibula, usually 2–3 in. above the tip of the malleolus

2. fracture of the lateral malleolus below the syndesmosis (tibiofibular ligament is not injured).

In both these injuries, lateral displacement of the foot occurs, but sometimes fracture of the posterior malleolus with posterior displacement of foot may occur.

Treatment

Abduction fracture with displacement requires open reduction under general anaesthesia and screw fixation of medial malleolus, followed by a padded above-knee plaster cast. If diastasis is also present, then screw fixation of the syndesmosis must be carried out (figs 91a and 91b).

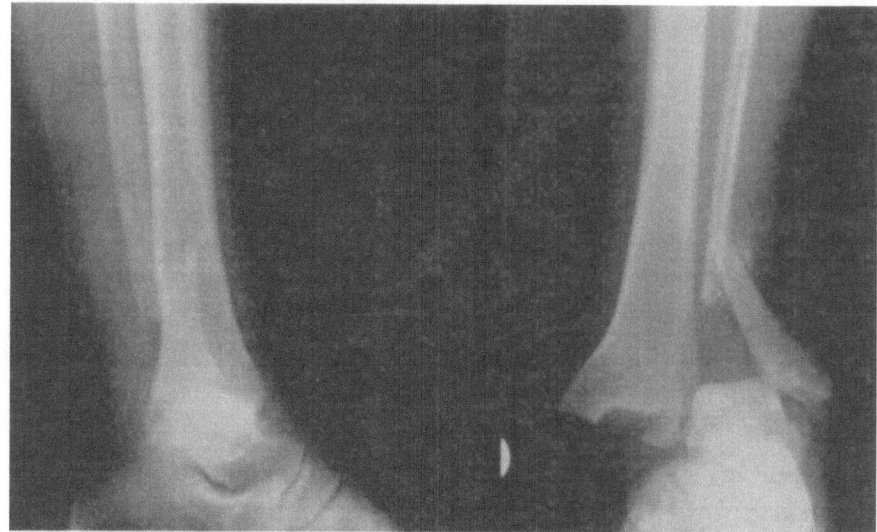

Fig. 91a: Abduction-type fracture of the fibula and medial malleolus with complete disruption of the tibiofibular syndesmosis and upward dislocation of the talus.

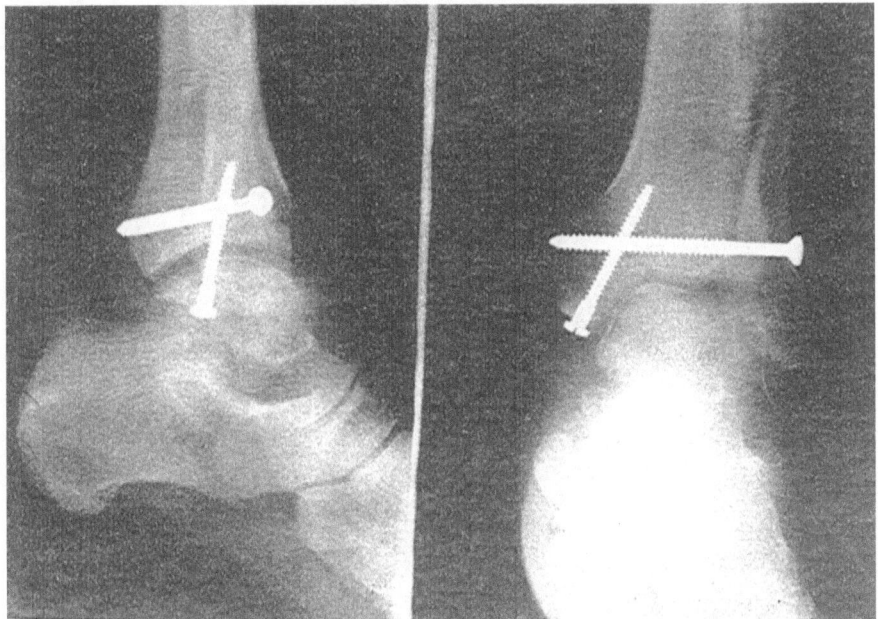

Fig. 91b: After reduction and screwing of medial malleolus, together with cross-screwing of the tibia and fibula.

Union of this fracture is slow; therefore, plaster immobilization is required for three months. The plaster cast may get loosened when the swelling has subsided; hence, a tight-fitting plaster cast must be reapplied. No weight-bearing should be allowed for six weeks from the time of injury.

Prolonged rehabilitation is required, but still, some residual limitation of movements may remain.

Adduction Injuries

Adduction injuries occur in about 10% of the cases.

Mechanism

Forcible adduction or inversion of the foot can cause:

1. a sprain or rupture of the fibular collateral ligament

2. a transverse fracture of the lateral malleolus at or below the main portion of the tibia

3. a fracture of the lateral malleolus along with a vertical fracture of the medial malleolus (fig. 92).

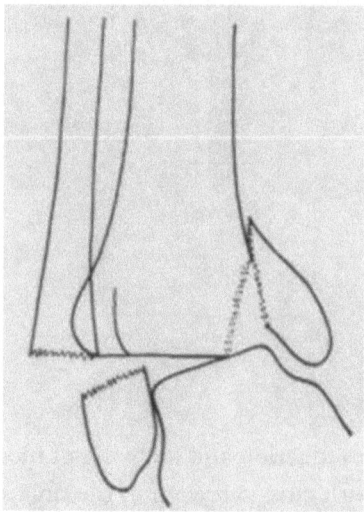

Fig. 92a: Adduction injury showing fracture of the lateral malleolus at joint level and vertical fracture of the medial malleolus.

These injuries commonly occur in young persons. Often, the damage to the articular surface of the tibia is more marked, and post-traumatic arthritis is not uncommon. Amongst the injuries of the ankle, this type is the most common, but adduction injuries are often combined with some degree of internal rotation.

Treatment

Simple first-degree fracture of the lateral malleolus is stable and can be treated by strapping, but it is better to give below-knee plaster cast for six to eight weeks, followed by early weight-bearing. Slight displacement of fracture of the lateral malleolus can be treated by immobilization in a plaster cast for at least eight weeks. When there is marked displacement of the lateral malleolus, the screw fixation is indicated and should be done, followed by padded below-knee plaster cast for 8–10 weeks. After four weeks, non-weight-bearing walking with crutches may be allowed. If joint surface has not been damaged, results are usually good.

Vertical Compression Injuries

Mechanism

Vertical compression injuries usually result from a fall from a height, and the pattern of the fracture depends on the position of the foot at the time of impact and the direction of the compression force.

With the foot in neutral position, the articular surface of the tibia is comminuted and displaced upwards (fig. 92b). If the main force falls on the forefoot, the foot is pushed into dorsiflexion, and the fracture of the anterior margin of the tibia occurs. Sometimes the anterior tubercle of the tibia is split off and displaced laterally. If at the time of injury inversion or eversion of the foot is present, the medial or lateral malleolus may be split off. Both malleoli may also be split off by the dorsiflexion type of injury, where the body of the talus may burst them open. If the foot is forced into plantar flexion, the main injury will be to the posterior margin of the tibia. This can occur from falls but can also occur from football injuries when the player kicks forcibly into the ground.

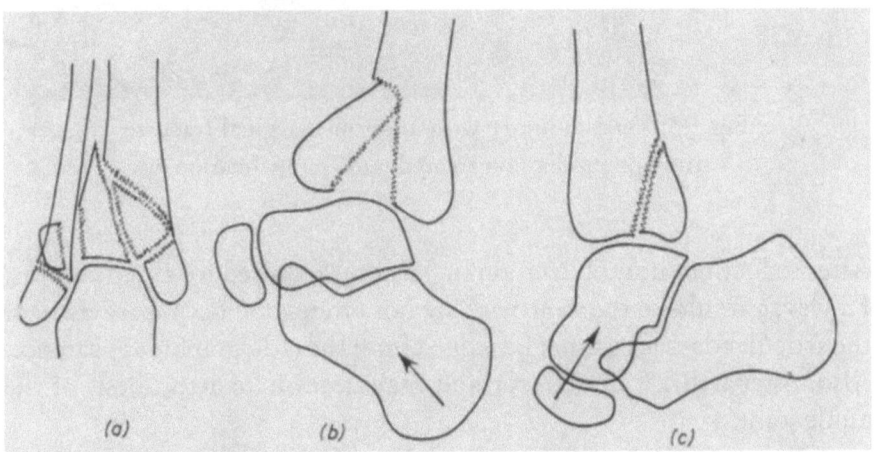

Fig. 92b: Vertical compression fractures: (a) fracture of the articular surface of the lower end of the tibia with lateral displacement and burst fracture of both malleoli, (b) anterior marginal fractures with anterior subluxation of the talus, and (c) isolated posterior marginal fracture of the tibia (slight anterior step is present).

Treatment

The aim of the treatment must not only be to replace the talus accurately into the ankle mortise, as with all fractures of the ankle, but also to restore the mortise itself as accurately as possible. Manipulation under anaesthesia followed by application of a well-moulded padded plaster cast may give good results, but large anterior or posterior marginal fragments requires open reduction and screw fixation (fig. 93).

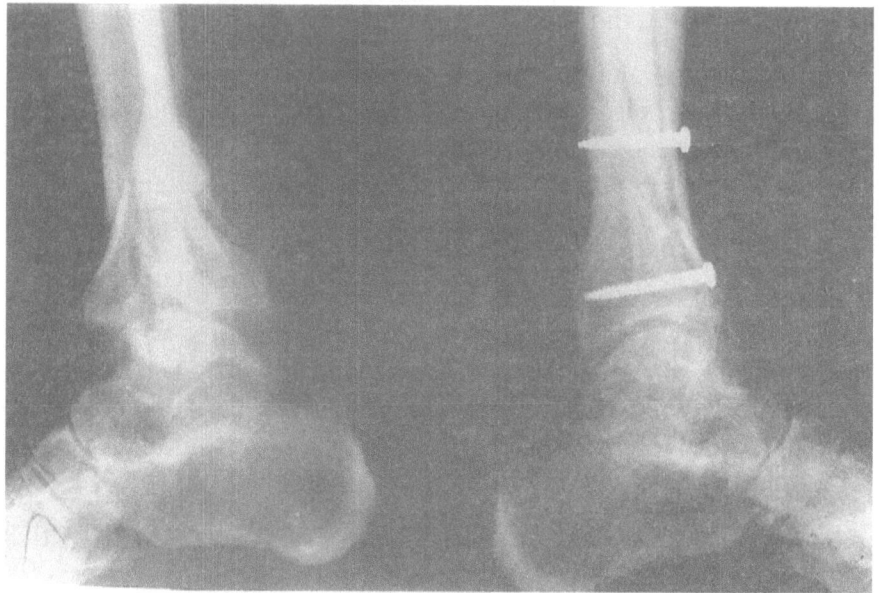

Fig. 93: Vertical injury with anterior marginal fracture and open reduction treated with screw fixation.

After reduction, immobilization in plaster is required for three months. However, results of the treatment are not often good because severity of the articular damage cannot be judged from the radiographic appearance. Also, osteoarthritis does occur and may necessitate arthrodesis of the ankle joint.

Shearing or Sideswipe Injuries

Shearing or sideswipe injury occurs from a direct blow with considerable force on either side of the ankle and is often seen in miners and motorcyclists. The injury is often compound, and the fracture is usually of the bimalleolar type and often comminuted (fig. 94).

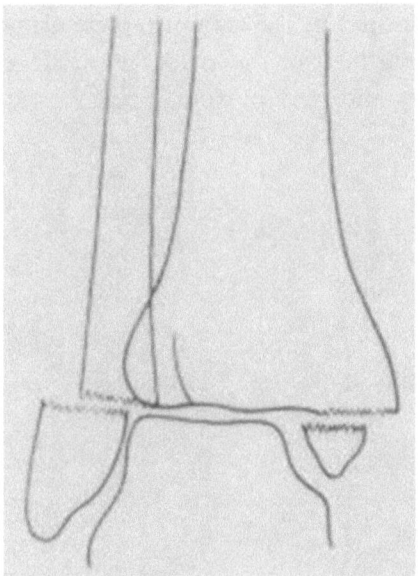

Fig. 94: Bimalleolar fracture due to shearing or sideswipe type of injury.

Treatment

Shearing or sideswipe injuries are usually unstable. Temporary fixation of the fractured malleoli by Kirschner pin wire may maintain stability and facilitate the inspection of the wounds, skin grafting, and treatment. If no open wound is present, screw fixation of both malleolus should be carried out, followed by immobilization in a below-knee plaster cast. The end result will depend upon the degree of soft-tissue damage and articular damage, but injuries of this severity are likely to result in some degree of permanent disability.

Fracture of Medial Malleolus

Avulsion fracture of the tip of the medial malleolus indicates complete avulsion of the deltoid ligament and is caused by abduction. Transverse fracture at joint level may result from abduction, external rotation, or shearing strain. In this type of fracture, the medial malleolus is often displaced forwards by the tibialis posterior tendon, and the soft tissue may be interposed in the fracture, preventing proper reduction. Sometimes small fragment of the articular cartilage is driven between the main fragments and may prevent a perfect reduction unless they are removed (fig. 95).

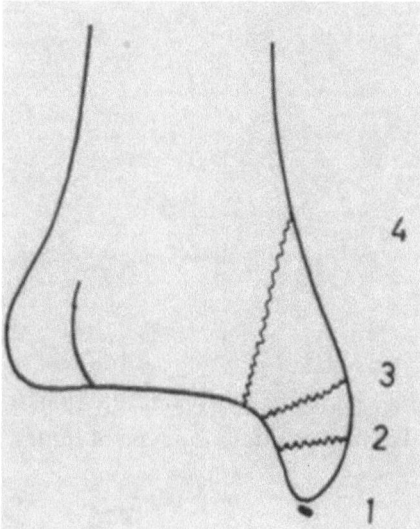

Fig. 95: Different types of fractures of the medial malleolus: (1) avulsion of deltoid ligament with the tip of the medial malleolus abduction, (2) fracture below the joint level (abduction), (3) fracture at joint level (abduction, external rotation, or shearing strain), (4) vertical fracture abduction.

Fracture of the Posterior Margin of the Tibia

Posterior marginal fracture of the tibia can occur in three ways. Most commonly, it occurs in association with external rotation injuries, where the body weight, combined with the rotation of talus, splits off the posterior margin of the tibia, and the lateral malleolus is also fractured, thus allowing posterior displacement of the foot.

Less frequently, it is caused by abduction injuries, but the marginal fragment is usually small.

Also, it occurs with vertical compression injuries when the foot is in plantar flexion. This is the only way in which an isolated fracture of the posterior malleolus can occur, but displacement is often minimal.

A small fragment may be left to unite itself, but if the fragment is large and involves over one-third of the joint surface and if satisfactory reduction cannot be obtained by closed methods, open reduction and fixation by a single screw is indicated.

Injuries of the Lower Tibial Epiphysis

This is the commonest fracture in the region of the ankle in children in the age group of 10–15 years. The epiphyseal plate separates from the metaphysis, taking with it a triangular wedge of the bone, usually on the posteromedial side, usually accompanied by spiral fracture of the fibula. Anterior or lateral displacement is rare (fig. 96).

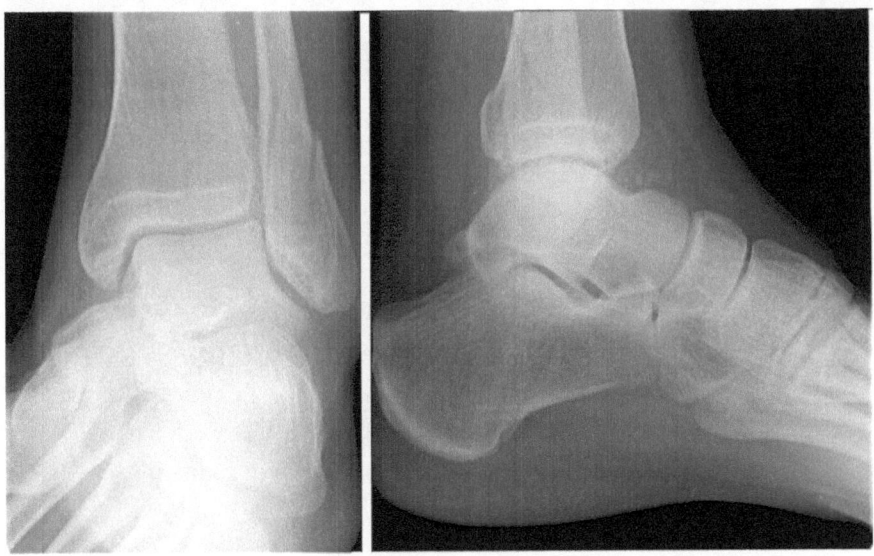

Fig. 96: Injury to the lower tibial epiphysis with posterior displacement. A large triangular fragment of the tibia is attached to the epiphysis and the spiral fracture of the fibula.

Treatment

Reduction can always be obtained by manipulation under general anaesthesia, but strong force is required to do so. The presence of a triangular fragment makes over-reduction impossible. After reduction, the leg is immobilized in an above-knee plaster for six weeks. Healing of fracture does occur quickly.

With adduction type of injury, a vertical fracture of the medial malleolus may occur which crosses the epiphyseal line, and fragment is displaced upwards. Damage to the epiphyseal plate may result in premature fusion on the inner side and an increasing varus deformity of the ankle (fig. 97).

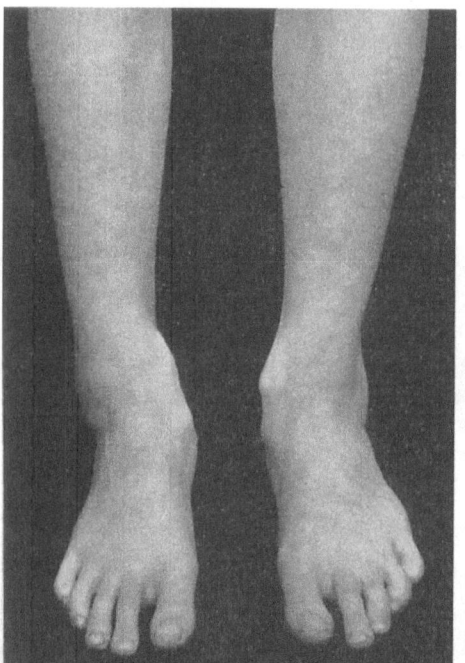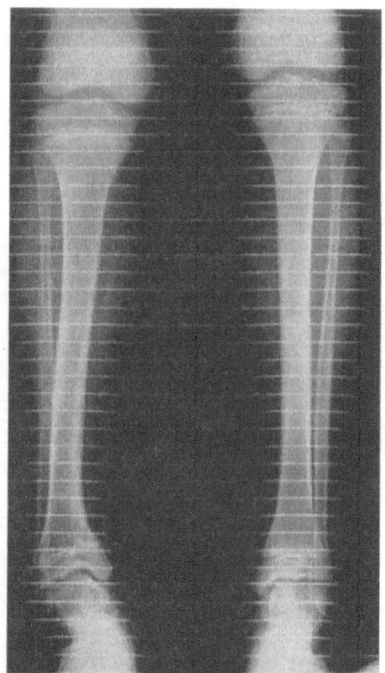

Fig. 97: Varus deformity of the right ankle joint following an injury to the medial aspect of the lower tibial epiphysis.

This can be prevented by accurate reposition of the medial malleolus by open operation. The position can be maintained by soft-tissue suture. However, screw fixation may be required, and transfixation of the epiphyseal line carries little risk of premature fusion, provided that the screw is removed as soon as union has taken place.

Epiphyseal Arrest

The varus deformity resulting from this requires osteotomy of the lower end of the tibia and is repeated at intervals till growth ceases. Alternately, an epiphysiodesis of the outer part of the epiphyseal plate can be carried out, but this will cause shortening of the limb. To avoid this complication, an accurate initial reduction of fracture is the best method of treatment.

Stress Fractures of the Fibula

Stress fractures of the fibula occur in cross-country runners, army recruits, and sometimes middle-aged women who stand for long hours. The onset is typical—a sudden severe pain during activity occurs over the site, at the lower end of the fibula, followed by local tenderness and swelling, increased local temperature, and redness. The condition may be bilateral. X-ray film shows no fracture for two weeks, but then it shows a zone of density or a transverse crack 1½–2 in. above the tip of the lateral malleolus.

Treatment

A supporting bandage with non-weight-bearing walking plaster cast for four to six weeks will relieve the symptoms, but vigorous sport activities must be avoided for three months.

CHAPTER 26

INJURIES OF THE FOOT

Fractures and Dislocation of the Talus

Chips and Avulsion Fractures

Small fragments of bone are sometimes avulsed from the neck of the talus when the anterior capsule is damaged by forcible plantar flexion of the foot. This is also called footballer's ankle. The posterior process of the talus can be avulsed by the pull of posterior talofibular ligament, which is fractured by forcible plantar flexion of the foot.

The dome of the talus is fractured either at the lateral margin or at the medial margin. These fractures are easily missed in radiological examination.

The mechanism of the injury varies for the above two fractures. The first occurs due to inversion and dorsiflexion strain, forcing the lateral margin of the talus against lateral malleolus, and second occurs due to a combined plantar flexion, inversion, and rotation strain.

The fragment is usually incompletely separated, but sometimes it is detached completely, and it lies upside down. The loose fragments should be removed, but cases with incomplete separation should be immobilized in a below-knee plaster cast for six to eight weeks till complete union takes place.

Crack Fractures of the Neck and Body of the Talus

Crack fractures occur occasionally without subluxation or dislocation of the subtalar joint. Crack fracture of the neck of the talus unites well and seldom causes disability, but fracture of the body of talus involves the articular surface of the talus in the weight-bearing area, and if displacement is also present, it may lead to traumatic arthritis.

Fracture–Dislocation of the Talus

These talar injuries can be further subdivided (fig. 98):

1. fractures of the neck or body with subtalar dislocation
2. fractures of the neck or body with dislocation of the body out of the ankle mortise.

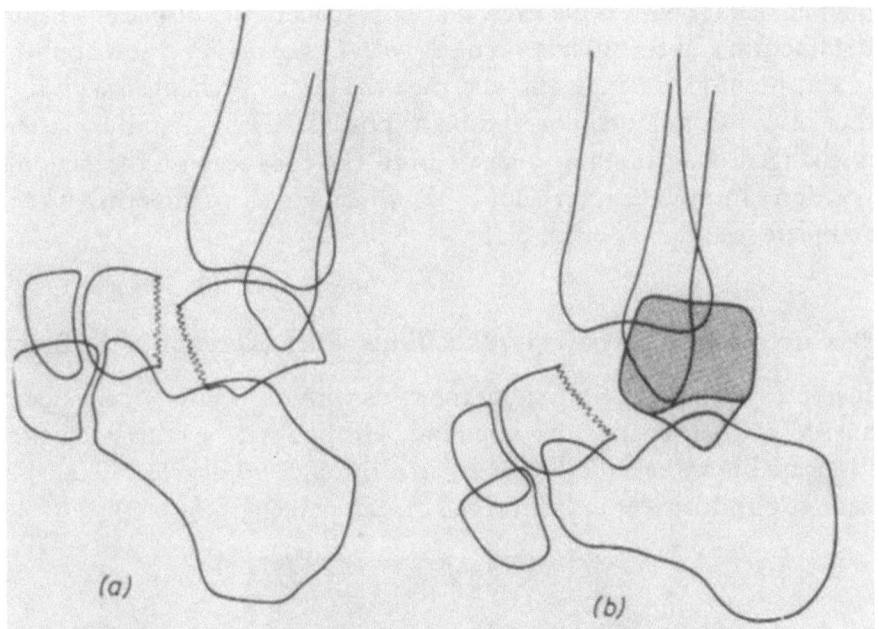

Fig. 98: Fracture of the neck of the talus: (a) subtalar dislocation and (b) complete dislocation of the body and rotation through 90 degrees.

Both these injuries are caused by forcible dorsiflexion injuries of the foot, with impingement of the neck or body of the talus against the sharp anterior margin of the tibia.

Fracture of the Neck or Body with Subtalar Dislocation

When a fracture occurs through the neck of the talus or through the anterior third of the body, there is an upward displacement of the head of the talus with dislocation of the posterior compartment of the subtalar joint and the calcaneus is displaced forwards with the rest of the foot. The same displacement occurs with fracture through the body.

Treatment

In both cases, the foot must be forcibly plantar-flexed under general anaesthesia, and plaster must be applied. The foot should be in full plantar flexion with some eversion. This reduces the displacement of the fracture and the subtalar joint. A below-knee plaster cast is applied in this position for six weeks, and then the plaster is changed with the foot placed in as much dorsiflexion as possible. Thereafter, the plaster is changed at fortnightly interval until the foot reaches the neutral position. Immobilization should continue for three months, when complete healing has taken place.

Fractures of the Neck or Body of the Talus with Dislocation of the Body

Fractures of the neck or body of the talus with dislocation of the body are serious injuries and are compound. The body of the talus is usually dislocated posteromedially and rotated through 90 degrees; it can be palpated under the skin behind the medial malleolus (fig. 99).

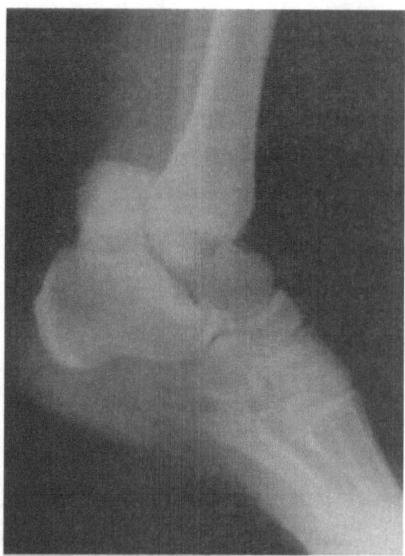

Fig. 99: Fracture of the talus with displacement of the body out of the ankle mortise.

Treatment

In closed injury, manipulative reduction can be done by applying strong traction to the foot, with a Kirschner nail through the calcaneus and foot held in dorsiflexion and eversion. Firm pressure is then applied over the displaced body to force it back into place. If this method fails, the displaced fragment should be transfixed with a Steinmann pin to facilitate manipulative reduction. If neither of these methods are successful, then open reduction is carried out. Sometimes it may be necessary to break the medial malleolus to reduce the body of the talus into ankle mortise with the help of a transfixed Steinmann pin. The fracture can be fixed back by a screw. The ankle is immobilized in below-knee plaster cast for three months so that union takes place.

Total Dislocation of the Talus

Total dislocation of the talus is an uncommon injury. The intact talus is displaced from the mortise and can be found in any position, of which anterolateral is most common. Secondary fracture, particularly of the medial malleolus, commonly occurs.

Where talus is displaced out of the mortise, reduction is a great urgent matter in order to prevent sloughing of the skin, which becomes tightly stretched over the displaced bone.

Complications

In the injuries of the fracture–dislocation of the talus, avascular necrosis of the body of the talus may occur. It can be diagnosed by increasing radiological density of the body, which can be detected within two to three months of the injury. The incidence is highest with the dislocation of the body, but it also occurs in one-third of the cases of fractures through the neck with subtalar dislocation. It is not a quite serious complication, and if immobilization is continued for four to six months, in the majority of cases, revascularization takes place. If this does not occur, and painful arthritis has taken place, the treatment is pantalar arthrodesis.

Dislocation of Subtalar and Midtarsal Joints

The common dislocation is medial dislocation produced by a forced inversion strain on the foot. It is easily recognized by marked inversion deformity of the foot, and the head of the talus is prominent on the dorsum of the foot. Reduction can be easily done under anaesthesia, and it should be done as soon as possible to avoid damage to the skin. The foot and ankle should be immobilized in a plaster cast for four to six weeks.

Fracture of the Calcaneus

Fracture of the calcaneus usually results from a fall from a height on to one or both heels. This fracture is often bilateral and may occur in association with fractures of the spine. The usual mechanism is a combination of compression and shearing strain. They may be subdivided as follows:

1. Isolated fractures not involving the subtalar joint (fig. 100). This is a small group which includes (fig. 101):

    a. fracture of the medial tuberosity

    b. beak fracture of the tuberosity

    c. fracture of the anterior process.

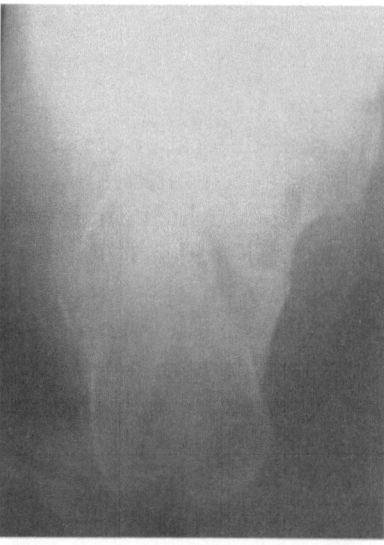

Fig. 100: Isolated fracture of the calcaneus.

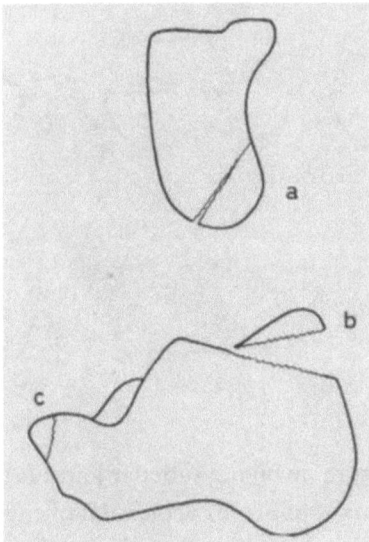

Fig. 101: Isolated fracture of the calcaneus not involving the joint: (a) fracture of the medial tuberosity, (b) beak fracture of tuberosity, and (c) fracture of the anterior process.

2. Fractures involving the subtalar joint. Majority of fractures fall in this group, which include:

   a. involving but not displacing the posterior articular facet
   b. involving the posterior articular facet with depression of the lateral fragment which usually includes nearly over half of the joint surface
   c. uniform depression of the whole posterior facet
   d. complete disruption of the subtalar joint
   e. isolated fracture of sustentaculum tali (fig. 102).

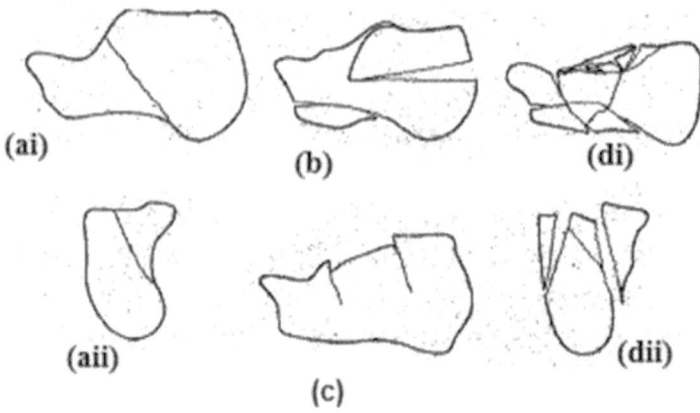

Fig. 102: Fracture involving subtalar joint: (a) fracture with no displacement of joint, (b) depression of the lateral part of the joint surface, (c) depression of the whole of joint surface, and (d) complete disruption of the joint surface.

In majority of cases, the fracture line runs from medial tuberosity forwards and laterally, leaving the posterior joint surface into two equal fragments. There is compression and comminution of the lateral fragment. Lateral displacement of the lateral fragment commonly occurs.

Diagnosis

This fracture is often missed due to inadequate history, clinical examination, or radiography, but diagnosis is easy on the basis of following points:

1. A complaint of pain in the heel after a fall from a height.
2. On clinical examination, tenderness and broadening of the heel with a characteristic bulge beneath the lateral malleolus (after two to three days, bruising is usually visible on the sole of the foot under the long arch). In all severe fractures, the patient is unable to stand or tiptoe on the affected side, and movements of the subtalar joint are limited and painful.

3. Adequate radiograph, which must include:
   a. a lateral film of the ankle and heel
   b. axial view of the calcaneus
   c. an oblique view of the foot
   d. anteroposterior view of the ankle and midtarsal joint.

A comparative view of the other foot is often helpful.

Treatment of Isolated Fractures Not Involving the Subtalar Joint

Initially, the treatment required is compression bandaging and elevation of the foot until the swelling subsides. Then it may be followed by plaster cast for four to six weeks. After two weeks, weight-bearing may be allowed. The treatment usually gives good results.

The beak-type fracture can be reduced by manipulation and immobilization in a plaster cast, but sometimes operative replacement may be required.

Treatment of Fracture Involving the Subtalar Joint

Fractures involving the subtalar joint are difficult to be treated, and disability as a result of it runs into many months.

   a. Fractures involving but not displacing the posterior articular face: These fractures do not require reduction but should be treated in a plaster cast for three months. This will prevent displacement to occur. When the swelling and pain have subsided, the plaster may be changed after two weeks, and the patient may be allowed non-weight-bearing walking with the use of crutches. The results are generally good, but it takes five to six months before the patient becomes fit for work.

   b. Fractures involving the posterior articular facet with depression of the lateral fragment: When the outer fragment is large, reduction can be achieved by the use of Steinmann pin, levering the fragment down to restore the joint surface and then immobilizing the foot in plaster, incorporating the pin for six weeks (fig. 103).

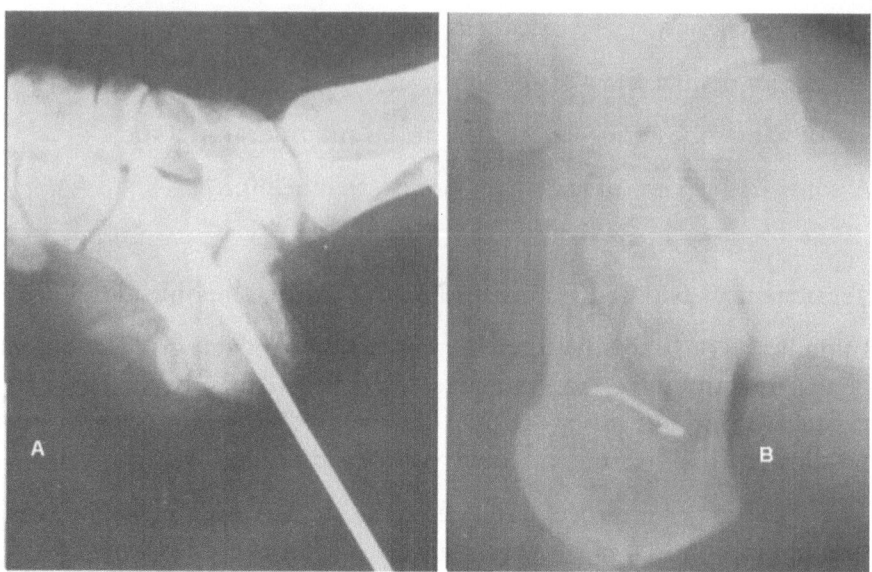

Fig. 103: Fractured calcaneus treated by elevation with a pin and staple fixation.

A fresh radiograph must be taken. If it shows that healing has taken place, the pin may be removed, and a new plaster may be applied, but weight-bearing must be avoided for further six weeks.

If this treatment is not successful, open reduction and replacement of the fragment should be undertaken. After the operation, a plaster cast is worn for three months.

If untreated, these fractures unite badly, and due to distortion of the subtalar joint, they lead to secondary arthritic changes and valgus deformity of the foot. The treatment is arthrodesis of the subtalar joint with restoration of the proper position of the foot and correction of the valgus deformity of the foot.

c. Uniform depression of posterior facet: It will require an operation to do the elevation of the fragment, and it gives good results. If depression is a minor one, it may be treated by a plaster cast for six weeks. After the operative treatment, a plaster cast is to be applied for 10–12 weeks.

d. Complete disruption of the subtalar joint: In this case, the subtalar joint is damaged beyond repair, and decision is required to adopt conservative treatment and spontaneous ankylosis or, better still, to do subtalar arthrodesis. This must be done within four weeks of the injury, and good results are obtained. If it is delayed, residual disability along with pain occurs. The disability may take the following forms:

  i. lateral submalleolar pain and tenderness, usually over the outer side of the calcaneus, probably due to scarring around the peroneal tendons

  ii. persistent pain under the heel

  iii. rigid valgus flat foot

  iv. excessive dorsiflexion of the foot

  v. inability to take weight on tiptoe on the affected side, resulting in the inability to run or climb stairs

  vi. pain from secondary arthritis of subtalar joint.

Injuries of the Forefoot

Dislocation of the Tarsometatarsal Joints

Dislocation of the tarsometatarsal joints results from forcible lateral rotation of the forefoot. The damage is usually greatest at the level of first interosseous space, and various degrees of separation occur between the first and second metatarsals. Extensive damage to the soft tissue occurs, including all the ligaments of the metatarsals and cuneiform and cuboid joints, and the bases of the metatarsals are displaced laterally. Occasionally, damage to the dorsalis pedis artery occurs, and if damage is severe, gangrene of the forefoot may occur. Sometimes the base of the metatarsal remains intact. Cuneiform is dislocated at its articulation with navicular, and it may be rotated completely.

Treatment

Closed reduction should be attempted, but sometimes it is not successful. Then open reduction and internal fixation are carried out to prevent redisplacement. This can be easily done by Kirschner pin/nail (fig. 104), and fixation of the first to the second metatarsal base is the key to a stable reduction, which may require the use of several pins. A plaster cast is applied, incorporating the pins and is retained for eight weeks, although pins may be removed after three weeks. Usually, good results are obtained.

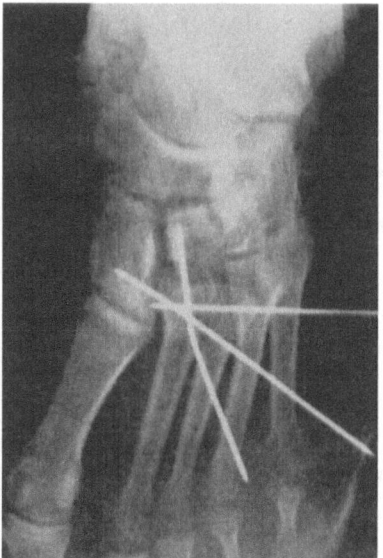

Fig. 104: Fracture of the metatarsals with displacement treated by cross pins.

Fractures of the Metatarsals

Avulsion Fracture of the Base of the Fifth Metatarsal

Avulsion fracture of the base of the fifth metatarsal results from forcible inversion of the foot. The base of the fifth metatarsal is torn off by the attachment of the peroneus brevis tendon.

Treatment

A below-knee plaster cast for four to six weeks will make the fracture to unite, and it gives good results. Sometimes infiltration with local anaesthesia, followed by adhesive strapping for three to four weeks, is sufficient and produces good results.

Fractures of the Neck of the Metatarsals

These fractures are usually stable, but sometimes the head of the metatarsal may be displaced downwards and may cause metatarsalgia (fig. 105).

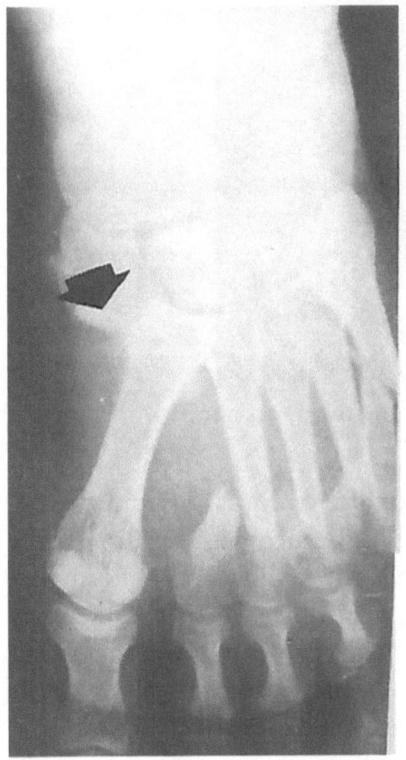
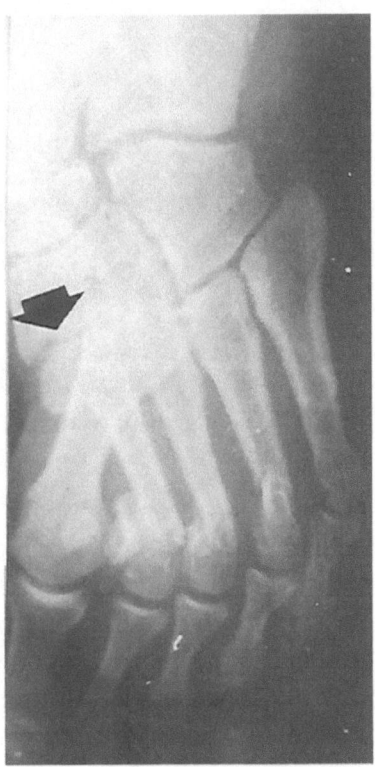

Fig. 105: Fracture of the neck of the metatarsals.

Treatment is by manipulative reduction when displacement is there, followed by a plaster cast for four to six weeks. Walking may be allowed after 10–14 days.

Stress Fracture of the Metatarsals

Stress fracture of the metatarsals is also called march fracture because it occurs in army recruits after route marches. The second or third metatarsals are often affected (fig. 106).

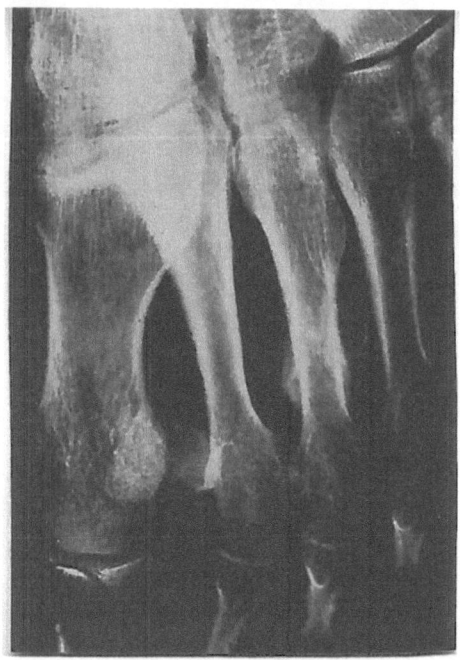

Fig. 106: March fracture of the third metatarsal.

There is sudden onset of pain during or after the activity, and there is tenderness over the affected metatarsals, associated with swelling of the dorsum of the foot and redness as well. X-ray shows no abnormality for the first two weeks, but after this, a fusiform mass of callus may be seen around the affected metatarsal, with or without a crack on the neck of the metatarsal. Immobilization in plaster for four to six weeks is required, and weight-bearing must be avoided for three weeks.

Some patients can be treated by simple bed rest with avoidance of weight-bearing for three weeks, followed by a metal bar support to the shoe for one month.

Fractures of the Phalanges

Fractures of the phalanges usually result from a heavy weight being dropped on the foot. No splintage is necessary except for the big toe. In some cases, strapping of the forefoot is beneficial, along with walking in broad-based shoes or shoes cut open in the front portion.

Fractures of the terminal phalanges are usually accompanied by a subungual haematoma, and prompt decompression by trephination with a red-hot needle or wire paperclip may save the nail.

CHAPTER 27

CHEST INJURIES

Injuries of the Ribs and Sternum

The twelve ribs on each side of the thorax are encased in their own soft-tissue structure. Anteriorly, ribs 1 through 10 are attached to the sternum through costochondral cartilage. The twelfth and occasionally the eleventh rib have no attachment to the sternum. The ribs have enormous plasticity, allowing considerable distortion in shape before reaching the limit of this elasticity and fracturing.

Mechanism of the Injury

The mechanism of the injury in rib fracture in a non-pathological situation is invariably one of a direct blow. The direct blow will fracture one or more ribs but usually leave them within their soft tissue case. If the force of the injury is not expended at this point, however, the fractured rib may be forced internally through the parietal pleura and possibly even into the lung tissue itself. It may happen, but it is rare for the fractured ends to penetrate the skin and communicate with the air.

Simple and Multiple Fractures

Little bleeding occurs with the simple rib fracture within the soft-tissue structure of the thorax cage. Occasionally, a rib or several ribs are fractured at two different points. Because of the negative pressure within the pleural cavity, such circumstances create the flail chest that has the paradoxical motion of moving inwards when inspiration occurs.

Examination

In a true fractured rib, the pain is created when the patient's sternum is compressed towards the spine with counter-compression against the spine. The patient can usually point to the site of the fracture.

X-ray Examination

The definite interruption of the cortices of the fractured rib(s) may or may not show on the X-ray film (fig. 107). Rotational views are often helpful in visualizing the fracture(s).

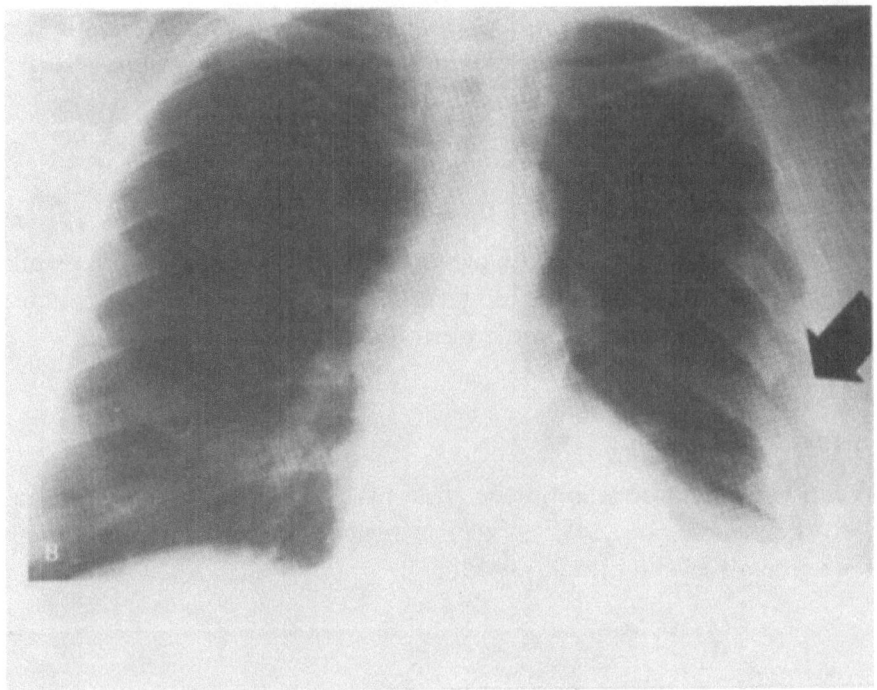

Fig. 107: Fractured ribs (4 to 7). Arrow points to the fracture of the sixth rib.

Treatment

Elastofoam or elastocrepe: An elastic bandage coated on one side with polyurethane foam is useful to maintain immobilization when ribs are fractured. Strapping of the involved side of the thorax with a tape may be helpful, but this should extend past the midline anteriorly and posteriorly. However, this strapping must be applied in position of deep inspiration and withholding of the respiratory movements. Intercostal nerve blocks proximal to the fracture may also be beneficial and will completely finish the pain pattern caused by the fracture. The Elastoplast wrapping diminishes the pain which occurs with inspiration and expiration to such an extent that it becomes tolerable within several days to a week. There is a tendency by the patient to do shallow breathing in an attempt to splint the fracture and prevent pain. This may lead to atelectasis, and patient should be instructed to do deep breathing in order to maintain adequate aeration of the lungs.

The most effective method of managing the flail chest is to use endotracheal intubation with positive pressure breathing. The positive pressure of the endotracheal system provides a better gas exchange.

Tearing of the Pleura and Puncture of the Lung

In the event of a tearing of the pleura, a chance exists for blood to spill into the pleural cavity. If the lung has been injured by the rib fragment, the air may also escape into the pleural cavity.

X-ray Examination

A fluid level will be seen on the chest plate if there has been bleeding into the pleural cavity. When air has escaped into the cavity, one may see a free-air level on the X-ray film.

Treatment

The patient with haemothorax and fractured rib(s) may be treated by wrapping the thorax with an elastic bandage. If the fluid level is too high, it may be aspirated, following the use of local anaesthetic. However, this procedure must be used only when there is evidence of increased pressure within the pleural cavity from haemorrhage. In the event of pneumothorax, the patient may require the insertion of tubes through a suction seal to accomplish the re-expansion of the lungs.

Costochondral Separation

Costochondral separation is another injury to the ribs. This is the separation of the bony end of the rib from the cartilage structure joining it to the sternum. The costochondral separation occurs from a direct blow just like in a rib fracture. It tends to occur in a person who infrequently engages in contact sports. It is a painful process, with the pain being severe with inspiration and expiration.

X-ray film will not show the injury since the cartilage is radiolucent.

Treatment

The most effective treatment is the use of elastofoam or elastocrepe. Usually, by a week's treatment, the intense pain subsides and gives way to tolerable discomfort, and by the end of two weeks, the patient is comfortable without external support. Sometimes it may take three to four weeks to recover completely.

Fracture of the Sternum

The sternum consists of three segments superimposed on the manubrium, which is attached to the clavicle at a notch on each side. The manubrium of the sternum attaches to the body of the sternum at the second rib level by a synostosis. The lower extension of the body of the sternum has attached to it a small segment of cartilage which is called xiphoid process. An injury to the sternum occurs by a direct blow. The sternum is primarily of cancellous bone with broad surface so that significant displacement seldom occurs. Just posterior to the superior sternum lies the arch of the aorta. Behind the lateral margin of the sternum, at its junction with the rib cartilage, lie the internal mammary vessels. This close relation must be reckoned with any significant displacement injury.

Examination

The patient may or may not be able to give an adequate history. When he does, it is usually one of being stuck on the anterior thorax by an object, such as the steering wheel. Palpation will show pain and tenderness at the area of fracture. There may or may not be palpable displacement or angulation. In any sternal injury, a closed heart injury or aortic injury is possible. Auscultation of the heart or aorta may reveal harsh murmur at the aortic or pulmonary area. Such murmurs are distinctly abnormal and must be explained and investigated. X-ray examination and, if required, angiography must be done. If angiography shows tear of the aorta, surgical repair of the aorta must be undertaken immediately.

X-Ray Examination

In a plain chest X-ray film (fig. 108a), one may see some haziness of the arch of the aorta, either at its cardiac origin or as it starts its decent in the intercostals arteries (fig. 108). Angiography can reveal the tear, either at the origin of the aorta or in its course.

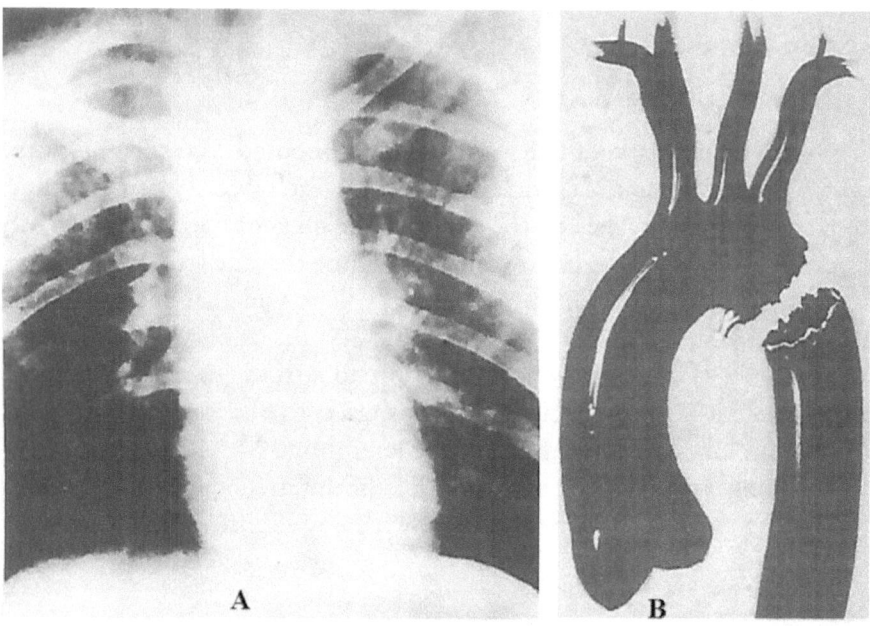

Fig. 108: (A) X-ray film shows haziness of the aortic arch and widening of the superior cardiac shadow. (B) Illustration of the tear in aortic arch of the patient. Prompt surgical correction is necessary upon recognition of this entity.

A fracture of the sternum may or may not show itself on the X-ray film. A true lateral view may show interruption of the anterior and posterior cortex, and it is most likely to give indication of a fracture. Direct injury to the xiphoid process also occurs, and the tip of it may be seen displaced towards a posterior direction.

Treatment

The uncomplicated fracture of the body or manubrium of the sternum seldom requires treatment, although the patient is more comfortable if the chest is wrapped in a bandage. Even though the direct injury to the xiphoid process is symptomatic, it is of no long-term consequence and only requires symptomatic treatment.

Sternoclavicular Dislocation

The mechanism of the injury in the sternoclavicular dislocation may be a direct blow to the medial clavicle which forces this head posterior in its relationship to the sternum. This is, however, an uncommon injury. The sternoclavicular dislocation is not a common injury, but when it does occur, it usually results from a force driving the shoulder posteriorly and leaving the head of the clavicle anteriorly and a little superiorly. This dislocation can occur only with tearing of a portion of the ligamentous attachments.

Examination

On examination, a comparison with the opposite uninjured side, a variation in the position of the clavicle can be seen. In the more typical type of injury, the upper margin of the clavicle is palpable, more anterior and superior than its fellow of the opposite side. Often, ecchymosis is present over the joint area. On palpation, local tenderness is also present.

X-Ray Examination

X-ray examination of both the injured and normal side should be taken, but in general, rotational views are necessary, including oblique views from the anterior to posterior side.

Treatment

Anaesthesia must be given. Then it may be possible to direct the head of the clavicle back into its normal relationship with the sternum. This method is usually applied first by increasing the anteroposterior force against the outer shoulder with one hand while directing the head of the clavicle with the other hand. As soon as the clavicle begins to fit into its relationship with the sternum, the shoulder is brought forwards. Should reduction occur and stability be established, the arm is bandaged to the chest (fig. 109). Elastic wrapping is often used for this dressing, and 6 in. plaster should be used over the soft padding to keep the bandage from shifting.

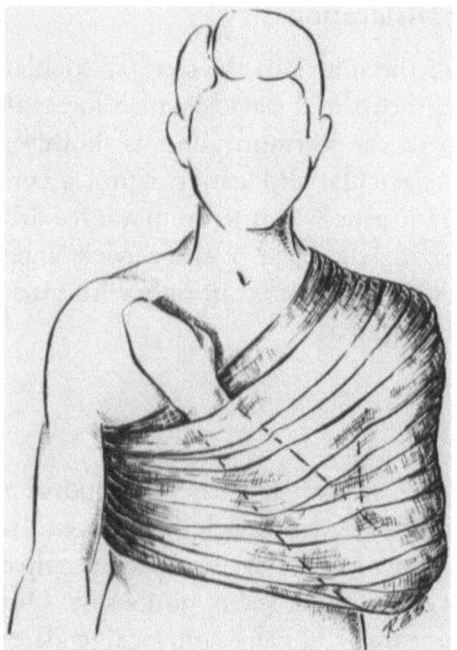

Fig. 109: Bandage used to immobilize the shoulder girdle.

If closed reduction fail, open reduction may be performed, and fixation of the clavicle with sternum may be done with a threaded Kirschner wire. It should be remembered that vital structures are lying just posterior to the area of the injury.

Sometimes these remain painful for many months or years after the injury and would require appropriate treatment.

Fractures of the Ribs and Sternum in Children

Rib fracture generally occurs in children after a crush injury. Because of marked elasticity of children's rib, the usual fracture in a child is greenstick type. It may be difficult to see it on an X-ray film (fig. 110), but oblique X-ray of the thorax with bony detail may be of great help.

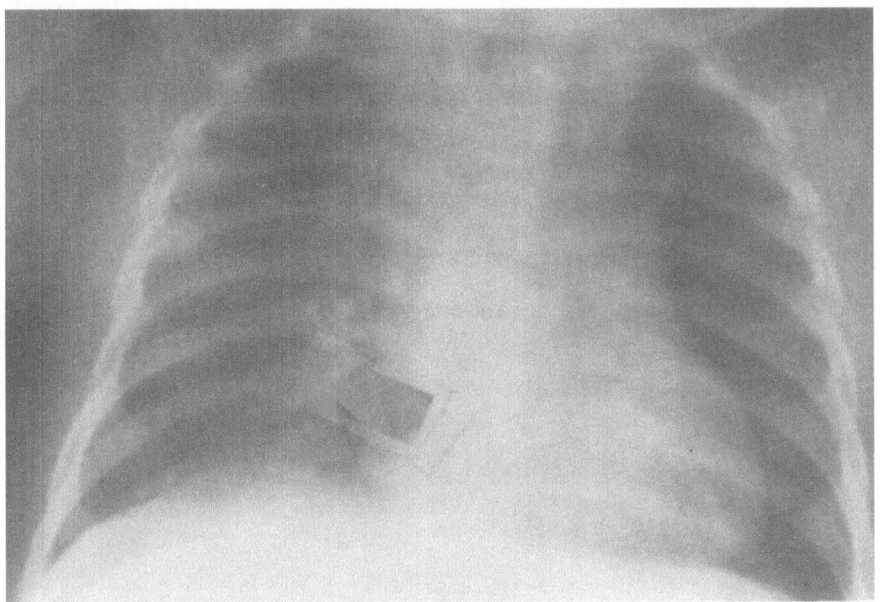

Fig. 110: Fracture of ribs with arrow.

The use of elastocrepe bandage may be helpful in providing great comfort to the patient in early days, and the child gets well soon. Many children can be treated by simple analgesics.

Fractures of the sternum occur rarely in older children, but if it occurs, it can be treated by simple body jacket.

CHAPTER 28

FACIAL FRACTURES

The face skeleton consists of bones of the jaws, nose, and cheeks. These include the mandible, maxilla, and zygoma, the palatine nasal and lacrimal bone, lateral orbit and zygomatic processes of the frontal, and temporal bones. Their borders are not well demarcated from other bones of the skull, and these bones are light, thin, and fragile.

The facial bones are important socioeconomically as well as functionally, and accurate reduction of the fracture segments is very important.

If the fractures of facial bones are open or associated with laceration, the laceration should be closed carefully and early. A delay of a week or so in the treatment of facial fractures will usually not impair the facial result.

Fortunately, facial fractures are rare in children. However, nasal fracture should be treated accurately as deformity may become marked as the nose grows.

Physical Examination

A careful examination of the facial fractures is very important for diagnosis. Almost all facial fractures can be diagnosed accurately by four areas of the examination. They are mandibular, maxillary, nasal, and malar. Gross displacement and dissymmetry will be easy to detect.

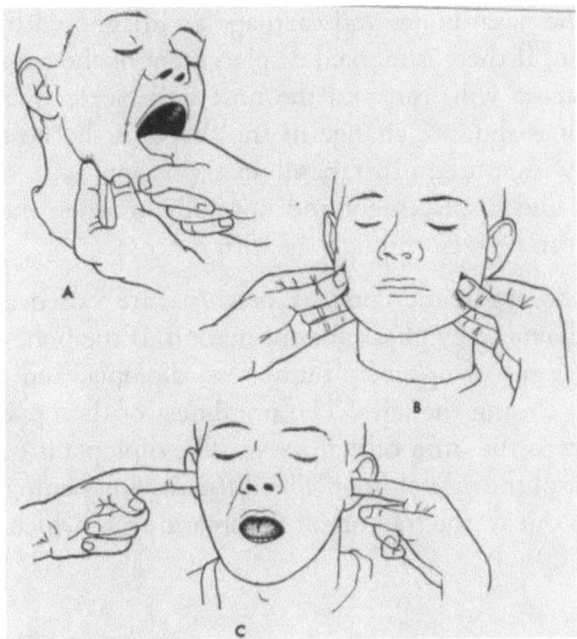

Fig. 111: Physical examination of the mandible.

If the fractures involve the jaws, the teeth will not occlude properly. If the mandible is injured, this will deviate on the opening, on closing, or on both. The body of the mandible can be palpated best with one examining finger along the lingual side and the other used externally. The angle and posterior edge of the mandible can be felt simultaneously. The mandible has got the shape of a horseshoe and is bent in the middle with the ends fixed against the heavy bone of the skull. The circular effect is such that if stress is applied, causing one fracture, another fracture in the same line of force or a dislocation at the temporomandibular joint will occur. For example, a blow directly on the chin may cause fractures of both condylar ends, a bilateral fracture at the angle, or a bilateral body fracture.

Injuries to the maxilla or portions thereof are easy to diagnose. The key to diagnose is motion. If bones cannot be moved intraorally, the fracture is probably not significant. If the teeth cannot resume pre-injury occlusion, it shows that the maxilla is involved.

Injuries of the nasal bones and cartilage are diagnosed by inspection and palpation. If there is marked displacement of the nasal bones, the adherent mucosa will tear, and the nose will bleed. If inspection of the nasal bones shows a change in the shape of the nose, the bones are probably fractured. Intranasal examination will reveal septal haematoma, and displacement and normally an open fracture of the nasal bones can be seen through the torn mucosa.

Injuries to the zygomatic complex or cheek are varied and are very difficult to diagnose by physical examination. If the bone is fractured, it will show signs of upper-lip numbness, diplopia, and difficulty in opening and closing the jaws. The numbness of the upper lip occurs due to injury to the infra-orbital nerve. The diplopia is caused by the displacement of the orbital floor. The difficulty in opening and closing the mouth is due to the fracture of zygomatic arch, which is displaced inwards.

X-Ray Examination

X-ray examination of facial bones is often difficult but is necessary.

The X-ray examination of the mandible requires anteroposterior, lateral, and right and left oblique views. This is also necessary for maxillary fractures because maxillary fractures are hard to be seen by anteroposterior and lateral views. If there is a fracture of the zygoma or the orbital floor, there may be blood present in the maxillary sinus. Nasal fracture can be seen in lateral view and anteroposterior view. However, the functions of these bones and facial contour are more important, and X-ray appearance is not.

Anaesthesia

All facial fractures can be reduced under general anaesthesia. Fractures of the mandible, maxilla, and nose can be reduced satisfactorily under nerve blocks and infiltration of the fracture site. The nasal mucosa can be anaesthetized by local application of xylocaine or similar agent.

Treatment

Mandibular Fractures

The fracture fragments are usually displaced because of the pull of strong muscles attached to them. The mandible is the most massive of the facial bones, and the strong methods of fixation are required to maintain the reduction of most injuries of this bone. Since the goal of treatment is to restore the teeth to their original position, teeth can be used to assist in maintenance of the reduction. As a general rule, the more teeth a patient has, the more reduction can be maintained by the use of these teeth. It is important to achieve accurate reduction so that the teeth will occlude properly. If there is a single fracture with good dentition, the fracture can be held by the use of interdental wiring, and the correct occlusion can be maintained by a few weeks of intermaxillary fixation (fig. 112). For intermaxillary fixation, wire loops are placed on the maxillary teeth, and jaws are wired into occlusion. The intermaxillary fixation may be removed in four weeks' time, and loops may be kept for 7–10 days longer. The patient is allowed to progress from liquid to solid food. When the patient can chew actively without pain at the fracture site, fixation may be removed.

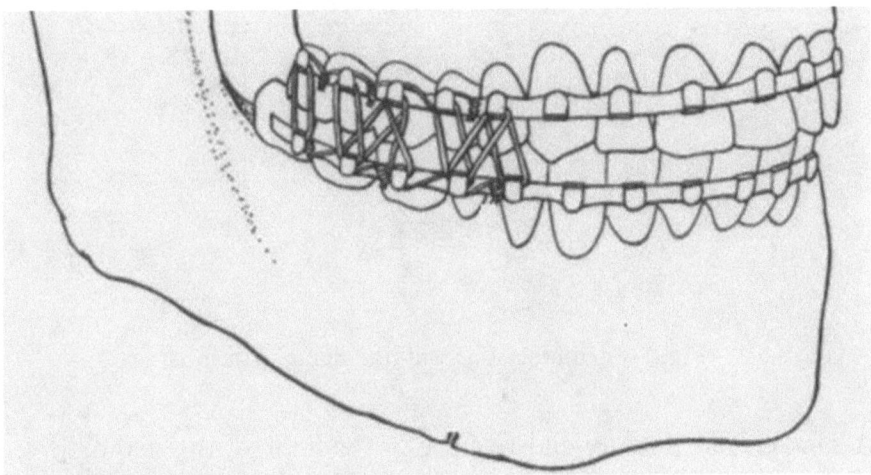

Fig. 112: Interdental fixation.

A liquid diet will suffice when the jaws are closed, but a simple basic diet consisting of milk, eggs, and sugar may also be given. Vitamin liquid should also be given based on the daily requirements. The diet may be supplemented or doubled when required. The patient is advised to watch his weight because, on an average, about 10 lb of weight is lost when jaws are wired for four to six weeks.

When two mandibular fractures are present, reduction and internal fixation can be done. A chosen method is to use figure-of-eight heavy wire through four drill holes in the lower mandible, below the roots of the teeth (fig. 113).

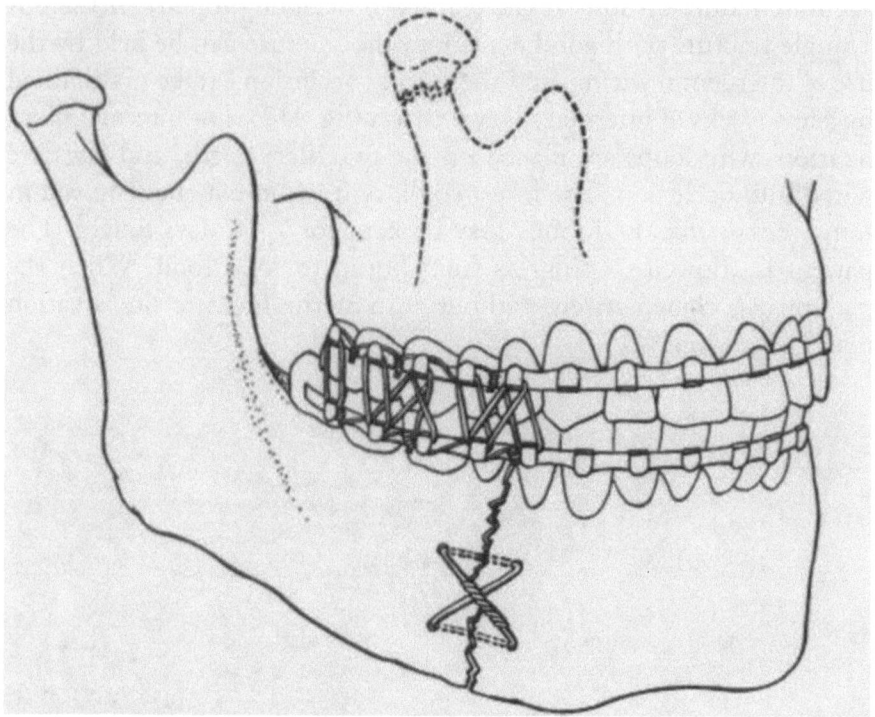

Fig. 113: Interosseous and interdental fixation.

A subcondylar fracture and fracture of the body of the mandible on the opposite side should be treated by direct interosseous wiring of the fracture of the body and intermaxillary fixation to hold the teeth in occlusion. Open reduction of the fractures of the body and rami is done often, but the approach is rarely required to be done for condylar fractures. If an open reduction of condylar fracture is necessary, the exposure of the bone should be done in such a manner that blood supply to it will not suffer.

Non-union is rare in mandibular fractures. Infection at the fracture site sometimes develops, which will require removal of internal fixation to allow the infection to heal. In case of osteomyelitis, the devitalized bone should be removed, and wound should be drained. If a defect develops, bone chips or bone chain can be used to fill the defect.

Maxillary Fractures

The maxilla is irregular in shape. Injuries to the maxilla involve the articulating bones and seldom of the maxilla alone. A significant injury to the maxilla results in instability of the upper jaw or a portion of it. The maxilla heals at a slower rate than most of the bones of the facial skeleton, but maxillary fractures are not greatly disturbed by muscle pull.

There are three common fractures of the maxilla (fig. 114):

i. The fracture includes the alveolar process, the palate, and pterygoid process in a single detached block.

ii. There is a transverse fracture line through the middle of the nasal bones, through the frontal process of the maxilla, across the lacrimal bone, through the orbital plane and infraorbital margin, and along the maxillary zygomatic suture line.

iii. The fracture occurs at the junction of the facial bones with the cranium. The bones of the face are detached from the cranium through orbits across the root of the nasal bones and at the zygomatic frontal suture line.

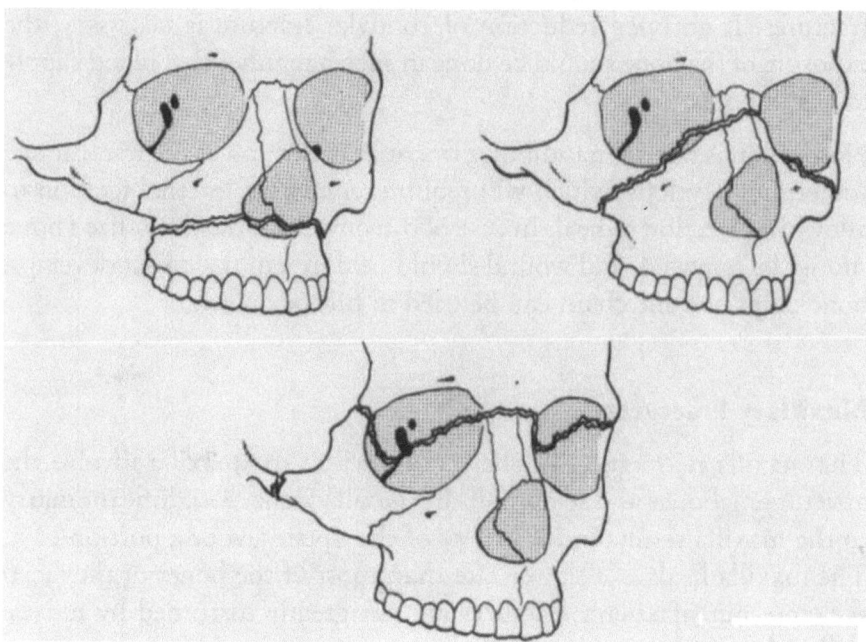

Fig. 114: Types of maxillary fractures.

Most maxillary fractures will involve one side or a portion thereof, such as the alveolar ridge. In the treatment of maxilla fracture, occlusion of the teeth may be used for stabilization of the fracture. Because of slow rate of healing, the fixation is maintained for 10 to 12 weeks (fig. 115). Non-union rarely occurs in this method of treatment of immobilization.

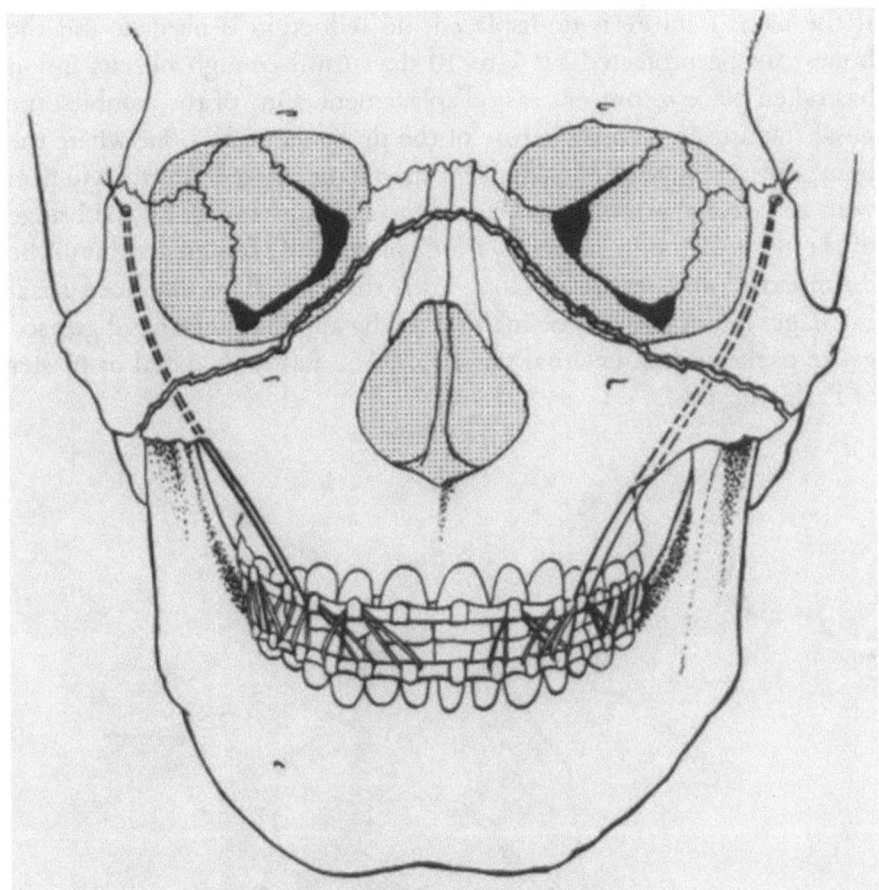

Fig. 115: Fixation of the maxillary fracture.

Nasal Fractures

Nasal bones are most frequently fractured facial bones. The nasal cartilage, which forms the soft part of the nose, is very important in nasal injuries, especially the septal cartilage, which may be either dislodged from its insertion or dislocated from the vertical plate. The healing of an injured nasal cartilage is less certain than the healing of the nasal bones since deformities often develop.

Nasal fractures are treated in one of the three ways: no treatment, closed or open reduction with immobilization by splint, or external skeletal fixation.

If the nasal fracture is undisplaced, no reduction is needed, and the bones can be protected for 7 to 10 days until enough fibrous union has taken place to prevent easy displacement. One of the troublesome nasal fractures is a chip fracture of the tip of the nasal bone where the bony septum joins the cartilage septum. Often, these fractures will heal with an overgrowth of bone, resulting in a bony hump on the bridge of the nose. If the nasal bones are displaced, the fragments should be disimpacted and realigned along with the injured or displaced nasal cartilage. Reduction can be maintained by applying intranasal greased gauze packs and an external nasal splint of malleable metal or plaster of Paris (fig. 116).

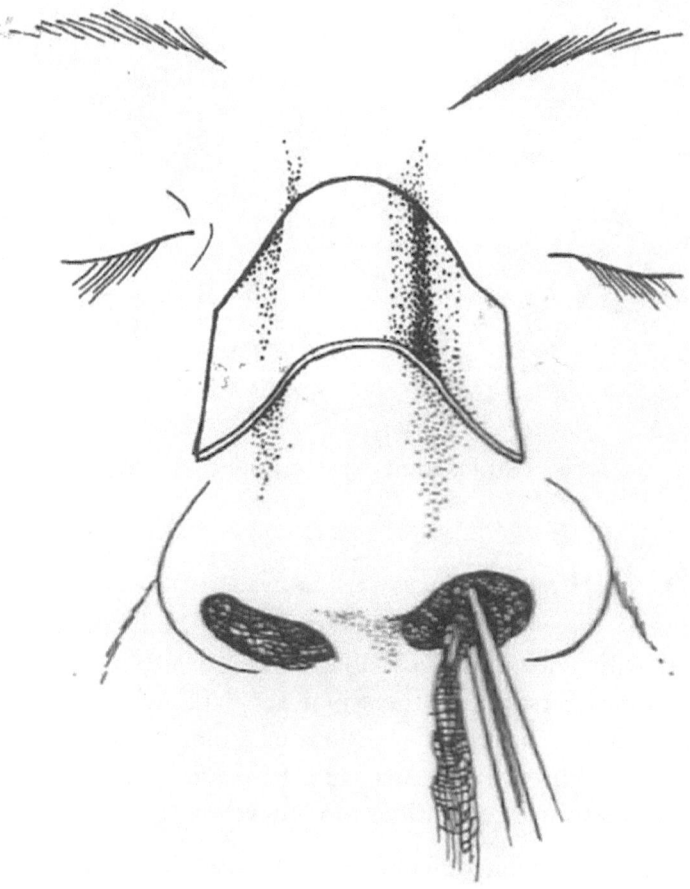

Fig. 116: Treatment of nasal fracture by nasal splint and intranasal greased gauze packs.

The intranasal packs may be removed in 24 to 48 hours, and the splint is removed in 7 to 10 days. The splint should be changed every two or three days till it is visible that the nasal skin is tolerating the splint well. Too much pressure by the splint against the bones will cause necrosis of the nasal skin. The unstable or severally comminuted nasal fractures are treated by applying two thin plates of aluminium on either side of the nasal bones and are wired to each other transnasally (fig. 117). They can be left for two or three weeks until the fragmented bone becomes firm.

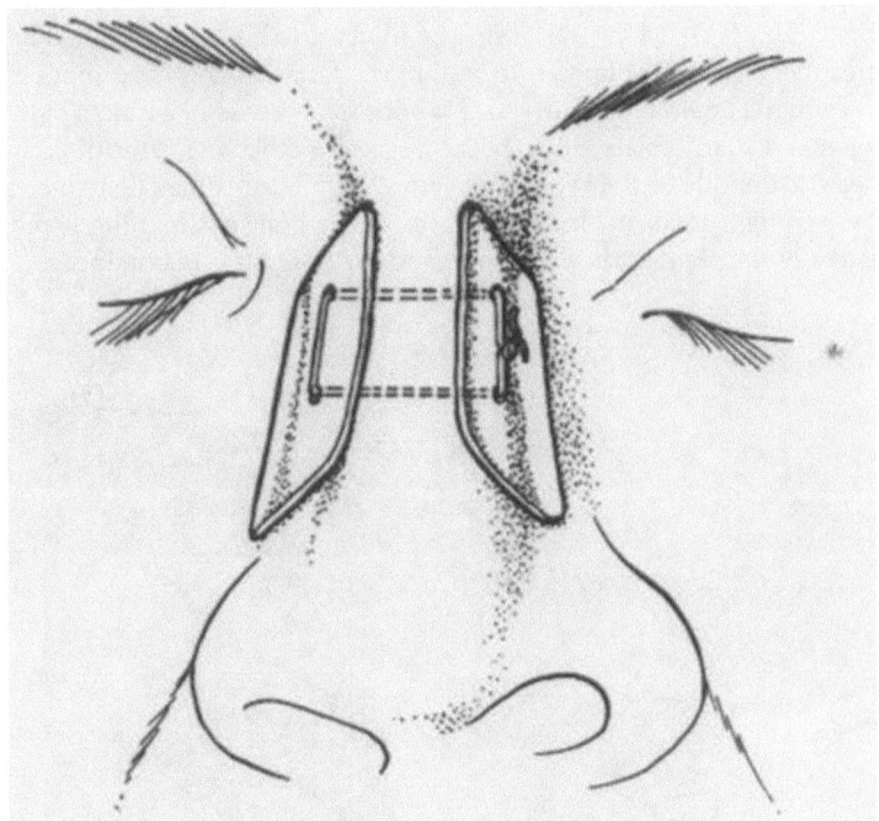

Fig. 117: Treatment by thin aluminium plates on either side and fixation by transnasal wiring.

There are a few complications from nasal bone fractures. The septal cartilage may buckle after trauma, causing obstruction, and will require partial resection for relief. If nasal bone heals with a disturbed contour, rhinoplasty may be required to restore the contour to normal. Infection rarely occurs. Occasionally, nasal fractures may be associated with a spinal fluid leak, but most of the leak will stop spontaneously.

Fractures of the Zygomatic Process

The zygoma also articulates with many other facial bones, and injuries rarely involve the zygoma alone. This bone is massive and forms the lateral wall and a portion of the inferior wall of the orbit. The zygomatic bone to be completely separated by fracture would involve three fracture lines (fig. 118). Many variations of injury to this bone occur. The treatment given is supposed to restore the facial contour and support the orbit. The simplest injury to this bone structure results from a blow against a sharp object, such as the edge of a table or a door directly against the side of the zygomatic arch. At times, this may be reduced by passing a small hook directly behind the bone and pulling it out laterally. The bone may spring out, and the position is maintained.

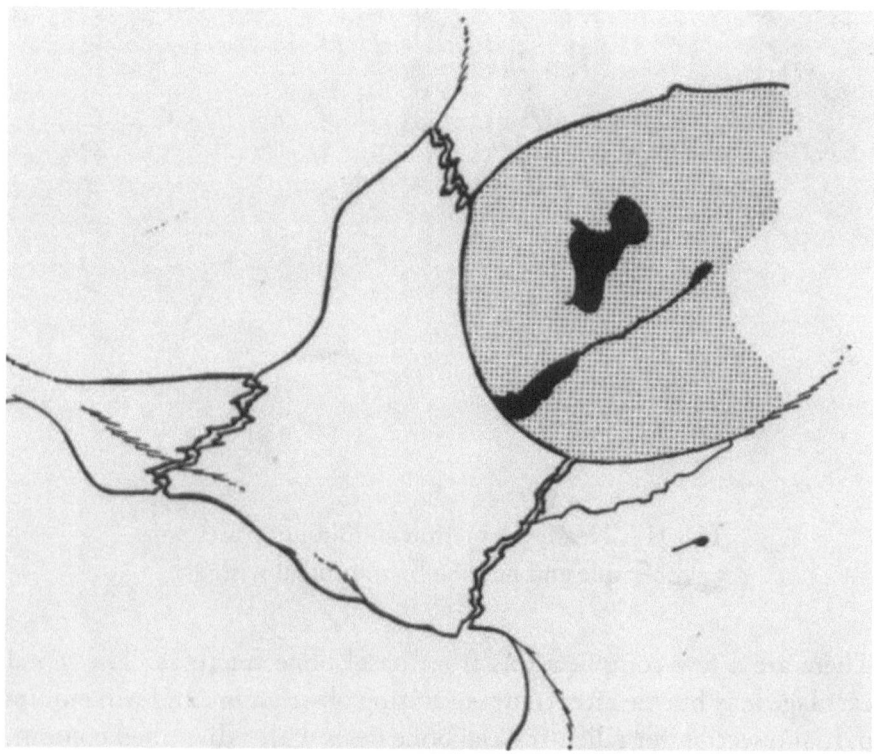

Fig. 118: Types of zygoma fractures.

Another approach is to make a small incision in the temporal region near the hairline. Open the temporal fascia and pass an elevator inferiorly to the coronoid process and then elevate the fracture. Care must be taken not to go below the temporal fascia to avoid injury to the frontal branch of the facial nerve. This technique can be used to reduce a complete fracture of the zygomatic bone (fig. 119).

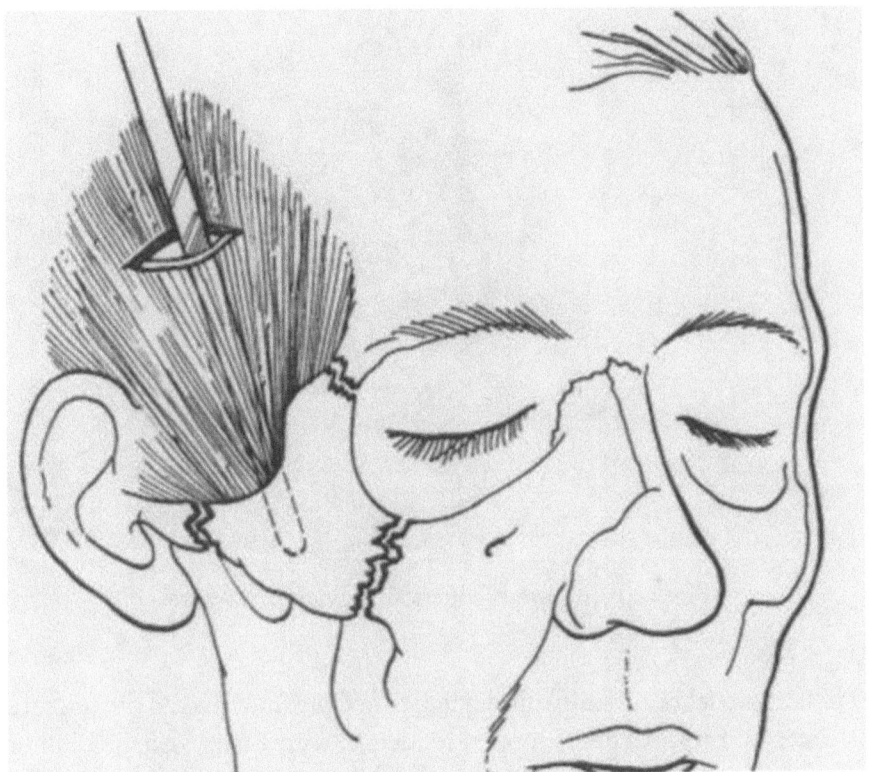

Fig. 119: Temporal reduction of zygoma fracture.

A similar approach to the fractured zygoma is made intraorally by incision in the buccal mucosa above the tuberosity of the maxilla and insertion of an elevator into the notch formed by the posterior border of the arch and lateral zygomatic wall, thus elevating the fragments (fig. 120).

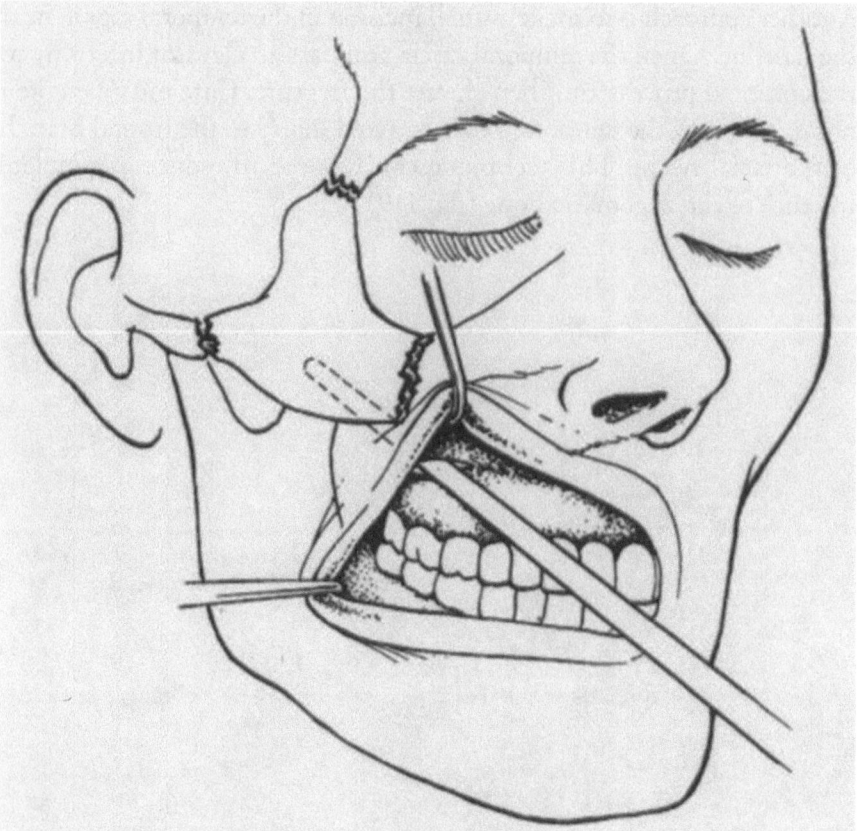

Fig. 120: Intraoral reduction of zygoma fracture.

These approaches are simple and quick to operate. However, if the fracture is complex and unstable, an open reduction with direct visualization of the zygomatic arch, especially the orbital floor, may be carried out. The orbital floor may be fractured and displaced, and if the eye muscles and ligamentous structures are not involved, there will be no enophthalmos or diplopia, but it must be watched carefully as these complications may develop later on and need to be treated by open reduction.

Multiple Facial Fractures

The patient with multiple facial fractures usually has associated injuries that have to be treated, either first or concomitantly. The principle of treating multiple fractures is to find the fixed point (which is usually the zygomatic process of the frontal bone) and then, by internal skeleton fixation or external skeleton fixation, to align the facial bones in relation to this fixed point and to one another.

All the facial bones are broken, maxillary fracture is freely movable, and mandible fracture is also present. The method of fixation is done. The zygomatic bone is fixed with wire to the frontal bone. The frontal bone is fixed to the maxilla by wire. The maxillary sinus are opened and packed. The nasal bones are moulded and fixed with two metal plates that are wired to each other. A Kirschner wire is passed from the malar prominence to increase stability. The mandibular fracture is not disregarded. In patient with full dentition, arch bars are placed on the maxilla and the mandible, and these bars are fixed to each other and to the zygomatic frontal suture line (fig. 121).

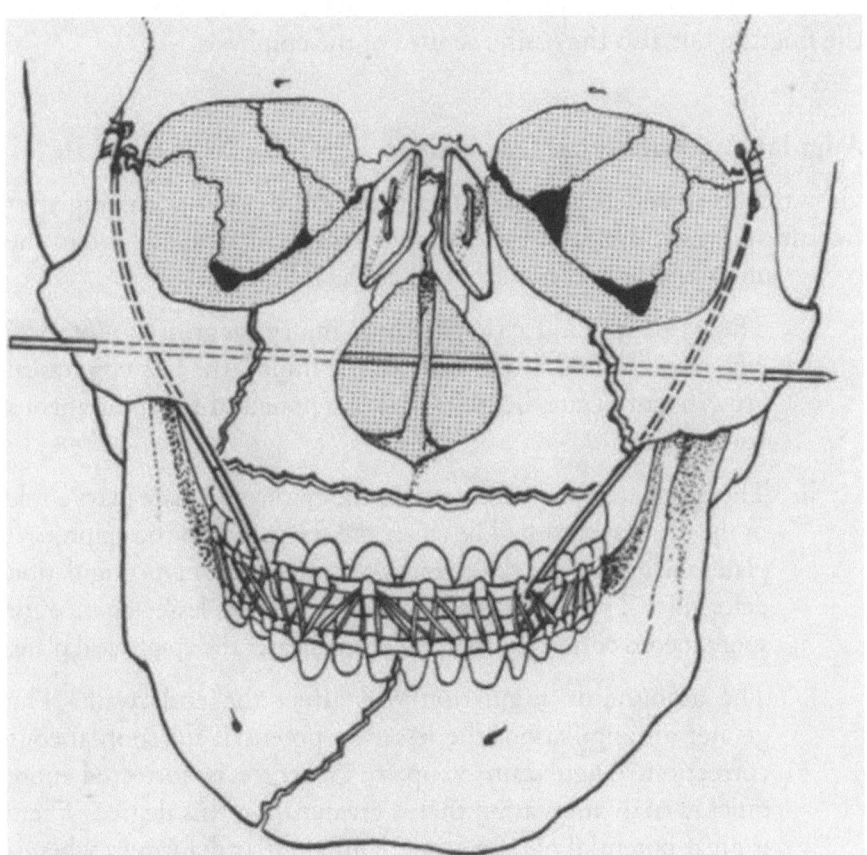

Fig. 121: Fixation of multiple facial fractures.

CHAPTER 29

FRACTURES IN CHILDREN

Fractures in children are different. The basic principle of treatment of fractures in children is to reduce it to an acceptable position and not cause potential damage to vital structures adjacent to the fracture.

In order to evaluate the fracture of the limb in a child, the X-ray must be taken at planes varying from one another by 90 degrees and must include the joint above and below the fracture. In addition, it may be necessary to take views of the opposite limb, which can be compared with the views of the injured limb. This way, one can assess not only the fracture but also the ossific centres of the epiphysis.

Angular and Rotational Deformities

Growth and remodelling can correct many deformities occurring after fractures in the child. There are many factors which contribute to the correction of angular deformity, such as the following:

i. The age of the child at the time of an injury has great significance. The older a child at the time of the injury, the less epiphyseal growth can occur; hence, less is the potential for spontaneous correction.

ii. The distance of the fracture from the epiphyseal plate plays a role in the ultimate result. The closer the fracture is to the epiphyseal plate, the greater are the chances of correction of any angulation deformity. Thus, a mid angulation will have lesser chance for spontaneous correction than a fracture nearer the epiphyseal plate.

i. The amount of angulation will affect the end result. The greater an angulation, the lesser its potential for spontaneous correction. Angulation of up to 15 degree is corrected more quickly than angulation that is greater than this degree. There is great potential of correction of an angular deformity when it occurs in the plane of motion of a nearby hinge joint

Rotational deformity of the longitudinal axis of a long bone must be corrected because the child has no growth mechanism to correct it. The rotational deformity can be identified by comparison of the X-ray film with that of the uninjured side. It can also be done by measuring the width of the proximal and distal fragments near the fracture site. These fragments should be equal. However, due to rotational deformity, one fragment may be wider than the other, and the bone near the fracture line will be oval and not round.

Injuries of the Epiphysis, Epiphyseal Plate, and Metaphysis

Epiphyseal injuries are classified into five different types (fig. 122).

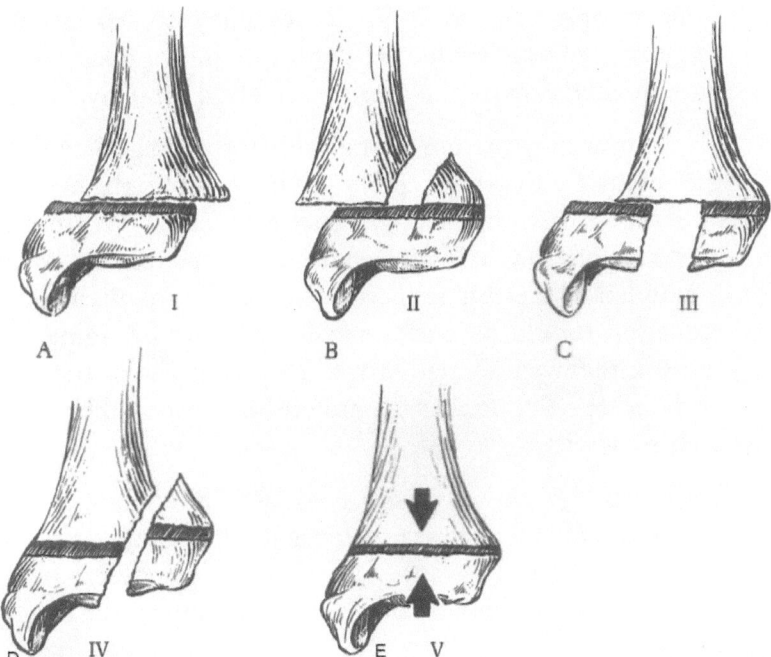

Fig. 122: Classification of epiphyseal injuries: (a) a slip through the hypertrophic layer of the cells, (b) partial separation of the hypertrophic layer of the cells of the epiphyseal plate between the segment of the metaphysis and epiphysis, (c) separation of the epiphyseal fracture and one segment across the plate, (d) fractures resulting from a shearing force across the epiphysis, across the plate, through the metaphysic, and into its cortex, and (e) an injury caused by compression force that crushes germinal potential of the epiphysis.

i. A slip occurs across the epiphyseal plate so that the metaphysis and epiphysis change their positional relationship. This slip occurs through the zone of hypertrophic cells, and no change in growth pattern occurs.

ii. A line of force causes a separation through a portion of the epiphyseal plate and then turns into the metaphysis, leaving a portion of the metaphysis with the epiphysis. Since the separation of the epiphyseal plate occurs through the zone of hypertrophic cells, no change in growth pattern occurs.

iii. A fracture splits the epiphysis and then completes its force across the epiphyseal plate. Displacement of one portion of the epiphysis occurs from the other part of the epiphysis as well from metaphysis relationship. This epiphyseal separation is at the level of hypertrophic cell, and this injury does not cause growth alteration once it has been reduced properly.

iv. Fractures resulting from a longitudinal shearing force through the epiphyses, across the epiphyseal plates, up to the metaphysis and the cortex should be reduced perfectly to prevent an alteration of growth. If the fracture cannot be reduced by closed method or if perfect reduction cannot be maintained, open reduction should be performed to reduce the fragments and transfix them with small wires. The wires across the interior of the plate will not alter the growth, but it should be removed after six weeks.

v. The injury to the epiphysis is caused by compressive force which, in effect, crushes the germinal cells. X-rays do not show any change. Swelling and pain over the epiphyseal plate are present. Time and failure of growth will confirm the diagnosis.

Most injuries to the epiphysis occur at the zone of hypertrophic cells, and if treated properly, it should provide minimal chance for growth irregularity. A crush injury to the epiphyseal plate will injure the germinal layer cell and retard growth.

The injury which occurs at the epiphysis of the child from infancy up to 6 months of age is typically of type 1 slip. This is difficult to diagnosis, but irritability, localized pain, and splinting of the limb of the child of this age group confirm the suspicion of this injury.

Immobilization for epiphyseal injury for six to eight weeks is required once it has been properly reduced. The growth potential consideration is of no great importance compared to the regard for the vascularity of the involved bone. The epiphysis receives its blood supply from the periphery of the periosteum. Few vessels penetrate epiphysis, so its nutrition depends upon adequate circulation from the metaphysis.

The intra-articular position of some epiphyses receives its blood supply from retinacular vessels. The typical example is the capital femoral epiphysis, where any displacement of the capital femoral epiphysis or of the femoral head could lead to loss of circulation. Similarly, a posterior dislocation of the hip joint may interrupt the circulation to the femoral head. Because of this fact, acute slipped capital femoral epiphysis, traumatic or otherwise, and the dislocated hip in a child are real emergencies. Restoration of the proper anatomic relationship is required as soon as possible. Other bones lying intra-articular are the humeral head, the odontoid process of the axis, and the carpal navicular.

Greenstick Fractures

A child's bone has got great elasticity, but it will produce an angular deformity when it is bent down after reaching the maximum limit. Thus, a greenstick fracture occurs (fig. 123).

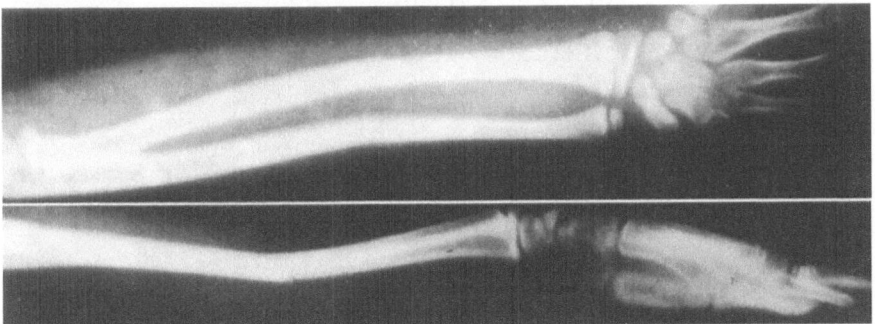

Fig. 123: Greenstick fractures of both bones of the forearm.

This fracture does not remodel itself quickly. Therefore, fracture angulation is reduced, and plaster cast must be applied until the fracture has united. The mid forearm is also a common site of greenstick fracture and should be corrected. Plaster cast should be applied till complete union of the fracture.

Another type of greenstick fracture is torn type, where buckling of the cortex takes place and occurs due to longitudinal compression force. This is a stable fracture and is treated in a plaster cast for four to six weeks.

Injuries to the Ligaments

In children and adolescents, injuries to the ligament around a joint are not common, but they do occur. The ligaments of the knee and ankle joint often tear, especially during competitive sports. More often, an avulsion bony injury may occur.

The ligament injuries are treated in a plaster cast for four to six weeks. No operative treatment is required.

Operations

Operative treatment should be avoided in fractures in children as much as possible. However, there are injuries in which operative treatment becomes absolutely necessary. They are:

    i. acute slipped capital femoral epiphysis

    ii. displaced femoral neck fracture

    iii. irreducible dislocation of the hip

    iv. open fracture of any bone

    v. avulsion fracture of the tibial tubercle

    vi. irreducible totally displaced radial head fragment

    vii. Volkmann's ischaemic contracture, developing

    viii. supracondylar fracture of the humerus with a deepening nerve deficit or weakening pulse

    ix. epiphyseal injury with displacement of fragment

    x. femoral fracture with marked displacement or shortening or reduction cannot be maintained

xi. avulsion of the tibial spine, if irreducible and closed

xii. fracture of the capitellum that is not well reduced

xiii. avulsion separation of 5 mm or greater in the medial humeral epicondyle which cannot be reduced or in which reduction cannot be maintained.

CHAPTER 30

FRACTURES OF THE LONG BONES

Fractures of the long bones include fractures of the shaft of the humerus, radius and ulna, femur, and tibia and fibula.

The vast majority are caused by obvious external violence. Sometimes difficulty arises on two occasions.

Stress Fractures

In an otherwise normal bone, repeated small strains may result in a stress fracture with aching in the limb and also localized swelling and tenderness. In the beginning, there may be very little radiological changes, but when periosteal reaction occurs, the question of infection or neoplasm may arise. While most often it occurs as march fractures in the metatarsal neck, less commonly it occurs in the tibia and femoral neck. Usually, these fractures are transverse fissures in the bone with some sclerosis on each side and subperiosteal thickening of the cortex. Sometimes with serial radiograph taken over several weeks, the diagnosis is established.

Pathological Fractures

If the bone has become weaker than normal because of some disease process, it may fracture as a result of minor strain or even moving in the bed. The causes may be primary or secondary tumour and also include a variety of general and local bone disease and infections, hormonal defects, blood and reticuloendothelial diseases, and malabsorption syndromes.

Anatomy

A major fracture is always accompanied by some injury of the surrounding soft parts and haemorrhages in the muscles, but important structures may also be injured along with it.

Humerus

The radial nerve is at special risk in fractures of the middle third, and brachial artery may be affected by traumatic spasm, contusion, thrombosis, or rupture. If impaired circulation is not restored within a few hours, Volkmann's contracture is likely to occur.

Radius and Ulna

Vascular insufficiency and Volkmann's contracture are real risk more often due to tight bandage or splintage. However, at the elbow, the cause is more likely to be the trauma of the original injury. The normal rotation of the forearm depends on the movements of the upper and lower radioulnar joints and the ability of the radius to rotate around the ulna. Slight malunion of these bones causes much more functional disturbance than in other shaft fractures and may cause limitation of the supination and pronation. Unequal shortening of the bones or angulations will cause subluxation of one or another radioulnar joint. For these reasons, perfect reduction of the forearm fracture is required for full functional recovery.

Femur

The mass of thigh muscles makes external splintage inefficient, and the natural muscle tone will cause shortening of the limb if not treated by continuous traction for some weeks. Shortening of ½ in. is of little importance, but angular deformity, valgus deformity, or varus deformity will result in degenerative changes in the knee joint in due course of time.

Tibia

The bone is subcutaneous, and fractures are often compound from within. Often, damage to the shin or skin loss occurs. In displaced fracture of the upper tibial shaft, the popliteal vessels may be injured. Ischaemic contracture of the calf and short muscle of the foot will result in clawing of the toes.

Diagnosis

1. History of the injury: The nature of the accident may give a clue to the type of fracture. For example, a twisting injury to the leg will produce a spiral fracture rather than a transverse fracture, but usually, the patient has little knowledge of the accident.
2. Continuous pain is present.
3. Loss of function occurs.
4. Swelling and local tenderness, bruising, and blood blisters appear within a few hours.

Particularly with injuries near the elbow and ankle joints, deformity of angulation, shortening, or rotation may by present. Abnormal mobility is detected.

Soft-Tissue Injury

Muscles, vessels, and nerves may be injured. Multiple injuries must be considered if pain is present elsewhere. X-ray examination must be done in two planes, and if required, oblique X-ray must be taken.

Treatment

The aim of the treatment is to restore patient's normal function and normal appearance. The general principles of treatment are few and can be made to appear simple, but no dogmatic decision is required to be taken, considering the pros and cons of the problem.

All Fractures

Treatment of recent open fractures:

i. excision of devitalized tissue at the earliest possible time in view of the general condition of the patient
ii. skin cover as soon as possible to avoid the risk of wound infection

1. Reduction of the deformity:
    a. by closed manipulation
    b. by continuous traction
    c. by open operation

2. Maintenance of the reduction:
    a. by external splintage
    b. by internal splintage with or without external splintage (with or without traction)
    c. exercise of all joints
    d. periodic review of progress
    e. estimation of union
    f. final rehabilitation

Open Reduction and Internal Fixation of Shaft Fractures

Advantages:

1. Interposed soft tissue can be separated from the bone ends, and the deformity fully can be corrected.
2. Internal fixation can be applied.
3. The internal fixation is adequate. External fixation is not required, and joint stiffness is minimized.
4. Skin cover may be more easily obtained if graft is required.
5. Associated vessels and nerve injuries can be examined and, if required, can be repaired.
6. In case of multiple fractures, internal fixation of one or more fracture may greatly help the nursing care of the patient and reduce his discomfort.
7. The patient stays in bed, and hospital stay may be shortened.

Disadvantages:

1. The operation may be technically difficult and may fail due to comminution of the bone.
2. The internal splint may bend or break.
3. Introduction of metal screws and plate may cause aseptic inflammation due to chemical or electrical reaction.
4. The heat generated in drilling the bone or even the insertion of a screw may burn the bone cells and cause local necrosis.
5. If the internal fixation is not rigid, the slight movement will soon loosen the hold of the screws further.
6. The stripping needed to reduce and fix the fracture may devitalize the bone ends.
7. The accurate reduction of the fracture may bring two dead bone ends together.
8. The stripping and plate and screws fixation may increase adhesions and cause greater joint stiffness.
9. The wound may get infected with serious effects by way of pain, toxaemia, delayed union, sequestration of bone, multiple operations for draining abscesses and removal of foreign bodies and sequestra, and possibly bone grafting later on. The results may be prolonged stay in the hospital, muscle-wasting, joint stiffness, economic loss to the patient and community, and psychological suffering to the patient, his family, and the surgeon.

Metal Corrosion

The risk of metal corrosion in fracture treatment is always present. Hence, it is necessary to remember that the lesser metal used in the wound, the better. It is also necessary that the internal fixation to be used should be so rigid that external splintage is not required and it allows immediate mobilization of the limb. But the thicker, longer, and more numerous the plates and screws, the greater the risk of corrosion.

Infection

When using open method of treatment for closed fractures or internal fixation for compound fractures, the chances of infection are increased. However, with non-corrosive materials like vitallium and antibiotics, the situation improves, but it is a fact that increased operative exposure decreases the blood supply to the bone ends and increases the risk of wound infection.

Due to fear of infection, the routine use of internal fixation should be avoided because wound infection complicating the fracture is a very serious matter requiring prolonged treatment. But surprisingly, the fractures which benefit most from internal fixation are the fractures which are seen for second time after some interval one, which include most of the compound fractures.

CHAPTER 31

INTERNAL FIXATION OF FRACTURES

Routine use of internal fixation is not recommended, but if used in general for closed fractures or open fractures when the wound has healed, it gives considerable benefit to the patient.

Indications

1. Failure to reduce the fracture by closed manipulation: This is chiefly due to interposition of the soft tissue, muscle periosteum, or tendons between the fracture fragments. Muscle interposition occurs in fractures of the shaft of long bones particularly in femur. Interposition of the tendon occurs in hand fractures and in widely displaced fractures of the ends of long bones while periosteal interposition is found in avulsion fractures of the malleoli at the ankle joint.
2. Failure to maintain a satisfactory position in fractures of the shaft of long bones following closed reduction.
   a. Injuries of the forearm require accurate reduction.
      i. isolated fractures of the shaft of the radius
      ii. fractures of the shafts of the radius and ulna
      iii. Monteggia fracture–dislocations are unstable injuries which require internal fixation when good position cannot be maintained in plaster cast.
      iv. Unstable oblique and spiral fractures of the lower half of the shaft of the tibia.
      v. Comminuted and double fracture of the tibia (fig. 124).

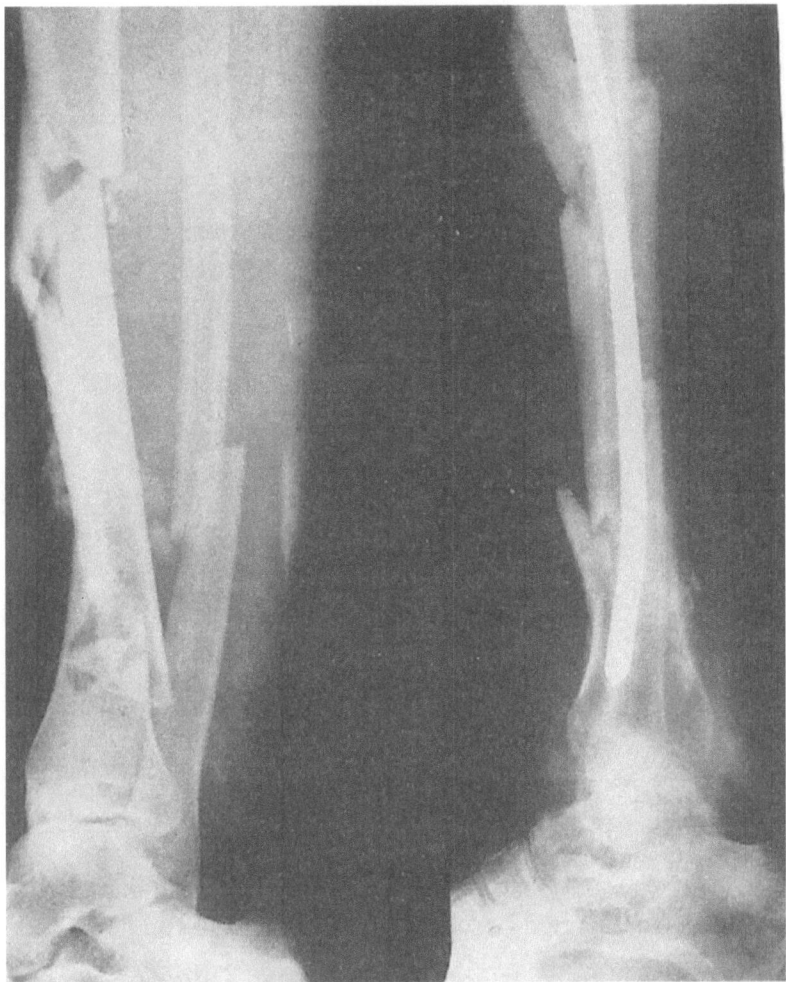

Fig. 124: Double fracture of the tibia union in a good position following intramedullary railing.

vi. Fracture of the upper one-third of the femoral shaft.
vii. Fractures of the forearm and the hand (fig. 125).

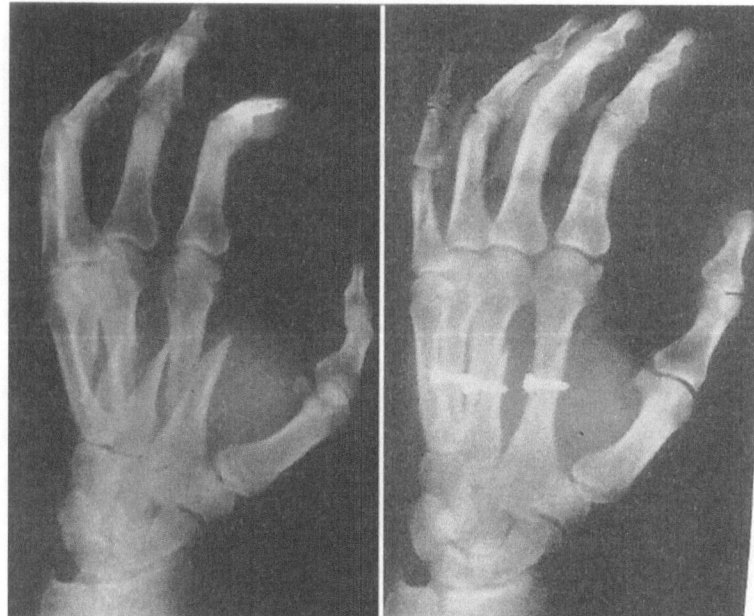

Fig. 125: Fracture of the metacarpals treated by open reduction and screw fixation.

b. Fractures involving joints: An attempt should be made to restore the joint surfaces, such as:

   i. in fracture of the malleoli of the ankle joint and of the posterior margin of the lower end of the tibia

   ii. when a large fragment is split off in abduction fractures of the external condyle of the tibia

   iii. in posterior or central dislocation of the hip joint, which should be considered when there is sciatic nerve palsy or when acetabulum is disorganized (fig. 126)

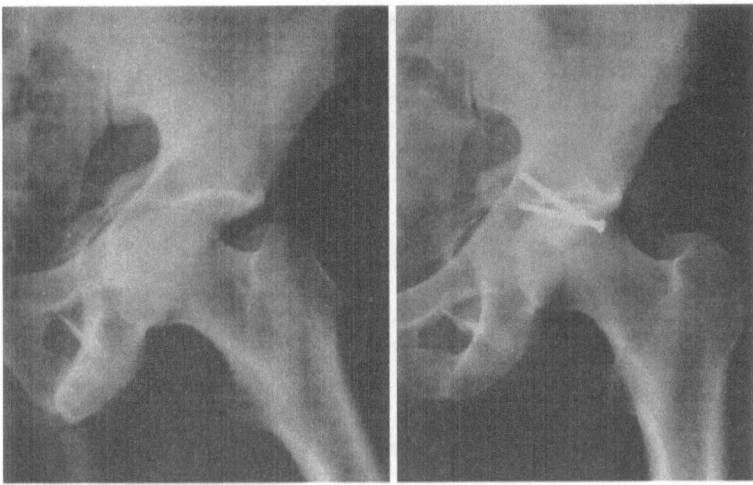

Fig. 126: Fracture of the acetabulum reduced and fixed by two screws.

iv. in fractures of the lower end of the humerus: *T*-and *Y*-shaped fractures of the shaft, avulsion of internal epicondyle, fracture (fig. 127) separation of the external condyle, and fracture of the articular surface of the external condyle.

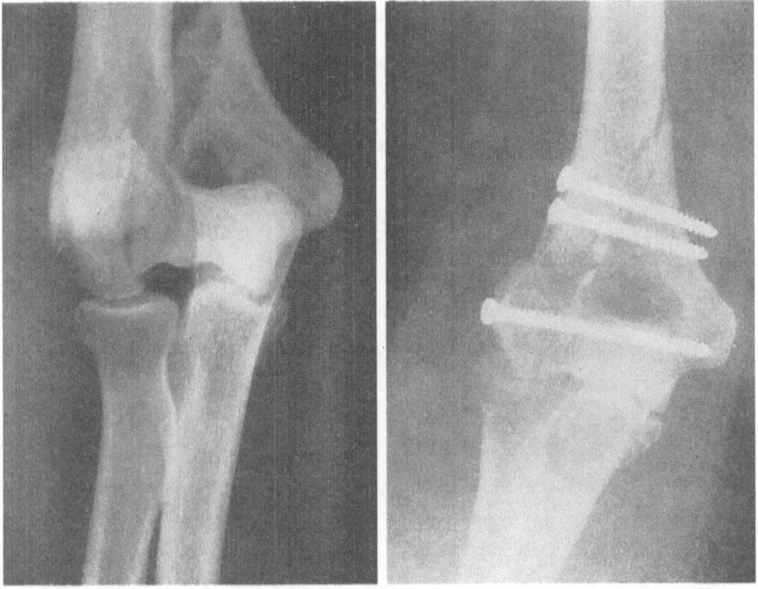

Fig. 127: Y-shaped fracture of the lower end of the humerus treated by open reduction and screws fixation.

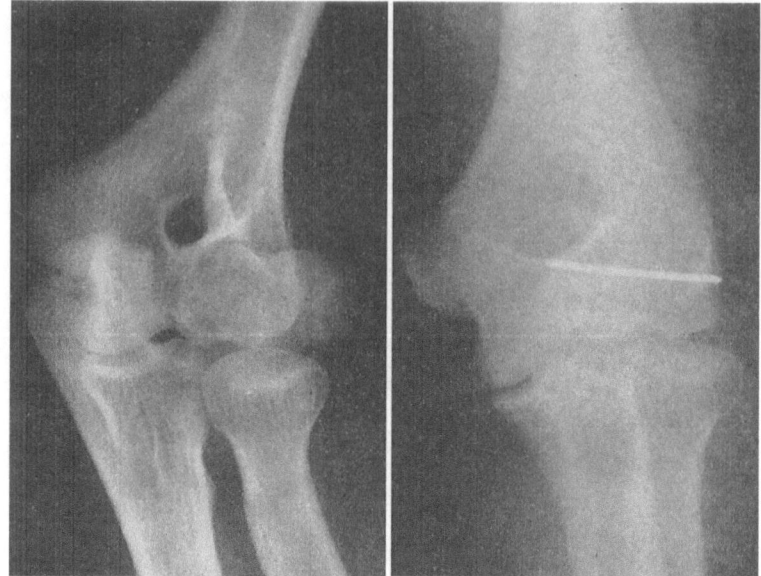

Fig. 128: Fracture of the articular surface of external condyle of the humerus treated by open reduction and internal fixation with a steel pin.

    v. in fractures and dislocations of the metacarpophalangeal and interphalangeal joints of the hand

    vi. when blood supply of one fragment is impaired and the fracture is displaced (union will not take place unless the fracture is accurately reduced and firmly fixed).

Internal fixation is required in the following:

    A. Fractured neck of the femur.

    B. Displaced fracture of the carpal scaphoid.

    C. Multiple injuries, such as injuries where there is a fracture of the shaft of the femur and tibia. Sometimes fractures are complicated by severe injury to the neighbouring structures. The fixation treatment of the fracture by internal fixation will help in the treatment of the injury to the skin, major vessels, and nerves. In such cases, even in open wound, internal fixation can be carried out.

D. Displacement of the spine: These injuries are very unstable and recur after conservative treatment. In dislocation of the cervical and thoracolumbar spine, there is a risk of injury to the cord or cauda equina, and stabilization by internal fixation should be considered.

E. In pathological fracture of the shafts of long bones, internal fixation is often required in secondary metastasis, particularly in the humerus and femur.

F. In delayed union or non-union of fractures of the shaft of the long bones, internal fixation with or without bone graft may be required.

Timing of the Operation

It has been proved that open reduction and internal fixation, if delayed for a week, give better results. This is because the capillary circulation is re-established within a week and healing of the fracture is better. Callus formation is good in three months' time when the operation has been delayed for six or more days.

There is sufficient evidence that incidence of non-union in fractures of the shafts of the long bones after open reduction and internal fixation is reduced when the operation is performed at the end of the first week or during the second and third weeks after the injury. This is due to the time allowed for the re-establishment of circulation.

In fractures of the ends of long and short bones (particularly involving the joints of the ankle, knee, elbow, and hand), early fixation is advisable, and risk of non-union is very much reduced.

Operative Technique

In operation of open reduction, the soft tissue around the fracture site should be disturbed as little as possible. The periosteum stripping should also be avoided, and if possible, the plate should be applied over the periosteum. In a comminuted fracture, the soft-tissue attachment of the fragments of the bone should not be removed. Perfect reduction can be achieved with minimal damage to the soft tissue. This is especially true in fractures involving the joints.

Fixation Methods

There are three principal materials used at the present time for surgical implants. They are stainless steel, vitallium (cobalt–chromium alloy), and titanium.

Stainless steel was the first to be used. It is a corrosion-resisting material for the production of surgical implants. Though used often, occasionally corrosion develops at the point of contact of two separate pieces of material, such as plate and screws.

Vitallium has proved to be good from the point of tissue tolerance and mechanical strength.

Titanium has been introduced recently, but it is completely tolerated by tissues and has proved to be very successful because of its good mechanical properties.

A. Steel pins: These are employed for intra-articular fractures and in repositioning small bony fragments around the joints (fig. 129). The pins can be cut after insertion so that their tips lie beneath the shin or they can project outside the skin. In each case, the pin should be removed when the fracture has united.

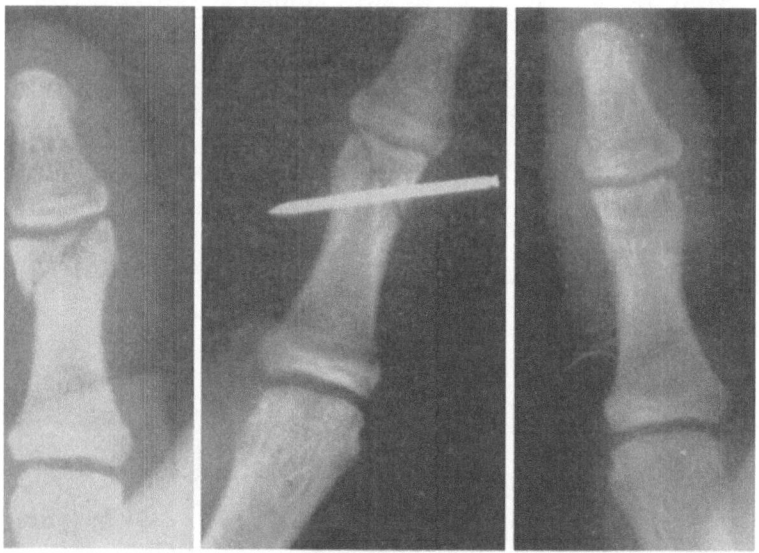

Fig. 129: Open reduction and internal fixation of the fractures of the phalanges of the hand.

B. Screws: Single screw is used for fracture to fix displaced fragments around the joints which are too large to be fixed with a pin. One or more screws may be used for the fixation of oblique or spiral fractures of the shaft of the radius and ulna, humerus and tibia. While making a hole for the screw, the drill of the correct size should be used. Usually, it should be small in size so that screw fixation is firm and rigidly done.

C. Lag screws: These are used for fixing large fragments in fractures of the ends of the long bones. They are larger than a normal screw and have a coarse-thread end.

D. Plate: In oblique and spiral fractures of the long bones, the plate provides more secure fixation. Only plates of good quality, which provide rigid immobilization, should be used.

E. Nail and plate: A combination of nail and plate is required for certain fractures such as trochanteric fracture of the femur. The nail and plate may be separated or in one piece. A disadvantage of two-piece nail plate is that the screws holding it may get loosened.

F. Intramedullary nails:

  i. Trifin nail for fixation of fracture of the neck of the femur is used. It is better to introduce it in such a manner at the lower border of the greater trochanter so that it almost lies vertically and has got fixation at three points—in the femoral head, on the calcar femoral, and in the lateral cortex of the femur. The results are better with this procedure.

  ii. Küntscher nail: It is used for fixation of fractures of the shafts of the femur, tibia, humerus, and radius and ulna. It is often introduced into the bone under X-ray control without exposing the fracture site. But it is safer and easy to expose the fracture and introduce the rail under direct vision after reducing the fracture. In fracture of the femur and ulna, the rail is first driven into proximal fragment in a retrograde manner so that it projects through a small incision above the great trochanter or olecranon. The fracture is then reduced, and the nail is driven into distal fragment. In fracture of the tibia, the nail must be curved, and it is introduced through the upper end of the anterior surface of the tibia behind the patellar tendon, or it is introduced through the upper end of the shaft above the tuberosity. In fracture of the humerus, the nail is introduced through the superolateral surface of the greater tuberosity. In fracture of the radius, the nail is introduced through the styloid process. The diameter of the nail is very important. It should preferably be of the same size at the narrow part of the medullary cavity of the bone in which it is introduced. If the nail is too large, it may split the shaft of the bone, or if it is too small, the fixation may be insecure. Reaming of the medullary cavity must be done as it is required but should not be overdone. After reaming, the nail will provide efficient immobilization, but it needs to be supplemented by a plaster cast.

iii. Rush nail: It is used for the treatment of fractures of the shaft of the long bones. The nail must be sufficiently rigid to allow it to be driven into the bone and to provide stable fixation, flexible enough to conform to the contours of the medullary cavity, and resilient enough to realign itself within the bone. To be effective for fixation, it must provide fixation at three points: at the proximal and distal portions and at the fracture site. The head of the pin with rounded hook grasps the cortex and control rotation, prevents migration of the pin into the bone, and assists in extraction. It is useful for fractures of the radius and ulna, upper and lower end of the humerus and tibia, and lower end of the femur.

Post-Operative Management

It is often necessary to apply external support for internal fixation because fixation is insecure:

1. when the bones are osteoporotic
2. after intramedullary nailing of a transverse fracture of the shaft of a long bone when one fragment may rotate on the other
3. when screws are only used in oblique or spiral fractures of the long bones.

4. when single screws or stainless steel pins are used to fix fragments of the bone in or around the joints.

External fixation is usually provided by plaster cast or, for the lower limb, by traction. In some cases, a firm bandage over cotton wool is applied and removed when the wound is healed, and then a plaster cast is given.

When no plaster cast or external splintage is used, the patient should not be allowed to put weight on the limb, and undue strain should be avoided.

Complications

i. Infection: This serious complication is responsible for unpopularity of internal fixation. The end result of it is chronic osteomyelitis and non-union. In an open fracture, the risk of infection is reduced by delaying the internal fixation until the wound has healed or by rigid non-touch technique, gentle handling of the soft tissue, and simplicity of the surgery.

ii. Mechanical breakdown: Fracture of plates, intramedullary nails, and screws is not uncommon. It is usually due to incorrect post-operative management, especially inadequate protection until union has taken place. Often it is attributed to inadequacy or weakness of the internal fixation device.

iii. Non-union or delayed union: It is a fact that internal fixation rarely expedites the union of the fracture; rather, it often delays it. This complication in fractures of shafts of the long bones is often reduced when the operation is carried out during the second and third weeks after the injury.

CHAPTER 32

REHABILITATION

Rehabilitation is concerned with the restoration of joint movements and redevelopment of muscle power which are lost as a result of soft-tissue damage. Immobilization is necessary to allow fractures and dislocation to heal. It is not the fracture itself but the immobilization used in the treatment that causes joint stiffness. Realization of this fact has led to increasing use of internal fixation and early mobilization.

The following are the general principles:

i. Maintenance of mobility of those joints, not immobilization for treatment of fractures.

ii. Preservation of the muscle power during the stage of immobilization.

iii. Restoration of the function when immobilization is discarded.

The basic techniques of rehabilitation are as follows:

i. Exercise: Exercise can be isometric or isotonic. An isometric exercise is static without joint movement. Quadriceps exercises are an example of isometric exercises. Isotonic exercises involve joint movement. They are most useful in regaining movements and control of muscle power throughout the range. The isometric exercises, if properly performed, are more useful for developing muscle strength.

ii. Either technique can be used freely, assisted by water or sling suspension if the muscle is weak. If the muscle is stronger, resistance can be offered by gravity, water, weights, or hand of the physiotherapist. Though judged by the muscle strength, the function depends on strength, endurance, speed of action, and coordination of the patient.

The best results are obtained by active voluntary exercises performed by the patient himself. Electric stimulation is of no value in increasing the muscle power.

All exercises and exercise routine must be adapted to the condition of the muscle, joints, and the patient as a whole. In an inflamed joint, the exercises are of no value; rather, it will irritate the joint further and cause further stiffness. In such cases, only static exercises are useful. In other cases, progressive resistance exercises are of great benefit to the patient.

Various apparatuses have been introduced for exercises to provide resistance to help develop muscle strength. It has two advantages:

i. It helps treat many patients at one time.
ii. With weight or spring balance techniques, the objective record can be maintained.

However, there are many disadvantages and dangers in the use of apparatus. Much of the apparatus is cumbersome and noisy, and the patient often does not follow the regime of exercises strictly.

Proprioceptive Neuromuscular Facilitation

The strength of contraction of a muscle depends on the number of motor units serving it that are stimulated. This depends on the degree of excitation of the anterior horn cells supplying those muscles. It is the principle of the behaviour of the central nervous system that maximum sensory input produces maximum motor output. Thus, if it is required to obtain maximum contraction in a muscle, maximum stimulation of the sensory nerves should be produced. This can be done by putting the muscle on stretch with the pressure and resistance of the hands of the therapist.

Another method is to stimulate the sensory nerve endings by irradiation. In such cases, stimulation of one muscle will work upon other adjacent muscles as well and improve the muscle power.

One other method commonly used is successive induction; this means that when there is maximum voluntary movement of an agonist, the antagonist is facilitated. Thus, if there is weakness of the flexors of the wrist, maximum activity is encouraged in the extensors of the wrist, and it will help the flexors to produce a better movement.

Technique

The movements of the upper limb take place in a diagonal plane. In this way, all muscles are put to stretch. In the upper limb, there are two diagonal patterns of movements and their antagonist patterns. At the shoulder joint, the flexion, adduction, and lateral rotation take place. Along with this movement, the elbow joint can he flexed and extended. With flexion, supination of the forearm can be done, and with extension, pronation can be performed. At the same time, the movements of the wrist and fingers can be done. In an antagonistic position, there is extension, abduction, and medial rotation of the shoulder. The movements at the wrist, fingers, and thumb take place similarly. It must be noted that rotation is very important as most muscles perform this rotatory action in normal function. There are definite advantages of giving multiple joint movements because many more muscles are activated and stronger muscles support the action of the weaker muscles as well. Sometimes maximal resistance is used to stimulate the muscles and increase the sensory inflow. Traction and compression are used—traction to improve flexion movements and compression to help extension movements. This can be done by placing the hand over the muscles and tendons which are contracting, and patient is also stimulated by the touch of the hand.

The patient can help himself if he follows the movements of his limb with his eyes and follows the instruction given to him precisely and firmly.

There are two techniques which work better, and they are divided into:

i. strengthening
ii. relaxation.

Strengthening Techniques

Strengthening techniques are repeated contractions, slow reversals, and rhythmical stabilization. Repeated contraction can be used, alone or combined with other methods. In addition, resistance is gradually offered to help the muscle to improve its function and power. The patient is instructed to continue these movements regularly.

Slow reversals depend on the fact that muscles will contract more strongly if the antagonist also contracts at the same time. This can be done by changing the hand from one side to the opposite side without giving a chance to the patient to relax.

Rhythmical stabilization is performed by asking the patient to maintain a given position against increasing resistance, which is maintained until good power has been gained, and then the resistance is transferred to the opposite side without relaxation. This is a difficult job but should be repeated three or four times.

Relaxing Techniques

The relaxation techniques are used to increase the range of movements. The techniques used are the following:

    i.   slow reversal–hold–relax technique

    ii. contract–relax technique

    iii. hold–relax technique.

Slow Reversal–Hold–Relax Technique

In this technique, the arm moves actively to the point where range is limited and muscle spasm occurs, then the patient maintains the contraction of the right muscle. When maximal contraction has been achieved, the patient is asked to relax and then encouraged to move against resistance into an increased range. This is repeated as often as required.

Contract–Relax Technique

In this technique, the patient is given passive movements to the point where no further range can be gained. After it the muscles are held in position and given contraction. When maximum relaxation has been achieved, the limb is moved passively into the increased range.

Hold–Relax Technique

In this technique, the patient maintains the position without movements taking place, and the limb is moved to the point where muscle spasm or pain occurs.

Rhythmical stabilization can also be used to gain relaxation. This technique can be used for patients in any position, such as lying, prone lying, or sitting, and it can be used as unilateral, bilateral, symmetrical, or asymmetrical movements. They can be adapted for use with weights or springs. These methods are not a substitute for functional activities but they can produce good results with all forms of active work.

Circuit Training

Circuit training consists of building an exercise programme which is planned to the individual physical activity. The programme consists of the following:

i. exercising the main muscle group with resulting increase in strength and endurance
ii. obtaining maximum general effect and improve stamina
iii. improving certain skills by practice.

Circuit training is the logical final stage of any exercise programme because it aims at a functional end result, and individual success is based on one's own capability.

Thus, exercise programme can be summarized into the following:

i. The only way to increase muscle strength and endurance is by active voluntary exercise.
ii. The precise method used is not of any value, provided the muscle is exercised maximally and the method used is adapted to the circumstances.

iii. There is no apparent relation between muscle strength and stamina.
iv. Strength and endurance are of little practical value without coordination.
v. In most cases, a combination of techniques will be appropriate, starting with simple development of strength and progressing to functional activity.

Heat

Heat can be provided in a variety of forms: infrared, radiant heat, short-wave diathermy, wax bath, and hot-water baths. The principle of treatment for all these is to relieve pain, relax muscle spasm, and improve circulation. Heat makes subsequent exercise or treatment more effective. Thus, after the removal of the plaster of Paris, the patient is encouraged to do exercise. It will work better if the heat treatment has been given first. Similarly, scarred soft tissue can be stretched more effectively after heat. The choice of heat depends on the requirement and convenience. Wax bath are useful in treating the hand, ankle, and foot. Heat is retained longer to improve the condition of the skin. Short-wave diathermy is of little value because it is a complicated and expensive treatment. Infrared and hydrotherapy are more valuable, effective, and convenient.

Electric Stimulation

Electrical stimulation of the muscles can be of value when its use is inhibited by pain, disuse, or over-action of stronger muscles. One or two sessions of stimulation can be of great value in demonstrating the viability of the muscles to the patient. This is of value after tendon sutures or grafts after long periods of immobilization and sometimes after tendon transposition and to re-educate the quadriceps after patellectomy. The patient should be instructed to work the muscles with the current. The current can be stopped occasionally, and the patient does movements himself. This treatment is an addition to the recovery of active movement, and it cannot replace it.

Massage

Massage has many advantages, such as increasing circulation, reducing muscle spasm, and relieving pain. Massage has one definite effect on the muscles, and it is the softening on soft-tissue scarring. There are many situations where scarring and adhesions are the sole bar to function. Intensive oil massage and slow stretching are of great value in such cases.

Passive Movements

There is a little place for the use of passive movements in the aftercare of fractures, except in the later stages of stiff shoulders and, occasionally, in stiff knees and ankles.

Hydrotherapy

Hydrotherapy requires a large heated pool. The size of the swimming pool with adequate facilities will help the patient in the rehabilitation far better than otherwise. Hydrotherapy, in fact, provides assisted movements. It can provide all forms of activities— Resistance offered by the outside air disappears in the water.

The warmth and comfort are an excellent media for mobilizing stiff joints, whether stiff from prolonged immobilization, disuse, or intra-articular damage. There is no contraindication for hydrotherapy except the recent presence of infection and recent cardiac ischaemia.

Rehabilitation after Fractures of the Upper Limb

The problems associated with rehabilitation of fractures of the upper limb are stiffness of the shoulder, elbow, wrist, or hand; redevelopment of the power of the muscle controlling these joints; and coordination of neuromuscular function.

Shoulder

Simple fracture of the clavicle and scapula not involving the shoulder joint does not produce joint stiffness of the shoulder. In any fracture of the humerus which requires more than four weeks of immobilization, the shoulder becomes stiff from it. The shoulder should be exercised as soon as possible.

Fracture involving the shoulder joint produces more disability resulting in stiffness and loss of muscle control. Fracture of the greater tuberosity of the humerus, fracture of the neck of the humerus in old persons, and fissure fractures of the glenoid are the most troublesome.

The shoulder becomes stiff early in old people; therefore, quality of re-education is not very important as early movements are to be started soon. The injury to the rotator cuff can cause a painful arc movement between 70 and 120 degree abduction due to the inflammation of the supraspinatus tendon, which impinges against the acromion process.

Injection of ICC, IML prednisolone into the tender spot, repeated three times at weekly interval, will relieve the pain of this complication.

Simple Dislocations of the Shoulder

The movement returns quickly when the immobilization is finished. The problem arises in recurrent dislocation of the shoulder joint, which is treated by an operative procedure. Active exercise and hydrotherapy with the addition of resistance exercises can help in recovery of good movements of the shoulder joint in about 12 weeks' time.

Stiff Shoulder

Stiff shoulder responds well to repeated gentle stretching and mobilization, but it may be noted that the elbow and finger joints react badly to such treatment. The aim of the treatment is relief of pain, reduction of muscle spasm, restoration of joint movement, and redevelopment of muscle power. External rotation and abduction are the most important movements to be restored.

Relief of Pain and Spasm

Ice packs applied to the shoulder are the most effective in relief of painful muscle spasm and are useful in all cases of stiff shoulder. The first treatment should be for 10 minutes, progressing to 20 minutes after third or fourth treatment.

Restoration of Movements

Active exercises for all ranges of movements can be supplement by sling suspension method and can help in the recovery of movements. Self-assisted exercises using pulleys are valuable. Wall-climbing is a useful technique for the recovery of the patient's shoulder. Hydrotherapy is most valuable for restoring shoulder movements. The shoulder should be exercised in all ranges, lying, side-lying, and sitting. In late stages, swimming is very helpful in recovery of function. When movements cease to return by active exercises, passive methods can be utilized. In general, passive movement should be delayed for three weeks. Active movements are assisted by passive stretching as well, but sudden force should be avoided. If these methods fail, manipulation under anaesthesia must be carried out. An injection of Icc prednisolone into the joint can help relieve the pain.

Later on, volleyball and other methods of occupational therapy, such basketry, stool seating, weaving, and cord-knotting, are all useful. At a later time, weaving, printing, carpentry, and gardening can be used. Then cross-cut sawing, log-splitting, heavy carpentry, cement-mixing, polishing, wood-finishing, and digging are valuable. For women, general homework (window-clearing, polishing furniture, interior-cleaning, interior decoration) is a useful activity.

Fractures Associated with Nerve Lesions

The circumflex nerve lesion is a common complication of the fracture or shoulder dislocation.

Traction lesion of the upper trunk of the brachial plexus is also common, but recovery does take place. Paralysis of the deltoid is caused by lesion of the fifth cervical nerve root, but it is also accompanied by wasting of infraspinatus muscle. Exercises such as external rotation of the shoulder joint are beneficial. Paralysis of the deltoid alone is not a disability, but with both spinati and deltoid paralysed, abduction of the arm is not possible. In such cases, a reconstructive surgery or arthrodesis of the shoulder can be considered.

Elbow

Fractures in and around the elbow can cause more complications than other injuries of the upper limb. This is due to the complex nature of the elbow joint subserving flexion, extension, and rotation movements and the presence of a large number of structures in relation to the joint which are likely to be injured.

Fracture of the olecranon, supracondylar fracture of the humerus, and dislocation of the elbow, with or without fracture, are likely to cause limitation of flexion and extension.

Fracture of the head of the radius and fractures of the shaft of the radius and ulna are likely to cause limitation of rotation.

The danger of passive movements to the elbow after an injury is always there, and it causes stiffness, painful spasms, and myositis ossificans.

Stiff Elbow

Passive movements should never be given to elbow joint. The patient should also be told not do stretching of the joint on his own.

Active exercises only are allowed. The patient should extend the elbow joint against resistance. Occupational therapy can provide activities to encourage flexion and extension of the elbow joint. Basketry, light fretwork, sandpapering, light gardening, and carpentry are all of value.

Myositis ossifican may follow dislocations, fracture–dislocations of the elbow, or forced passive movements. The development of this condition will be suspected by the increasing pain in the elbow and loss of movement at the elbow joint (fig. 130). X-ray must be taken, and if the condition is confirmed, the elbow is rested completely in a sling until pain is gone and the X-ray film becomes negative. Subsequent mobilization must be done gradually.

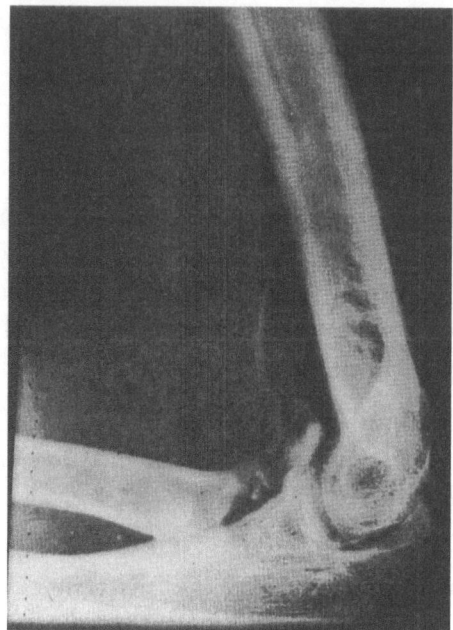

Fig. 130: Myositis ossificans.

Ulnar Palsy

The ulnar nerve is often injured in elbow injuries. Complete paralysis with clawing, paralysis of the interossei and lumbricals, and sensory loss are obviously present. Slight tingling in the little and ring fingers or a little weakness of the intrinsic muscles must be considered carefully if injury to ulnar nerve is suspected. Motor weakness may also appear slowly.

Some limitation of the extension is inevitable after fractures of the elbow. If no improvement occurs after three weeks' interval, then further rehabilitation may not likely to increase the range of movements. However, time and normal use will benefit the patient up to 20 degrees over a period of six months.

Rotation

Involvement of the superior or inferior radioulnar joint and malalignment of the bone ends in the radius and ulna fracture lead to restricted movements of pronation and supination. Even in fracture of the radius and ulna, stiffness does occur in prolonged immobilization (longer than eight weeks), and it may become permanent if not treated. Occupational therapy, such as carpentry, the use of the screwdriver, manipulation of loom by rotation movements, and games using rotation movements are all useful in the recovery of functions. For women, simple household jobs, such as food preparation (beating cakes, kneading dough) washing clothes, doing crafts (leatherwork, rug-making), provide a wide range of movements. Tennis, badminton, cricket, and table tennis utilize rotation.

Wrist

The most common fractures around the wrist are the Colles fracture and fracture of the scaphoid. Within 14 days after the removal of plaster, active exercises will help the patient to recover full range of movements, provided the patient has done exercises during the period of immobilization. If the fracture involves the joint, some stiffness is inevitable. The movements of a stiff joint can easily be restored by occupational therapy, such as basketry, weaving, light metalwork, and carpentry. In later stages, activities such as gripping, throwing, catching balls, and heavy work will improve the patient's functions. Other activities like peeling of vegetables, making pastries, bottling of fruits, and doing household duties which provide plenty of wrist movements are of great help in the recovery of functions. Crafts such as clay-modelling, pottery, and making tufted rugs are also suitable. In osteoarthritis of the wrist joint, intra-articular injection of steroid once a week for three weeks is to be considered. A leather support can be worn for it as well. However, these methods give temporary relief, and permanent relief is obtained by arthrodesis of the wrist joint.

Bennett Fracture–Dislocation

The usual methods of rehabilitation are resistance exercises, games, and occupational therapy. These are helpful in recovery of functions after the injury, but power returns gradually.

A fibreglass splint can be worn to relieve the pain. The patient can perform most of the duties while wearing the splint.

Fractures of the Hand

In fractures of the hand, the period of immobilization should be of minimum possible time. This will prevent stiffness and allow movements to recover early. If the fracture shows any degree of displacement, internal fixation and early movements are the best treatment.

Heat in the form of wax baths or warm saline soaks is valuable in early stages, followed by active exercises, neuromuscular facilitation, games, occupational therapy, and workshop activities.

Most simple fractures of the hand do not present much of a problem in rehabilitation, but when there is much soft-tissue damage and subsequent fibrosis (as in crush injuries, haemorrhage, and neglected oedema or sepsis), the problem is great, and results are not encouraging.

Severe fibrosis must be treated by oil massage several times daily to soften the fibrous tissue, and contracted structures are gently and slowly stretched. No sudden forced movement should be used, and manipulation is absolutely contraindicated. It does more harm, leading to worse fibrosis following excitation of inflammatory exudate. Success can be achieved in even the most severe deformities if the principle of 'slow, little, and often' is followed.

Rehabilitation after Crush Fractures of the Vertebrae

Simple crush fractures of the vertebrae are often caused by road traffic accidents and sporting accidents.

As soon as the symptoms subside (within 24–48 hours), spinal extension exercises are started and continued till complete recovery. At no stage should forward flexion exercises be allowed. In patients with fracture of the lumbar spine, spinal support may be fitted to the patient before getting out of bed.

Eight to ten weeks from the time of injury, majority of patients have normal living. The restriction is to avoid severe exercises for a further one month.

Rehabilitation after Fracture of the Hand

Rehabilitation after Lower-Limb Fractures

Rehabilitation after lower limb fractures falls in four stages.

1. exercises in bed
2. early mobilization (walking in plaster or caliper, correct use of crutches and sticks).
3. re-education in walking
4. retraining for works.

Exercise in Bed

Throughout the period of immobilization, the patient should practise static exercise of all those muscles acting across the immobilized joint and full active movement for all other joints. All exercises are carried out for five minutes every hour throughout the daytime.

Weight-Bearing

Weight-bearing is safe only if sufficient callus formation and healing have taken place; the degree and timing of weight-bearing depends upon the following:

1. the type of fracture
2. the adequacy of reduction
3. the degree and method of stabilization.

Rehabilitation in early stages consists primarily of static exercise, which varies from case to case. Mainly, static exercises of gluteal, quadriceps, and calf muscles form the basis of individual treatment. It is a fact that quadriceps muscles are the key to the function of the knee. They readily work after the injury to the knee or the adjacent structures. Calf muscles are the key to the recovery from injuries to the lower leg. Intrinsic muscles of the foot are important in the ankle, and foot injuries and glutei are the controller of the hip joint.

Before and during weight-bearing, active exercises of all muscles must be carried out to ensure the strength in them and to help in walking.

Unless the programme of treatment is carefully managed, strain of foot will develop in non-injured leg during the early stage of rehabilitation in middle-aged and old people who are kept in bed for several weeks or more.

Effect of Internal Fixation

The use of internal fixation lessens the problems of immobilization, whether used in early stages or later, due to delayed union. In case of fracture of the tibia, internal fixation eliminates the prolonged incumbency in bed and allows for early mobilization of the knee joint and ankle joint respectively.

In internal fixation, the weight-bearing is delayed for 6–12 weeks. The patient can return to works in 12–14 weeks after the fracture of the tibia, and in 20–24 weeks after the fracture of the femoral shaft, it is to be remembered that internal fixation does not affect the rate of clinical union. In majority of cases, the fractures of the femur and tibia unite in 12–24 weeks, but in many cases, the fracture line is visible in the X-ray film for many months in spite of good callus formation.

Walking with Crutches

Correct crutch-walking lays the pattern for all the walking re-education to come, from non-weight-bearing through partial weight-bearing to full weight-bearing. The essential feature of correct crutch-walking is the swinging of the injured leg through the air and the establishment of the correct rhythm of walking.

Many people prefer the elbow crutches instead of the axillary crutches. The elbow crutches must be adjusted to the correct length with comfortable handgrips. Later on, when the patient starts using the walking sticks, it is essential that they should be adjusted in length accordingly. It is better to use two sticks in place of one during rehabilitation.

Walking in Plaster

The common faults in plaster-walking are external rotation of the leg as the weight is taken on the injured limb and circumduction of the injured limb. Correct plaster-walking requires good power and spring of the sound limb and good power of the glutei on the injured leg to level the pelvis when rocking over the immobilized limb. For this reason, gluteal exercise, extension, and abduction of the hip are introduced in the early stages of the treatment.

In the elderly or in bilateral lower-lumbar disabilities, it may help to fit a shoe raise to the shoe of the non-plastered leg. When the patient can walk correctly and static quadriceps exercises are done, he can resume his work.

Weight-Relieving Caliper

Simple half-ring adjustable-length calipers will provide enough support and protection for weight-bearing and help the patient in walking around.

Rehabilitation after Removal of the Plaster

When the fracture has soundly united and the plaster and caliper have been removed, the problems of rehabilitation are the following:

1. redevelopment of wasted muscles, particularly the calf and quadriceps
2. mobilization of the knee and ankle joints
3. re-education in walking.

In the first week, it is important to establish the patient's confidence in his leg so that he can develop the normal rhythm of walking.

The exercise routines are practised, and a limp-free walking is insisted on at all stages.

The use of a pair of walking sticks is primarily to maintain balance and re-establish a walking rhythm. It does not provide protection.

Once confidence has been restored, the patient may be allowed to start walking normally. Gradually, the rhythm is sped up, and the power of movements is increased. The exercises develop the power to raise full body weight on the toes of the injured leg. Strong coordinated muscle action and coordinated movements develop the spring in quick walking and running. Then the patient develops limp-free walking with good movement, good power, and good coordination, which show good rehabilitation.

Delayed Rehabilitation

Some people would like to return to their work before the fracture is united. It is economically and psychologically better to allow them to work. If they later on, after a period of three to six months, develop muscle weakness or joint stiffness, sound rehabilitation procedure will help them to achieve maximum result.

The Trochanteric Region

The use of internal fixation provides early mobility and conserves the vitality of an elderly patient. Union of fracture is demonstrated radiologically.

During rehabilitation, mobilization of the hip and knee by non-weight-bearing exercises, with particular attention to the strength of the hip abductors, is the basis of good functional results.

The Hip

Dislocation of the hip and fracture involving the hip joint present a problem, and recovery of function is usually slow. Rehabilitation of these injuries consists of non-weight-bearing mobilization for a period of 12 weeks, followed by gradual increase of weight-bearing, whether surgery has been done not. If the clinical condition remains good at one year after injury, the long-term results are good.

The Knee

Recovery of knee flexion after fractures of the shaft of the tibia and fibula presents no problem. The patient usually regains movements up to 50 degrees in three weeks and full knee range in three month time. However, if immobilization in plaster has lasted for more than six months, knee movements are slow to recover, and full bending may take 19 weeks or more to recover.

Restoration of knee functions is the main problem after fracture of the femur. A large number of patients with fractures of the femur regain good knee movements up to 90 degree with good rehabilitation. With this range of movement, the patient can sit comfortably on a chair.

Early mobilization is the best way of preventing stiffness of the knee, and the end results depend upon the types of fractures, the method of reduction, and the duration of immobilization. Restriction of movements at the knee joint is due to the quadriceps' adherence, but a comminuted fracture of the femur always gives less range of movement, irrespective of how it has been treated.

The other major cause of restricted knee movement is the injury in and around the knee joint, producing intra-articular and periarticular adhesions.

Concurrent injuries of the knee joint, such as an associated comminuted fracture of the patella or intra-articular fracture, are almost certain to produce permanent stiffness of the knee joint.

Early mobilization is the keystone to obtain good results after isolated injuries of the knee joint, and haemarthrosis, if not aspirated and mobilized early, will cause stiffness of the knee joint.

The end result of patellectomy for comminuted fracture of patella are usually slower to achieve and less good than after patellectomy for chondromalacia, intra- and extra-articular damage, and adhesion tend to cause restricted knee movements. However, early mobilization and adequate rehabilitation can give excellent results.

Leg Length Differences

The incidence of differences in leg length may or may not present a problem, and it depends upon the individual. The usual method of calculating the leg length difference is to measure the leg length from the anterior superior iliac spine to the tip of medial malleolus. The overall degree of accuracy in clinical measurement of the leg length differences is such that a difference of ½ in. or more may be accepted as diagnostically significant.

If ½ in. is accepted as the criterion for short leg, then asymptomatic short leg occurs in a large segment of the population.

There is a small group of patients in whom this shortening of ½ in. may cause backache, often precipitated by unusual physical activity. The symptoms are reduced by fitting an appropriate shoe raise.

Short Leg Following an Injury

Post-traumatic short leg is a potent cause of persistent limp, and it may delay the recovery of a patient during the rehabilitation of leg fractures or, if uncorrected, may precipitate degenerative changes in weight-bearing joint, especially the knee joint, in later life. Post-traumatic short leg may also give rise to low backache. It can be assessed by temporarily giving a shoe raise, which may be given permanently if it gives relief.

Oedema

Oedema of the lower limb after the removal of the plaster is an important factor in delaying the recovery of the ankle movement and functional recovery.

There are two types of oedema:

1. a simple oedema, which is due to disuse and is controllable by simple antigravity drainage and wearing of elastic bandage
2. a resistant oedema, which is associated with osteoporosis, persistent muscle weakness, joint stiffness, and a cold blue foot.

In the initial treatment, there is a correlation between vascular damage and ischemia, osteoporosis and oedema. It has to be considered whether muscle-wasting, oedema, and joint stiffness are primarily due to disuse, placebo, thrombosis, or reflex neurovascular disturbances. The presence of patchy decalcification in the radiograph of the tarsus at the time of removal of the plaster increases the chances of subsequent oedema to nearly three times more than expected when radiographs are normal.

If marked osteoporosis of the ankle bones is found on the radiographs when the plaster cast is removed, post-plaster oedema develops more often than when osteoporosis is slight. Hence, disability period is also more prolonged unless intensive treatment is given.

The tendency to develop greater or lesser degree of oedema is present in all cases, and routine antigravitational treatment given helps in more rapid recovery of the movements and functions.

The incidence of post-plaster oedema following fracture of the tibia and fibula is about 25%. The incidence is higher in compound fractures and open reductions and lowest in simple shaft fractures treated conservatively.

Lack of exercise when in plaster and inadequate preventive measures taken immediately after the removal of the plaster increase the incidence of oedema.

Treatment of Post-Plaster Oedema

Post-Plaster Oedema can be treated using Viscopaste, Elastoplast, crepe bandage, a combination of Elastoplast for the foot and ankle and crepe bandaging above the ankle, and physiotherapy with elastic bandaging. However, the most effective methods are:

1. Vigorous and time-consuming physiotherapy, including centripetal massage and faradism twice daily and wearing crepe bandage at all other times.
2. The use of an elastic bandage applied from the metatarsal heads to the neck of the fibula. This should be applied immediately after the removal of the plaster and worn continuously. The routine use of elastic bandage is the most convenient and practical method of preventing and treating post-plaster oedema.

The Results of Intensive Rehabilitation after Fractures of the Lower Limb

Details of the end results of a fracture are rare, but the record shows the following:

1. final range and joint movement
2. time for clinical union
3. results in small series.

However, the following figures can be relied upon as shown by various series.

In fractures of the shaft of the tibia and fibula:

1. 95% of the patients return to duty
2. 95% of the patients regain good ankle movement and function.

The average time for the injury to return to active duty:

1. simple fracture: 25 weeks
2. compound fracture: 30 weeks
3. after open reduction: 35 weeks.

In fractures around ankle joint:

1. 95% of the patients return to duty
2. 95% of the patients regain good ankle movement and function.

The average time off duty depends on the severity of injury:

1. unimalleolar fractures: 12 weeks
2. bimalleolar fractures: 19 weeks
3. trimalleolar fracture: 20 weeks.

On the average, the time is increased by four to six weeks after open reduction.

Fractures of the Shaft of the Femur

In patients with fractures of the shaft of the femur, 72% return to duty in an overall average time of eight months. The average time off duty:

1. after early internal fixation: 26 weeks
2. after skeletal traction: 32 weeks
3. after non-skeletal traction: 42 weeks.

CHAPTER 33

OCCUPATIONAL THERAPY

The modern occupational therapy is essential for effective rehabilitation. There are three ways for doing it:
　　i. specific crafts to regain power, movements, and function
　　ii. vocational guidance and pre-vocational training
　　iii. manufacture of the temporary and permanent splints and production of prosthesis.

Specific Craftwork

Occupational therapy is particularly valuable in the rehabilitation of fractures of the upper limb and especially for the hand. One of the main objectives of occupational therapy is to encourage the use of purposive movements in graded manner to help in the stages of recovery. As the hand is used for functional activities such as handling tools, dressing, and writing; therefore, these activities are the best method of retraining after an injury, and it is also valuable in restoring the functions of the shoulder and elbow, whose main purpose is to position the hand for activities.

As soon as possible, activities of value should be introduced, not only to interest the patient but also to review his dormant movement patterns. The activities of the patient's job offer the best chance of success. Though it works well on morale, in many cases, this is not possible for many months after the injury or surgery. In some cases, it may never be possible, owing to the severity of disorder. If returning to the same pre-accident work is unlikely, then pre-vocational training can often be started for the occupational therapy.

At an early stage, the patient's interests, aptitude with tools, speed, and accuracy can all be tested, and a variety of crafts can be tried out. For these reason, light crafts, such as basketry, leatherwork, and weaving, may be given for the functional activities of the patient's upper limb in the first few weeks after the injury. Then the patient may be encouraged to do carpentry, which is ideal to build up power grip, increase the range of movements of stiff joints, and encourage coordination and stamina. It is a very valuable method since all men enjoy carpentry.

For women, housework and domestic duties are the daily duties, so training kitchen facilities for retraining in household activities is of great help for women's recovery.

Attached to occupational therapy should be well-equipped workshop with lathes, drills, and facilities for light metalwork, such as filing and welding.

As recovery progresses, a longer time may be spent in these activities, and gradually, harder tasks are given to the patient. The evaluation should be done at a weekly interval or in a day-to-day level so that the patient is encouraged to increase muscle power, range of movements, coordination, and stamina and to learn a new skill or writing with a deformed hand.

Occupational Therapy for Rehabilitation of Fractures and Dislocation of the Lower Limbs

The aim of occupational therapy in the lower limbs fractures is to help in the following:

i. re-education of the lower limb to the normal pattern of movement and coordination

ii. restoration of full range of joint movement

iii. restoration of power in weakened muscle groups

iv. maintenance of work habit and rebuilding tolerance to a fully active working day

In the lower limb, the place of occupational therapy is limited. Bicycle and treadle machines can be used or adapted to operating saw, lathes, or sewing machines. These machines help the flexion and extension movements of the hip, knee, and ankle. The more important movement of concern is walking as well as movements of the lower limb by means of workshop activities.

Woodwork is the most popular and adaptable occupation used for increasing joint movement and building muscle power. A well-designed bicycle machine can be used for sawing, sanding, polishing, and drilling. This machine is easily adjusted to give a graded range of required movements and to give strong repetitive movements of different muscle groups.

Other machines of value are the fretsaws for the use of calf muscles, lathe for the quadriceps and glutei muscles, printing presses adapted for all ranges of hip, knee, and ankle, and pottery wheel and large pedal loom for improving muscle power.

Amongst the simpler aids to daily living which are used to enable patients with lower-limb injuries to become independent soon are elastic shoelaces, a long-handled shoehorn, and a simple appliance to help put on stockings or trousers.

INDEX

A

acetabulum 164-5, 167-8, 170, 172, 174, 177-80, 183, 282-3
  aseptic necrosis 166, 169
  complications 166
  diagnosis 159
  dislocation 168
  femur displacement 165-8
  fracture above 167
  internal fixation 169
  posterior rim fracture 165
  prognosis 166
  treatment 166
Acromioclavicular Joint 70, 73, 75-9
  acromion fracture of 84, 89-90, 92
  diagnosis 73, 77
  dislocation 76
  strapping 75, 78-80
  subluxation 70, 76, 78
ankle joint:
  abduction fracture 222, 282
  adduction fracture 217, 223-4
  anatomy 214
  avulsion fracture 217
  bimalleolar fracture 227, 310
  congenital fusion 215
  deltoid ligament 216-17, 221, 228
  diastasis 220-2
  external rotation fractures 216-21, 228
  fibula 5, 19, 25, 30-1, 41, 209-12, 214-18, 220-3, 229, 231, 274, 307, 309-10
  fibular collateral ligament 214-15, 217, 223
  footballer's ankle 216
  fracture-dislocation 217
  hypermobile 215, 217
  immobilization 217, 219-20, 223-4, 226-7, 230
  mechanism 223
  socket and ball 216
  stress fractures 231, 244, 274
  treatment 216-18, 222, 224, 226, 230
arthrodesis 24, 127, 134-5, 142, 183, 226, 235, 240-1, 299, 301
  wrist after scaphoid fracture 127, 133-5
arthroplasty 135
avascular necrosis 13, 23, 182-3, 186, 192-3, 235
  hip joint 180-1
  neck of the femur 23
avulsion 9, 11, 15, 89, 93-4, 110, 139-40, 142, 214-17, 228, 232, 242, 272-3, 280, 283
  ankle 214-17, 232
  fingers 140
  greater tuberosity of the humerus 93-4
  medial epicondyle 110
  metatarsals 32, 170, 241-4
  posterior marginal fracture of the tibia 219, 225-6, 228
  shearing fractures 217, 227-8
  sideswipe fractures 217, 227
  sprains 214, 216
  talus 232

tibiofibular ligaments 216-17,
220-2
tilting talus 215
varus deformity 230-1
vertical compression 217, 225,
229
axillary nerve 17-18, 84, 101

B

Bennett fracture-dislocation 141
bone ends
  impaction of 54
  separation of 53
bone grafting 22, 30, 135, 155,
  213, 278
bone marrow 51
brachial artery 103-4, 116, 275
Bryant's traction 204-5
burst fracture 146, 225
butterfly-type fracture 160

C

calcaneus 30, 43, 170, 210-11,
  234-7, 239-41
  diagnosis 238
  fractures 236
  subtalar joint 232, 234
  treatment 235
caliper 303, 305
callus, organization of 54
callus formation 61-2, 68, 119,
  201, 285, 303-4
cancellous bone 22, 49, 120, 155,
  191, 249
Capitellum Fractures 110, 273
Carpometacarpal Dislocation 136
carpus 133, 135-6
  dislocation 135
  fracture-dislocation 135, 141

minor fractures 133
proximal row 135
scaphoid bone fractures 133
cast:
  above-elbow 28-9
  above-knee 28, 30
  arm 28-9
  below-elbow 28-9, 129
  below-knee 28, 30
  fingers 28-9
  hanging 100
  padded 38
cervical spine, dislocation 146
chest injuries:
  costochondral separation 248
  mechanism 246
  rib fractures 246, 248, 253
  sternum fractures in children 253
  tearing of the pleura 248
  treatment 247
children fracture:
  ankle 272
  forearm epiphyseal plate injuries
    269
  greenstick fractures 271
chip fracture 133, 177, 262
circular bandage 35
clavicular fracture 70, 72, 74-5,
  296
  in children 75
  figure-of-eight bandage 73-4, 76
  outer third 75
  treatment 73, 78
Colles fracture 34, 70, 127-8, 130,
  301
comminution 53-4, 108, 112, 119,
  141, 153, 238, 278
compound fracture, treatment 26
compression fracture 32, 159-60,
  225
  ankle 225

pelvis 160
condylar fractures 108-9, 255, 258-9
coracoid fractures 76, 89-91, 97
coronoid process fractures 71, 113-14, 116
Cortical bone 48, 51, 135, 213
costochondral separation 248
crepitus 2-3, 73
crutches 160, 164, 166, 169, 197, 201, 211, 213, 225, 239, 303-4
cuff-and-collar sling 74-5, 79-80, 90-1, 94, 96-7, 100-2, 108, 111, 115-16, 120

D

deep vein thrombosis 196
deformity 2-3, 14, 22, 30, 73, 128, 130, 137-8, 140, 200-1, 205, 230-1, 240, 268-9, 275-7
delayed union 13, 21, 31-2, 48, 50, 52, 61, 63-4, 198, 213, 278, 285, 289, 304
dietetic treatment 49

E

elastocrepe 247, 249, 253
elbow:
  aetiology 104
  complications 116
  coronoid process fractures 113
  crutches 304
  dislocation of 113, 115
  extension-type fracture 105
  flexion-type fracture 107
  fracture 31
  fracture treatment 114
  lateral condylar fractures 109
  stiff 117

supracondylar fractures 18, 20, 70, 104-8, 117, 203-4, 272, 299
ulnar palsy 117, 300
Electric Stimulation 291, 295
epiphyseal displacement 229-31
external fixation 28, 30, 213, 277, 289

F

facial bones 254, 256-7, 259, 261, 264, 267
  anaesthesia 256
  examination 254
  fracture 254-74
  manibular fractures 257
  maxillary fractures 259
  multiple fractures 266
  nasal fractures 261
  zygomatic complex 256
Fascial arthroplasty 135
fat embolism 12-13
femoral head 174, 177, 179, 185, 191, 193, 198, 271, 287
femoral neck fracture:
  extracapsular fracture 187
  intracapsular fracture 187
  mechanism 185
  mid-cervical abduction 194
  muscles 196, 205
  sex incidence 185
  Smith-Petersen nailing 191
  subcapital fracture 23, 186-7, 189
  subcervical fractures 187, 194-5
  trans-articular nailing 131
  transcervical fractures 186-7, 189
  un-united 194
  upper end 183, 185, 187
  vascular factor in the healing 192

weight-bearing 185, 192, 197, 201, 208
femur:
  abduction type 192
  age incidence 204
  anatomical reduction 190, 200
  avascular necrosis 186, 192
  basal fractures 186-7, 189, 194-5, 197
  bony structure 191
  classification 195
  clinical features 186
  complications 191, 193
  deep vein 196
  fixation device 193, 196
  fractures in children 197
  intertrochanteric fracture 186-7, 194-5, 197
  intracapsular fractures 187
  pattern of fracture 195
  post-operative management 196
  thrombosis 196, 275, 309
  treatment 191
  vascular supply 53, 190
fibreglass splint 127, 301
fibula 209-12, 214-18, 220-3, 229, 231, 274, 307, 309-10
  rehabilitation results 310
  shaft fracture 209
fingers:
  avulsion fractures 140
  closed reduction 137
  condylar fracture 255
  displaced fractures 137
  malleable metal splints 138, 262
  mallet 140
  open fracture 141-2
  plaster of Paris 138
  shattered joint 142
  splintage 138
  strapping 137-8

subluxation 131
foot (*see also* forefoot) 191, 201, 214-19, 222-3, 225, 228-9, 232-6, 238-42, 244
  calcaneus 236
  dislocation 232-6
  fracture 232
  fracture-dislocation 233
  metatarsal fractures 241-4
  midtarsal dislocation 236, 239
  subtalar dislocation 232-41
  talus 232-5
  tarsometatarsal dislocation 241
forefoot 225, 241, 245
  dislocation 241
  metatarsal fractures 242
  phalange fractures 245
  tarsometatarsal joints 241
  treatment 242-3
fractures:
  avulsion 9, 11, 89, 93-4, 140, 217, 228, 232, 242, 272, 280
  comminuted 9-10, 129, 132, 142, 196, 199, 285, 307
  complicated 7-9, 202
  compound 8-9, 25-7
  double 5, 9-10, 280-1
  fatigue 9, 11
  greenstick 9-10, 119, 188, 271-2
  impacted 9-10
  infected 26, 56
  multiple 5, 9, 11, 65, 246, 266, 277
  oblique 9-10, 218
  pathological 9, 11, 201, 274, 285
  rate of healing 53, 55
  simple 3, 8, 55, 62, 140, 142, 296, 302, 310
  spiral 9-10, 62, 103, 212, 229, 276, 280, 287-8
  transverse 9-10, 62, 112, 119-20, 206, 213, 224, 228, 259, 276, 288

H

haematoma 15, 22, 48-9, 52-5, 58, 61, 63, 67-8, 158, 245, 256
hand:
  classification of fractures 136
  occupational therapy 127
hip dislocation:
  aftercare 182
  anterior dislocation 172
  in children 183
  complications 182
  fracture-dislocation 177
  mechanism 172
  operative approach 182
  traction 174, 183, 190-1, 196
  types of 177
hip spica 28-9, 164, 182-3, 191, 201
Hippocratic Method 84, 86
humerus:
  anatomy 92
  brachial artery injury 103
  displaced 94
  fracture in children 99
  fracture of neck of 96
  fracture with separation 97
  fracture without separation 96
  fracture-dislocation 100
  greater tuberosity fractures 101
  greenstick 99
  radial nerve palsy 103
  reduction 94-5, 97-8, 100
  surgical neck 96
  treatment 94
  undisplaced 92
hydrotherapy 295-8

I

immobilization, inadequate 58, 66-7
implants 286
infection 44, 50, 53-4, 56-7, 61-2, 68-9, 200, 202, 213, 259, 263, 274, 276, 279, 289
internal fixation of fractures:
  acetabulum 164-5, 167-8, 170, 172, 174, 177-80, 183, 282-3
  closed manipulation 98, 119, 122, 126, 180, 277, 280
  delayed union 13, 21, 31-2, 48, 50, 52, 61, 63-4, 198, 213, 278, 285, 289, 304
  intramedullary nails 26, 99, 116, 121, 125, 205, 287, 289
  lag screws 116, 287
  nail plate 287
  non-union 13, 21-2, 36, 48-50, 52, 54, 61, 63-9, 73, 109, 119-20, 202, 259-60, 285, 289
  plates 67-8, 155, 194, 263, 267, 270, 278, 287, 289
  post-operative management 288-9
  rehabilitation and effect of 290
  satisfactory position 120, 219, 280
  Smith-Petersen 191
  stainless steel 286, 289
  steel pins 284, 286, 289
  titanium 286
  vitallium 279, 286
  Y-shaped fracture of lower end 108, 283
Intertrochanteric fracture 186-7, 194-5, 197
intra-articular adhesions 13-14
intra-articular fracture 157, 164, 286, 307
intracapsular fracture 187
intramedullary nails 26, 30, 99, 116, 121, 125, 201, 205, 212,

281, 287-9
ischaemia 20, 104, 296

J

joint stiffness 13-14, 16, 31, 79, 90, 95, 277-8, 290, 296, 306, 308

K

Kirschner wire 44, 136, 140-2, 252, 267
knee 15, 19, 24, 28, 30, 32-3, 41, 165, 172, 174, 201-3, 205-7, 210, 218-20, 303-8
  flexion recovery 307
  stiffness of 202
knee dislocation 205
Kocher's method 84
Küntscher nail 287

L

lag period 49-50, 55-6, 61, 63
lag screws 116, 287
laminectomy 156
lateral popliteal nerve 18-19, 45
leg length 201, 307-8
lesions 156, 298
limp 194, 305-6, 308
long bone fracture:
  aetiology 274
  deformity 275-7
  diagnosis 276
  infection 279
  metal corrosion 278
  open reduction 277
  radiological examination 274
  soft-tissue injury 276
  traction 275
  treatment 276
lunate bone 134-5
Luxatio Erecta 83-4, 88

M

malleolus abduction fractures 214-25, 227-32, 234-5, 238
mallet finger fracture 140
malunion 13, 22, 119, 130, 138, 205, 275
mandible 254-8, 267
  diet with treatment 258
  examination 254
  treatment 257
march fracture 32, 244, 274
maxilla 254-7, 259-61, 265, 267
median nerve 17-18, 104, 129-30
metacarpals 29, 44, 70, 137-41, 282
  displaced fractures 141
  fractured head of 140
metal, malleable 262
metal corrosion 278
metal plate 67, 267
metalwork 301, 313
metatarsals 11, 32, 170, 241-4, 274, 309
mid-cervical fracture 194
midtarsal dislocation 236
mobilization 31, 117, 127, 156, 196, 201, 278, 290, 297, 299, 303-7
Monteggia Fracture 70, 123-4, 280
muscular adhesions 13, 15
myositis ossificans 15-16, 117, 126, 182, 299-300

N

nail plates 287
necrosis 13, 23, 32, 50-3, 67, 69, 166, 169, 182-3, 186, 192-3,

235, 263, 278
neuritis 116, 130
  frictional 116
neuropraxia 17
non-union 13, 21-2, 36, 48-50, 52, 54, 61, 63-9, 73, 109, 119-20, 202, 259-60, 285, 289
  cancellous bone 22
  causes of 64
  definition 21-2
  diagnosis 64
  distraction 193
  fibrous union 22, 64, 262
  fracture gap 49, 67
  grafts 21-2, 30, 213
  internal fixation 26, 30, 68, 101, 103, 120-2, 191-4, 196-7, 201-4, 212-13, 258-9, 277-80, 284-6, 288-90, 304
  mechanism 69
  operative technique 285
  rigid fixation 102, 121, 186, 192
  sites in long bones 69
nose bones 254, 256, 261-2

O

occupational therapy 127, 298-9, 301-2, 312-13
odontoid process 271
oedema 31, 33, 39, 45, 211, 302, 308-9
  calcis fractures 32
olecranon, fracture of 7, 31, 43, 70, 104, 112-17, 287, 299
open reduction 100-1, 107-11, 116, 119-22, 125-6, 131-2, 140-1, 154-5, 203-5, 212-13, 221-2, 226, 258-9, 284-6, 309-11
orbital floor 256, 266

ossifiable medium 50, 53-4
osteoarthritis 23-4, 127, 169, 226, 301
osteotomy 130, 198, 231

P

palsy 45, 103, 117, 159, 182, 202, 282, 300
  radial nerve 103
  sciatic nerve 18-19, 158-9, 162, 164-5, 169, 172, 182, 282
  ulnar 117
patella fractures 31, 33, 206-8
Pelvic Ring 19, 157-9, 161, 166, 168-9
pelvis 29, 32, 157-60, 162-4, 166-8, 174, 305
  acetabulum 164-5
  blood transfusion 158
  diagnosis 159-61, 165, 167
  displacement of head 166
  disruption of pelvic ring 157
  fracture into the roof of acetabulum 167-8
  fracture lines 168
  fracture of posterior rim 165
  intra-articular fractures 158
  intrapelvic injuries 158, 162, 164-5, 169
  osteoarthritis 23-4, 127, 169, 226, 301
  prognosis 163
  pubis-ischium fracture 157, 160-1, 163, 169
  radiography in 160
  rupture of urethra 159
  sciatic nerve palsy 159, 182, 282
  shock 158
  sidewall fracture 164, 166-7
  skeletal pelvic injury 159

solitary fracture of bones 169
torn vessels 158
traction 169
treatment 160, 162, 164, 166, 169
vertical fracture 159, 163
periarticular ossification 13, 15
pertrochanteric fracture 194
phalanges 7, 29, 32, 44, 70, 137, 140-1, 170, 245, 286
  condylar fracture 109, 258-9
  fingers 15-16, 18, 28-9, 44, 86, 88, 98, 101-3, 117, 129-30, 136-8, 140, 292, 300
  fractures 245
  stable fracture 150, 272
  terminal fracture 140, 245
  toes 32, 210, 213, 275, 306
pins 80, 107, 121, 198, 242, 286, 289
  rush 121
  steel 284, 286, 289
plaster application 30-1, 33, 36, 220
plaster of Paris 6, 27-8, 115-16, 138, 152-4, 160, 163, 191, 205, 208-9, 216-17, 262, 295
plaster:
  padded 27, 33-5, 113, 120, 125, 129-31, 133-4, 210, 226
  unpadded 33-4, 129
plates 67-8, 155, 194, 263, 267, 270, 278, 287, 289
post-plaster oedema 309
posterior dislocation 19, 82, 84, 88, 113-14, 172, 175-6, 178, 271
posterior rim 164-5, 183
Pressure Bandage 32
prone method 87
prosthetic replacement 193-4
pseudarthrosis 64, 69

R

radial nerve 9, 17-18, 103, 116, 275
radiocarpal joint 132-3
radiography 16, 89, 136, 238
radioulnar joint 111-12, 119, 123, 126, 275, 300
radius:
  closed reduction 120
  Colles fracture 127
  fracture 111, 119
  head of 70, 110-11, 117, 132, 299
  open reduction 121
  persistent dislocation 126
  rotation movement 126, 300
recurrent dislocation:
  elbow 108
  shoulder 83, 88, 297
  splinting method 90, 196
  stable fractures 150
rehabilitation 37, 118, 127, 150, 223, 277, 290, 296, 300-8, 310, 312-13
  basic techniques 290
  Bennett fracture-dislocation 301
  carpentry 301
  circuit training 294
  clavicle 296
  craftwork 301
  delayed 306
  electric stimulation 295
  exercise in bed 303
  exercises 298
  hand fractures 302
  heat 295
  hip 306
  hydrotherapy 296
  ice packs 297
  knee 307

leg length differences 307-8
lower-limb fracture 303
massage 296
myositis ossifican 299
nerve lesions 298
oedema 308
osteoarthritis 301
pain relief 297
paralysis 298, 300
passive movements 296
proprioceptive neuromuscular facilitation 291
relaxation techniques 293
results 310
rotation injuries 126, 300
scapula fractures 296
shoulder dislocation 297
spasm relief 297
splint 301
stiff shoulder 297
strengthening techniques 292
successive induction 291
trochanteric region 306
walking in plaster 305
walking with crutches 304
weight-bearing caliper 305
roentgenographic examination 63-4
rotator cuff injuries 97, 297
rush pin 121

S

scaphoid bone 134-5
  arthrodesis 135
  bone grafts 22, 135
  carpal fracture 133, 135
  distal pole 133-4
  fascial arthroplasty 135
  rehabilitation 301
  removal of lunate bones 134
  treatment 134
  un-united 134
sciatic nerve 18-19, 158-9, 162, 164-5, 169, 172, 182, 282
sclerosis 22, 53-4, 64, 274
screws 26, 30, 68, 103, 116, 121, 123, 125, 136, 141, 180-2, 203-5, 278, 283, 286-9
secondary sepsis 66, 68
sequestrectomy 213
Shaft Fracture 204
  blood loss 4-5
  compound 26
  crepitus 2-3, 73
  fat embolism 12-13
  first aid 4, 30
  indications 32
  infected 26, 44
  internal fixation 26, 30
  intramedullary nail 26, 30
  Küntscher nailing 201, 287
  shortening correction 200
  Steinmann pin 44
  stiffness of knee joint 44
  subtrochanteric fracture 170, 203
  supracondylar fracture 18, 20, 70, 104-8, 117, 203-4, 272, 299
shearing fractures 147, 154
shock 4-5, 12, 158-9, 169
shortening of the limb 112, 137, 160-1, 163, 165, 191, 199-200, 231, 272, 275-6, 308
shoulder:
  after treatment 88
  anterior dislocation 83
  diagnosis 84
  Hippocratic reduction 84, 86
  humerus 84, 86
  immobilization period 83
  Kocher's reduction 84-6

    luxatio erecta 83-4, 88
    mechanism of injury 82
    pathological anatomy 83
    posterior dislocation 82, 84, 88
    prone method 87
    Putti-Platt operation 88
    recurrent dislocation 83, 88
    subcoracoid 83
    treatment 84
shoulder spica 28-9, 95, 102
skeletal traction 41, 43, 164, 166, 168-9, 196, 198-200, 311
Smith-Petersen nail 191
Smith's fracture 131-2
spine:
    abrasions over scapula 149
    ankylosis 241
    cervical dislocation 154
    cervical fracture 194
    classification 148
    cord damage 145, 147, 156
    diagnosis 149
    dorso-lumbar fracture-dislocation 146, 148-9, 155
    extension injuries 145
    extension-rotation 156
    flexion injuries 144
    flexion-rotation 145-6, 148
    immobilization of fractures and dislocations 150
    inspection 149
    internal fixation 150
    laminectomy 156
    longitudinal violence injuries 146
    lumbar facets of 145, 237, 239-40
    lumbar fractures 153, 155
    lumbar nerve roots 143, 146-9, 155
    odontoid fractures 271
    palpation 149
    pathological anatomy 144
    reduction 149
    rehabilitation after crush fractures 302
    rotational injuries 146
    shearing violence 147
    stable injuries 150
    thoracic shearing fracture 147, 154
    treatment 150
    unstable injuries 154, 280
    wedge fractures 150
splintage 30, 32, 129, 136-8, 169, 209, 213, 245, 275, 277-8, 289
splints 19, 28, 59, 138, 156, 312
    fibreglass for Bennett fracture-dislocation 127, 301
Sprains 214, 216
stable fractures 150
stainless steel 286, 289
steel pins 284, 286, 289
sternoclavicular dislocation 70, 251
sternum 246, 248-53
strengthening techniques 292
stress fractures 231, 244, 274
styloid process fracture 71, 132
subcervical fractures 187, 194-5
subungual haematoma 245
Sudeck's atrophy 13, 16, 38, 64, 68, 130
supracondylar fractures 18, 20, 70, 104-8, 117, 203-4, 272, 299
syndesmosis 216, 220-2

T

talus 23, 171, 215, 217-19, 221-2, 225-6, 228, 232-6
    avulsion 232

chip fracture 232
complications 235
crack fractures 232
fracture-dislocation 233, 235
midtarsal dislocation 236
subtalar dislocation 236
total dislocation 235
tarsometatarsal dislocation 241
  Kirschner wire fixation 44, 136, 140-2, 252, 267
tibia:
  compound fracture 213
  delayed union 213
  displaced fracture 210
  grafting 213
  non-union 69
  open reduction 212
  posterior marginal fracture 219, 225-6, 228
  shaft fracture 209
  skin loss 213
  tibiofibular syndesmosis 220-2
  titanium in internal fixation 286
  undisplaced fracture 210
  weight-bearing 209, 211, 213
tibiofibular ligaments 216-17, 220-2
titanium 286
traction 40-6
  pelvic fractures 159
  pulp traction 41, 44, 139
  skeletal traction 41, 43, 164, 166, 168-9, 196, 198-200, 311
  skin traction 41-2, 45, 199-200
  trauma 1-2, 11, 22, 34, 52-3, 55, 61-2, 64, 213, 263, 275
tuberosity:
  greater 71, 92-4, 96, 101, 288, 297
  lesser 71

U

ulna:
  anatomy 119
  dislocation of head 123
  shaft fracture 123
ulnar nerve 18-19, 111, 116-18, 300
Ulnar Palsy 117
ulnar palsy, rehabilitation 300

V

varus angulation 99-100
varus deformity 201, 230-1, 275
  epiphyseal arrest 231
vertical compression 217, 225, 229
vitallium 279, 286
Volkmann's contracture 105, 275

W

walking:
  with crutch 304
  in plaster 303, 305
Windowed Plasters 39
wound infection 213, 276, 279
wrist 2, 16, 18, 20, 33-4, 96, 100, 103, 121, 127-31, 133-6, 292, 296, 301
  carpus 135-6
  Colles fracture 34, 70, 127-8, 130, 301
  osteoarthritis 127
  rehabilitation 301
  Smith's fracture 131
  stiffness 134

Z

zygoma 254, 256, 259, 264-7